Nursing in Serbia with Lady Paget in 1915
The Adventures of Flora Scott of Leicester

Jess Jenkins

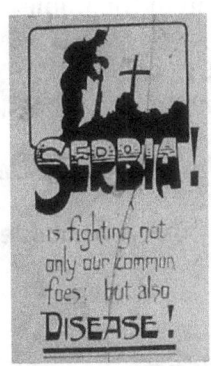

Nursing in Serbia with Lady Paget in 1915

For all those, women and men, who risked their lives to fight disease in Serbia, 1914-1919

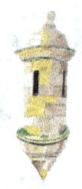

First published in the United Kingdom in 2022 by **The Lookout Press**, 31A Victoria Street, Fleckney, Leicester LE8 8AZ.

www.heritageco.co.uk

©Jess Jenkins and Robin Jenkins 2022

All rights reserved. No part of this publication may be reproduced, stored in a retrieval system, or transmitted, in any form or by any means, electronic, mechanical, photocopying, recording or otherwise, without the prior permission of the publisher and copyright holders.

The views expressed in this publication are those of the author, and are not necessarily endorsed by the publishers.

British Library Cataloguing in Publication Data.

A catalogue record for this book is available from the British Library.

ISBN 978-1-7395815-0-3

Typeset in 12/16 point Calibri.

"Probably no group of women have given so much of themselves under such tremendous odds, and emerged so magnificently - and so unsung in their own country"

from
The Quality of Mercy
Women at War, Serbia 1915-1918
by
Monica Krippner
1980

Nursing in Serbia with Lady Paget in 1915

Acknowledgements

This story began as the simple tale of one Leicester woman's experiences nursing in the First World War. However, the more I learnt about Serbia and the British nursing units, of which Flora was a part, the more important it seemed to tell the wider story. Little has been written about Lady Paget and her hospital and indeed most of the work of the Serbian Relief Fund has been neglected and overshadowed by the more glamorous tales of Mrs St Clair Stobart and the Scottish Women's Hospitals' all-women units. That the work and sacrifices of the women and men who risked their lives in order to relieve suffering in a distant foreign land, should be overlooked in this way is an injustice which I hope this little book will do something to address.

I am grateful to many for their help in researching this book. I would like to thank particularly the staff of the Imperial War Museum and the School of Slavonic and Eastern European Studies of University College, London. I am also indebted to David Newman of the Historic Ryde Society for his great kindness in seeking out Flora's various homes in Ryde and Richard Smout of the Isle of Wight County Record Office for his much appreciated help and advice in finding an obituary for Flora. I am also very grateful to Nicholas Rogers, archivist of Sidney Sussex College, Cambridge for supplying me with elusive details of the biography of Rex Jackson.

Finally, I would like to thank my family who have put up with my mutterings about nurses in Serbia for far longer than should have been necessary. In particular, I thank my husband Robin for all his guidance and support, not least in directing me to the memoirs of Konstantin Maglic which he uncovered in his own research on the history of Leicester's military hospital.

Contents

Introduction	1
1. Early Years	5
2. The Serbian Relief Fund- Lady Paget's Mission	7
3. Journey to Serbia	23
4. Lady Paget's Hospital	52
5. The Typhus Epidemic	76
6. Home to Leicester	118
7. Lady Paget's Return to Serbia	129
8. Nurse Scott after Serbia	160
9. Cast of Characters	178
Appendix 1: The Serbian Relief Fund 1914-1920	250
Appendix 2: Staff of Lady Paget's Hospital	262
Sources	272
References	276
Staff of Stobart's Unit	292
Index	294

Nursing in Serbia with Lady Paget in 1915

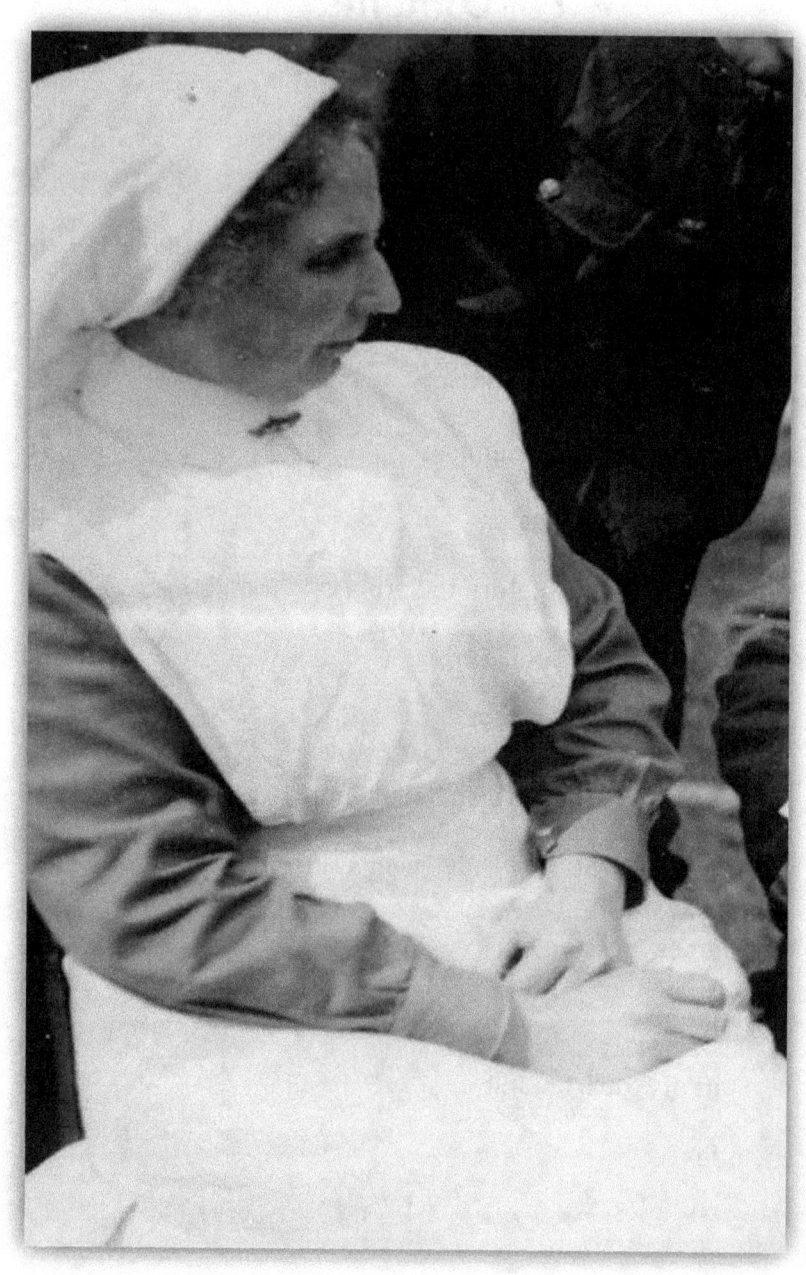

Introduction

'Willing to Go!'
Nursing in Serbia with Lady Paget in 1915

The Adventures of Flora Scott of Leicester

This is the tale of an ordinary woman in extraordinary times. It is the tale of one nurse who found herself alone, thousands of miles from home in an alien country and culture, nursing three hundred typhus stricken prisoners of war. Moreover, it is a tale which is part of a much greater story- that of the courage and commitment of a small band of women and men, now largely forgotten, who joined her in the uneven battle against disease and suffering and triumphed, sometimes at the cost of their own lives.

The former nursing home of Nurse Flora Scott, originally called 'Beausite', still stands in Leicester today. The street is no longer Victoria Road but is now known to all as University Road, after the founding in 1921 of the Leicester, Leicestershire and Rutland University College in the former county asylum buildings at the end of the road. This modest college, founded as a memorial to the dead of the First World War, now proudly proclaims itself as Leicester University and its modern campus has engulfed this once quiet avenue. Surrounding buildings have edged ever closer and the garden and greenhouse are no more but essentially little else has changed.

The fine imposing front door, as designed by Joseph Goddard (1840-1900) in 1875, still dominates the façade. The architect had planned the house to be both a home for his family and a means of impressing potential clients and he entertained there lavishly throughout the 1870s and 1880s. After his death, the family rented the house to the Clements School for Girls for a period before a certain Miss Flora Scott leased the property as a nursing home around 1910. Today, the house is divided into apartments and there is little to recall its former days. The blue plaque commemorating Nurse Scott has yet to appear...

Nursing in Serbia with Lady Paget in 1915

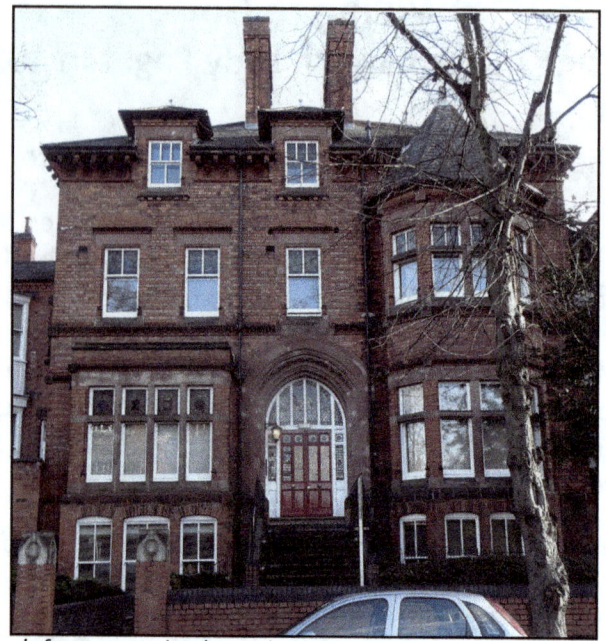

Flora's former nursing home in University Road, Leicester, 2019

'May God bless the women of Leicester...'

Amongst the many successful 'Flag Days' organised in Leicester during the First World War, the memory of one in particular stood out in people's minds. Perhaps it was the glorious sunshine. Perhaps the spectacle of three thousand school children packed before a platform in Town Hall Square, trained rather improbably to sing the Serbian national anthem or perhaps it was the outstanding achievement of a record breaking sum raised for the gallant Serbs.

Certainly the success of the day was sufficient to ensure that the Serbian Flag Day of 11 September 1915 was reported widely outside Leicester. On the platform that sunny afternoon alongside the Mayor, was the Bishop of Leicester, keen both to praise the Serbian nation for its courageous contribution to the Allied cause and to recall the recent work in that country of English doctors and nurses, noting with particular pride *'that Leicester had not been unrepresented in that noble band who had gone*

Introduction

out there to nurse and care for the sick and wounded'¹. To loud applause, he recalled *'Sister Scott and her nurses and the good work they had done'* declaring that the town was *'honoured in them'*. The people of Leicester, it seems, were already well aware of Sister Scott and her nurses.

In the evening, the Mayor and his party retired to the 'Cripples Guild' in Colton Street for the traditional tallying of the money raised during the day. The Flag days had been first organised as fund raising events, at the Mayor's request, through the Alexandra Rose Day Committee, a body formerly set up to support various town charities through the sale of roses made by disabled people on Alexandra Rose Day. In these more brutal times, it was deemed acceptable to dismiss those suffering with disabilities as 'cripples'.

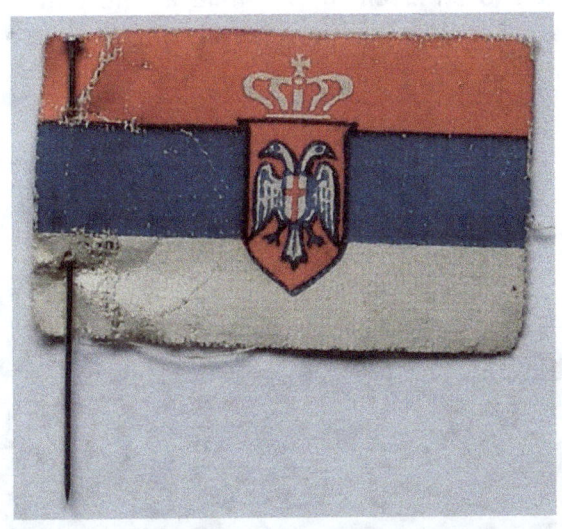

Serbian pin flag sold for fund-raising, c. 1915

After the inevitable rendition of the Serbian National Anthem, an excited audience received the final figures: the much admired 'lady

Nursing in Serbia with Lady Paget in 1915

collectors' selling flags on the streets, had raised £1,440, the sale of flags in elementary schools –by kind permission of the Education Committee- £132 and other contributions such as church collections had brought the total to a very impressive £2,128. When the august men had finished congratulating each other, Sister Scott thanked everybody on behalf of Serbia and moved a vote of thanks to the Mayor and Mayoress. Leicester was very pleased with herself and the Reverend J D Freeman was very pleased with the ladies of Leicester. He could not however, resist a sly swipe at the women's suffrage movement: *'He thanked God he had lived to see women in war – women administering to suffering humanity and rising to the heights of a gentle and thoughtful nature. The women of the land had given themselves to the great cause. All trivialities of twelve months ago had been swept away ....May God bless the women of Leicester and make us worthy of them (Applause)...'*

Did Sister Scott allow herself a wry smile at the enthusiasm of this rhetoric? It was all so very far from her experiences just a few months before....

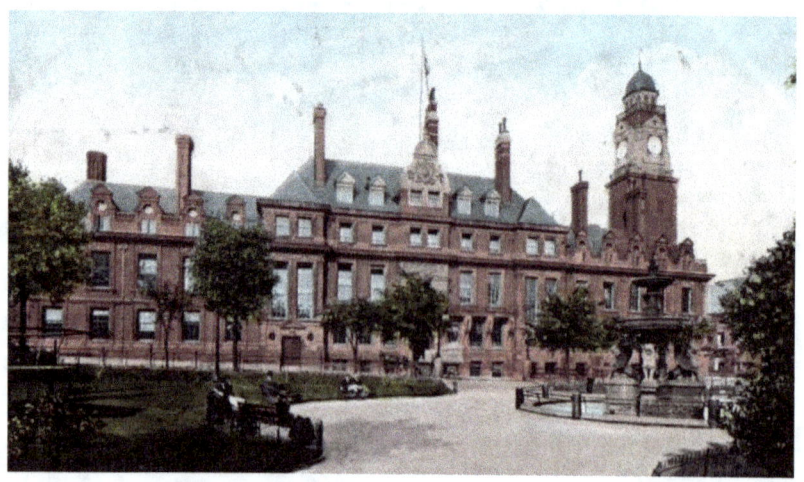

Postcard of the Town Hall Square, Leicester, c. 1907

Chapter 1

Early Years

'One of the best surgical nurses in the town'

Flora Martha Scott was born in Leicester on 11 September 1873 and baptised on 3 May 1874 at Christ Church in Bow Street, just off Wharf Street. Her father, William Scott (c1847-1903), was a tailor and draper from Scotland. His influence on his daughter can be perceived in odd elements of her vocabulary and stray dispassionate references to 'the English'. Her mother, Elizabeth (1845-1914) was the daughter of William Cotton, a butcher and his wife, Elizabeth and was born in Wilnecote in Warwickshire, the last child of a large family. Flora's mother was still a small child, when her mother died, and she seems to have spent much of her early life in Burton on Trent with Cotton relatives.

At the time of the 1871 census, William Scott, a draper, was a boarder at 24 Clyde Street in Leicester, living with John Gordon, a fellow Scotsman who was also a draper. Elizabeth Cotton meanwhile was in the Leicestershire mining village of Whitwick working as a school governess but more significantly, lodging with John Henderson, a Scotsman and draper. It may be significant that John's niece, who happened to be visiting at the time of the census was named Elizabeth Scot or it may simply be that the network of Scottish drapers in Leicestershire was particularly strong but it seems very likely that William Scott met his future wife in a draper's shop in Whitwick. The couple were married in Burton on Trent at the end of 1872 and set up home several doors down from William's initial lodgings in Clyde Street, with William now working as a travelling draper.

Flora has left no record of her parents but if her relationship with her siblings is any fair representation, they were a happy close knit family. The 1881 census recorded the family still living at 20 Clyde Street, off Humberstone Road with William's occupation given simply as draper. By this stage, Flora had been joined by a brother, Sydney, born in 1875,

Nursing in Serbia with Lady Paget in 1915

and a long line of sisters who were presumably a disappointment to Sydney if no one else: Jessie Sophia in 1877; Constance Annie in 1879 and Gertrude Mary in 1880. An afterthought, Agnes Morwood, would arrive in 1885. It is Flora's letters to her far flung siblings, now preserved at the Imperial War Museum, which form the most revealing source for her time in Serbia.

In 1891, when the census affords us our next glimpse of the family, William Scott, now describing himself as a draper's assistant, and his growing family, were resident at 43 Rutland Street, a rather more prestigious address. Flora, at the tender age of seventeen, was a dress maker and the young fifteen year old Sydney a clerk. All apparently was proceeding according to parental plans for the offspring but subsequent events suggest that Flora at least, was not content. The registers of the Royal College of Nursing record that Flora qualified as a nurse at the Royal Infirmary, Halifax in 1900. By this date, she had forsaken the dress trade for ever and entered the service in which she would be employed for the rest of her life. One can only speculate as to the struggle this had entailed in persuading her father of the wisdom of her own ambitions.

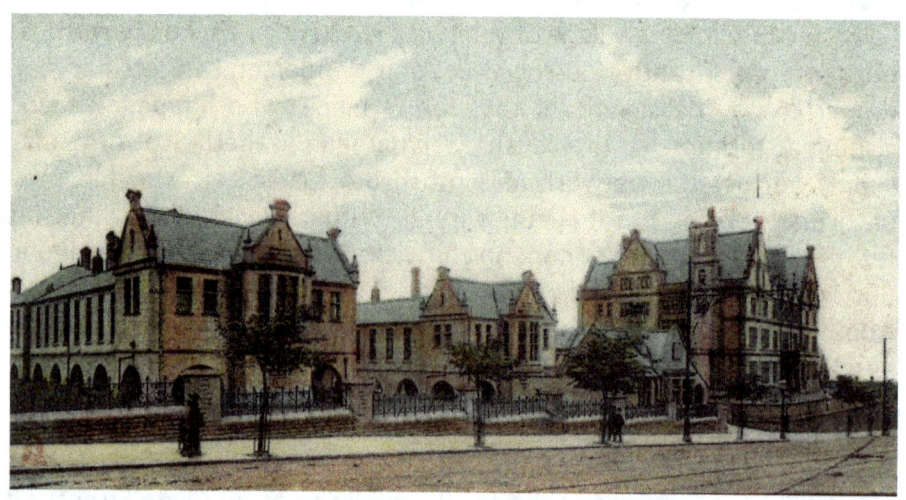

Postcard of the Royal Infirmary, Halifax, c. 1905

Early Years

By 1901, William was working as a tailor and draper and was himself an employer, resident at 60 Rutland Street. Sydney and Jessie worked with him whilst Constance and Gertrude now worked at typing and shorthand. Only Flora was absent. She was employed as a nursing sister at St Bartholomew's Hospital in Rochester, Kent. Her later career was outlined in an article in the *Leicester Daily Post* when it announced her departure for Serbia[2]. She had worked in four different hospitals before returning to Leicester c1906 when she joined Miss Pell Smith, a former matron at the Infirmary, in her nursing home, the well regarded 'Home Hospital', in Princess Road. According to the article, Flora stayed here only about a year before establishing her own nursing home at 28 Tichborne Street.

Wright's Trade Directory suggests Flora maintained close links with Leicester despite her regular absences, with Flora, Jessie, Constance and Gertrude all listed under 'Nurses', as resident at 8, Upper Tichborne Street in 1903. By 1909, Miss Flora Scott was recorded as running her own nursing home at 28, Tichborne Street. The enterprise must have prospered, for by the time of the 1911 census, she had moved her nursing home to 'Beausite' the large house in what was then known as Victoria Road, a leafy avenue leading out of the town towards the cemetery and County Asylum.

Meanwhile, Jessie Scott, was the proprietress of a Nurses' Home at 31, Highfield Street, supported by her sister Gertrude who acted as a stenographer. Constance in 1909 had made an interesting marriage, to a certain Sannyasi Charan Roy, known to Flora- inexplicably - as Frankie. Roy was a British citizen born in Calcutta who had qualified as a doctor at the Calcutta Medical School and Robertson Memorial Medical School in Edinburgh. His career in Leicester would seem to have prospered. By 1911, the couple were residing at Laurel Villa, in East Park Road with two servants. The medical directory for 1915 lists Roy at the same address with a practice at 109, Belgrave Gate, serving as District Medical Officer and Public Vaccinator for Leicester Union and late Resident Medical Officer at the Infirmary in North Evington. The couple were to have three sons: Philip Scott born in 1910; Keith Cotton in 1912 and Theodore

Nursing in Serbia with Lady Paget in 1915

Cotton in 1914.

Sydney had also married in 1901 to Grace Emma Bennett of Hinckley and in 1911 was working as a traveller in retail clothing living at 43, Long Street, Wigston Magna. The couple were apparently not settled, for in early 1914, they took the momentous and probably very wise step of emigrating to Canada. On 1 June of the same year Gertrude and Jessie also arrived in Quebec, intending to make their home there permanently.

Flora makes many references in her letters to *'the Canada people'* and clearly expected her letters to be shared around the family including those in North America. The only other sibling to marry was young Agnes, who in 1905, very much confirmed the theory that girls look for their father in a husband, when she married Neil Cook Stewart, a tailor and draper from the Isle of Arran. The couple lived at 8, Newstead Grove in Nottingham and had two children, Ellen and Alban who just happened to be staying with their Aunt Flora when she made the somewhat alarming decision to depart for Serbia.

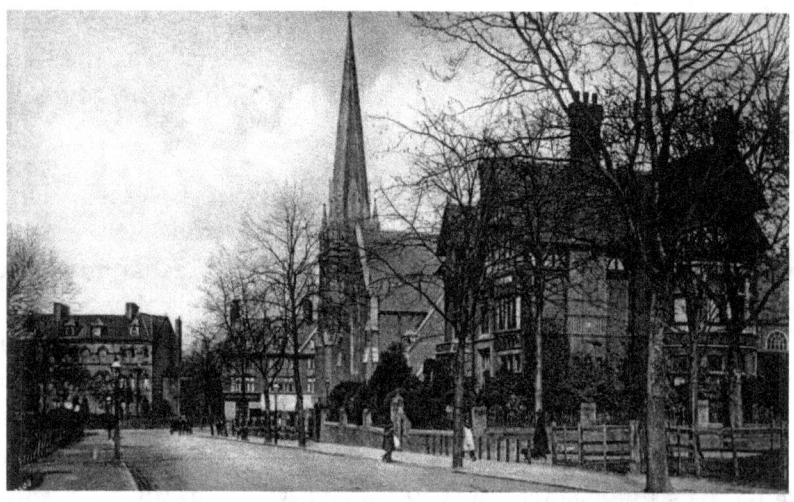

Postcard of Victoria Road and Church, Leicester, c. 1912

Chapter 2

The Serbian Relief Fund

Lady Paget's Mission to Serbia

'The members of Lady Paget's mission have left with us the happiest memories. Our thanks and gratitude for their work of devotion can have not limits, for they have done far, far more than we could ever have dared to ask or to expect'[3]

Few, before the catastrophic events of 1914 would have had even a vague idea of the whereabouts of Serbia. This small agricultural country of mostly mountainous terrain had the misfortune to lie in the way of the ambitions for expansion of two great empires. The main trading routes which led from the vast empire of Austria-Hungary [and Germany] south to Greece and the Aegean Sea and east to Constantinople and Asia Minor, crossed her territory. Her strategic position had made her a desirable prize first for the Turks as they sought to expand into Europe and then for the Austrians who had ambitions to fill the space left by the Turks.

As the Turkish Empire had begun to crumble, Serbia had, at the beginning of the nineteenth century, begun to wrest back her freedom, obtaining some degree of independence. Austria who had her own plans for hegemony within the Balkans, was resentful of an independent Slav nation active on its borders. As an empire that ruled over many Slavs not always quite so keen to be ruled over, she had good reason to fear the creation of a large Slavic alliance. In 1908, Austria made her aspirations fairly clear when she annexed the neighbouring country of Bosnia Herzegovina. Austria watched over this troubled region with undisguised avarice...

At the beginning of the twentieth century, Macedonia, today once more an independent nation, was still struggling to free itself from Turkish rule. As early as 1902, Charles and Noel Buxton, brothers sharing both

Nursing in Serbia with Lady Paget in 1915

parliamentary ambitions and, as good Liberals, an ardent interest in supporting the rights of small nations, had created a Balkan Committee with a view to sending aid to the beleaguered Macedonians. When a year later an insurrection and massacre took place, they founded the Macedonian Relief Fund [MRF] to raise finance to support the stricken population.

After the outbreak of the First Balkan War on 8 October 1912, the unlikely alliance of Serbia, Greece, Bulgaria and Montenegro won an even more unlikely victory over the Turks at Kumanovo sixteen days later. This hapless country of Macedonia, destined to be disputed over by Serbia and Bulgaria for many years to come, was then swiftly occupied by Serbia, keen to reclaim her ancient capital of Skoplje.

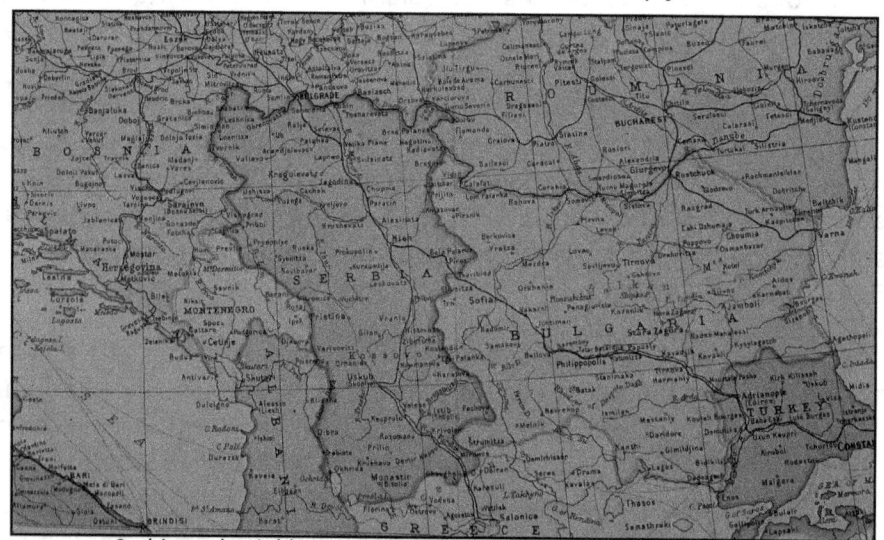

Serbia and neighbouring lands from The Great World War, *1916*

The MRF stepped in to aid not only the victorious Serbs but also the defeated, including the many Albanian refugees who had perversely fought on the side of the Turks. Miss Eglantyne Jebb (1876-1828), sister in law of Charles Buxton and future founder of the Save the Children Fund, was sent to administer the fund and travelled out in March 1913, via Vienna and Belgrade, with a Miss Hodges, a nurse.[4]

Miss Hodges planned to assist a fellow nursing colleague, Miss

The Serbian Relief Fund

McQueen, who was endeavouring to open a hospital supported by the MRF in Monastir. Miss Jebb quickly began to understand the complexity of passions with which she would have to deal. In Belgrade, the British Minister Sir Ralph Paget, *'a well known Turkophil'*, entrusted the pair of women with a bale of goods which was for *'Turks only'*, along with passes for free rail travel.[5]

In Skoplje, she met Mr Cahan, the young MRF agent, who like her was secretly disappointed that all was returning to normal life so quickly: *'Everything was in absolute order; there were houses, shops, restaurants, poplar trees... There was even in Uscub (Skoplje) a 'Bon Marché' and a tailor's shop 'Aubongu Turque'.'*[6] The First Balkan War was to end on 30 May 1913.

There had however, been quite sufficient excitement for the British consul, Mr Peckham. When the Turkish Governor had fled, he had gone out with other foreign consuls, to surrender the town to the victorious Serbs, equipped only with a white pillow slip on a broom. This action had brought an end to the looting and violence which had broken out in the town and prevented further bloodshed but had only drawn the disapproval of the British Government which thought it was no role for a consul. During the early years of the First World War, Mr Peckham would often regale British visitors with this tale, as he held court with the various medical personnel and distinguished visitors who passed through Skoplje. Miss Jebb talked with the Consul and found him *'the typical Englishman, with alas that official manner that all consuls acquire.'* She did not warm to him until she found that *'his chief amusement was sewing'.*[7]

At Monastir, where Miss Jebb found the two English nurses preparing an infirmary to receive large numbers of refugees, she found things to be rather different. The British Consul told her that there were around 11,000 refugees, mostly Moslem villagers who had fled the Serbian army. Amongst them, workers from the MRF were struggling to provide food for around 6000. It was to be Eglantyne's first experience of the plight of the refugee and it was not a lesson she would forget. She returned home

Nursing in Serbia with Lady Paget in 1915

eager to raise more funds to support the work but was rather overtaken by events. On 16 June 1913, Bulgaria made a surprise attack upon Serbia hoping to wrest back Macedonia. They were repulsed within a month but peace, when it came on 18 July 1913, was not destined to last long.

The small struggling nation of Serbia had been under Turkish rule since the disastrous battle of Kossovo in 1389. The date of the battle – 28th June – had been long regarded as a sacred national day, and young Serbs had been regaled from earliest days, with tales of the battle in much the same fashion as young Greeks would have once enjoyed Homeric tales of the battle for Troy. The selection of this date for Archduke Franz Ferdinand, the Austrian Crown Prince to visit Sarajevo in neighbouring Bosnia Herzogovina, was, to say the least, unwise. To many, it seemed deliberately provocative. It certainly seemed this way to a young Serb nationalist named Gavrilo Princip who promptly seized the opportunity to shoot him.

The assassination of the Archduke on 28 June 1914 provided the excuse Austria had long sought to attack Serbia. A reluctant Serbia found herself at war for the third time in three years and she was ill prepared for another conflict. She had no nursing service and many of her doctors had been lost in the previous wars. She was already exhausted economically and spiritually.

The Austrians attacked with great confidence but were shocked to meet stiff resistance. The image of gallant little Serbia holding its own against an aggressive neighbour was one with particular appeal to the Allied Nations and in particular their newspaper proprietors. With every intention of exploiting such sympathies, Mabel Grujic, the American wife of the Serbian Under-Secretary for Foreign Affairs set out for London to plead for help. She already had one good friend: Lady Leila Paget who had worked with her in managing a military hospital in Belgrade during the recent Balkan conflict (Oct 1912-May 1913). At the outbreak of war once more in August 1914, Lady Paget hurried back from holiday in California and hastened to throw herself into aiding Serbia.[8]

The Serbian Relief Fund

Louise Margaret Leila Wemyss Paget (1881-1958) had been born in Belgravia, into a world of privilege. Her father, Sir Arthur Fitzroy Paget, was an army officer and the grandson of the first Marquess of Anglesey who had lost a leg at Waterloo. Sir Arthur also had the dubious honour of being the General commanding the forces in Ireland at the time of the Curragh Mutiny in 1914. Her mother Mary, the daughter of Mr and Mrs Paran Stevens of New York, was well known in high society and expected her daughter to follow suit. Leila however, hampered by extreme diffidence, recoiled from the life of a debutante and was probably saved by marriage in 1907 to her cousin Ralph Spencer Paget (1864-1940), a career diplomat.

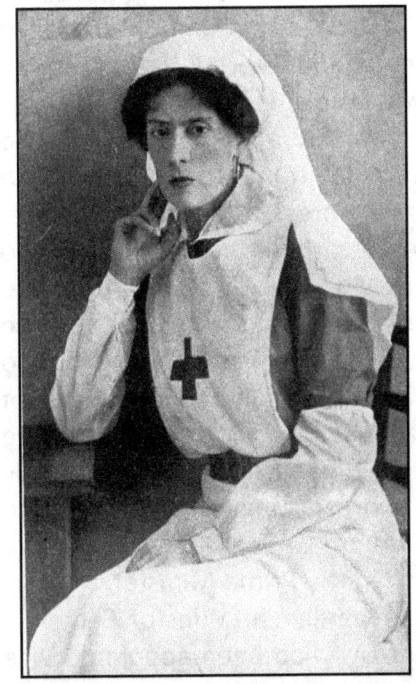

Whilst her husband was British Minister in Bangkok, Leila enjoyed exploring Siam but when, after his knighthood in 1909, he was posted to Bavaria, she found the life dull and urged him to accept a transfer to Serbia. The Pagets served in Serbia only from 1910 until 1913, but significantly, were there during the First Balkan War. Befriended by Mabel Grujić the American wife of the Serbian Under-Secretary for foreign affairs, Leila volunteered to assist in the management of a military hospital in Belgrade and is said to have worked so hard that her health gave way.[9] The experience of nursing in Belgrade clearly made a profound impression upon Lady Paget. Subsequent accolades of her as a 'born leader' and 'woman of indomitable heroism' suggest that she had discovered her true qualities during this period. Ensuing events certainly proved her a remarkable woman of great courage and determination.

In response to the plight of war-torn Serbia, a curious group of six

Nursing in Serbia with Lady Paget in 1915

'*experts in Balkan affairs*' was summoned to 22, Berners Street in London. The gathering which met on 23 September 1914, included men like the distinguished archaeologist Sir Arthur Evans (1851-1941) who had travelled in the Balkans in 1875 and Sir Ignatius Valentine Chirol (1852-1929) a journalist, author, historian and diplomat who had just returned from the area. Dr Robert William Seton Watson, a political activist, who was later to play a prominent role in promoting the cause of the new nation of Czechoslovakia and in establishing a school of Slavonic and Eastern European Studies at University College, London served as Honorary Secretary.[10] He was also joined by the journalist Bertram Christian, who acted as Chairman, and a Mr Fitzmaurice, who was probably Gerald Fitzmaurice, the chief translator at the British Embassy to the Ottoman Empire. The sole representative of the medical world at this stage seems to have been a certain Miss Mcqueen, who had evidently found her way back from Monastir. The group resolved to initiate a fund, modelled upon the Macedonian Relief Fund, to be known as the Serbian Relief Fund. Dr R W Seton Watson undertook to draft a letter for the press and it was agreed to approach a number of distinguished ladies and gentlemen to ask them to serve on an executive committee. Their number included Noel Buxton, Miss Jebb and Lady Paget and as the organisation grew, more distinguished names and patrons were regularly added. By February 1915, Queen Mary had agreed to serve as patron and no less than the Prime Minister, Herbert Asquith and the distinguished members of parliament Winston Churchill, Austen Chamberlain and Andrew Bonar Law had been appointed Vice Presidents.

By 1 October 1914, subscriptions already amounted to £1750. On the same date Lady Paget made a statement to the effect that she hoped to organise a unit of forty one persons for hospital work in Serbia. If transport could be secured, she hoped to start out on 15 October. A grateful letter was read out from a Serbian Minister stating that a hospital would be placed at the disposal of the Unit. It was estimated that the initial outfit would cost £1000 and its maintenance a further £600 per month. The Serbian Government undertook to supply rations.

The Serbian Relief Fund

A printed appeal to the public for funds, drafted by Seton Watson, was evidently successful and by 22 October subscriptions amounted to £4,983. Lady Paget was authorised to spend up to £500 on hospital equipment and a subcommittee consisting of Lady Grogan, Miss Macqueen and Lady Paget was set up to settle expenditure. Difficulties were clearly experienced in negotiations with Mr Morrison, a surgeon in Birmingham who was also planning to take a medical unit out to Serbia with the sponsorship of the Order of St John's, and in securing transport, but on 22 October, when the Admiralty confirmed its offer of transport from Southampton to Salonika via Malta on SS Dongola, Lady Paget was ready.

On 29 October 1914, when the first Serbian Relief Unit left Southampton bound for Serbia, it was natural - although not universally popular with medical staff and certainly not with Mr Morrison, her chief surgeon- that Lady Paget should lead the unit as administrator. The party consisted of four doctors, twenty four nurses, eighteen orderlies and 350 bales of equipment. The intention was to set up a hospital as close as possible to the front line, but since the Austrians were threatening to overrun Kragujevatz and the provincial capital of Nish, it was decided to install a hospital at Skoplje – better known by its Turkish name of Uscub- one of the chief towns in the territory of 'New Serbia', the area recaptured from the Turks in 1912.

Lady Paget was eventually joined by her husband, Sir Ralph Paget. His role of advisor was later formally recognised, when, on 29 March 1915, he was appointed British Commissioner *'acting on behalf of the Serbian Relief Fund and British Red Cross Society in Serbia'* by the Serbian Relief Committee. Although his role meant he travelled regularly between different units, he was frequently to be found with his wife in Skoplje.

Dismissing the offer of three tobacco warehouses, which were subsequently taken over by the British Red Cross, Lady Paget's unit chose as its hospital a former school which had recently been transformed by the Serbians into a hospital of 330 beds. The building was very dirty but offered good light and ventilation.

Nursing in Serbia with Lady Paget in 1915

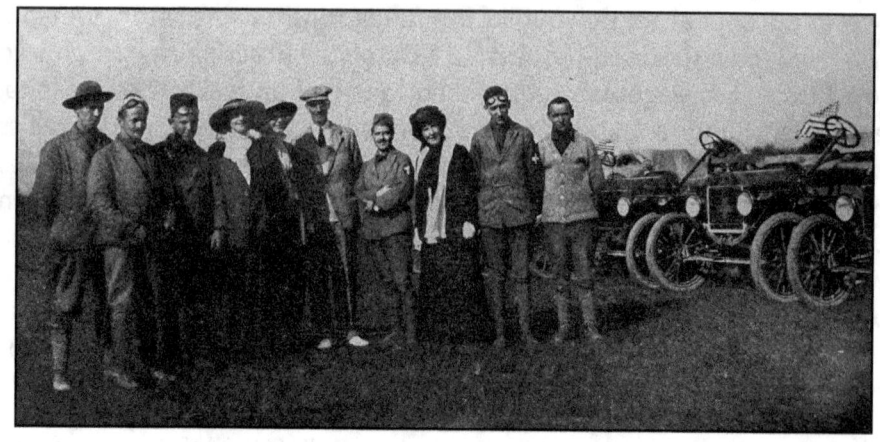

Sir Ralph Paget (in cap, centre) with relief workers from Paul Fortier Jones's With Serbia into Exile, *1916*

Dr Johnston Abraham, of the British Red Cross Field Unit viewed the preparations with undisguised envy:

'It seemed that the Paget unit which had arrived nearly a week in front of us, had appropriated the 'Gymnasium', a fine block of buildings used formerly as a technical school, and capable of accommodating three hundred beds. Previous to their arrival the Serbs had managed to overcrowd some five hundred patients into it. The first thing the English unit had done was to insist on all the patients being evacuated, and on having the whole place cleaned out in order that new beds, linen, and war equipment could be introduced, proper sanitary arrangements made, an operating theatre set up – in fact, all the essentials of a fully equipped English Hospital provided'...'[11]

After a heavy cleaning operation that lasted from 19th to 24th November, the number of beds was reduced to 272. The first batch of 180 wounded arrived at 6am on 24th November, consisting largely of serious cases with wounds caused by shrapnel and hand grenades. Many were in a bad condition, already suffering from gangrene and sepsis. A further 40 arrived the next day.

The Serbian Relief Fund

Sister Helen M Coleman who had been part of Mr Morrison's contingent from Birmingham, laid some claim to a connection with Leicester since she was the niece of the late Alderman G T Coleman. Her letter to friends in the town describing the early days of November 1914, was quoted in local newspapers in some detail:

'We are working very hard and have many worries and hardships and yet do not have to rough it nearly as much as some people, I think, for we have really good buildings, nice lofty rooms with good windows. It was the High School, quite a modern building, and if we had taken it over from the school people, it would have been all right; but the Serbs had used it as a hospital before our arrival, and it was filthy...The first few days we were here we simply cleaned and scrubbed until our hands were in a most awful state. Mine were so cracked and sore that it was positively painful to hold a pen or knife. Then one day over 100 badly wounded men arrived. Never have I seen such an awful spectacle...'[12]

When she returned to Leicester, in June the following year, Miss Coleman organised an exhibition of Serbian handwork to raise funds for the Serbians, and gave further details to the reporter from the *Leicester Daily Post* who interviewed her, as she posed for photographs in Serbian costume:

'I found a terrible state of things, when I first arrived in Serbia. The Serbians had had three years of war and in October last they were practically without nurses, doctors, dressings and surgical apparatus... Some of the men were in a fearful state when brought into hospital from the front... Some of the poor fellows had been on the train for ten days. Their wounds had been roughly bandaged on the battlefield, and when the bandages were removed in the hospital, sometimes a limb would drop off in consequence of mortification having set in, through want of proper attention...'[13]

Miss Alice Pell who also served with Lady Paget at this time, recounted similar memories:

'The wounded brought into our hospital were in the most appalling

Nursing in Serbia with Lady Paget in 1915

condition and, and most of them had been travelling for a fortnight. Their wounds were dreadful, and they were horribly septic. We had no clean cases at all. In one case I had we took a cupful of pieces of shrapnel from the man's leg. The bone was all shattered, and the wound very septic. Another man's leg was in the shape of a corkscrew when he was brought in. It was fractured, and had been twisted about so much on the journey. Both his feet were dropping off with gangrene, and he had a big gangrenous patch on his back. He lived about six weeks, and seemed quite hopeful of pulling through.'[14]

Whilst the surgeons worked non-stop, often forced to resort to amputations, Lady Paget found time to record her appreciation of all her workers. She was particularly impressed with the way the orderlies, with no medical experience, coped with the undressing and washing the patients: 'One can say that throughout the work of the hospital untrained and uneducated orderlies proved themselves to be extremely adaptable, quick to learn, conscientious in their duties and hard workers...'[15]

With notable exceptions, the unit seems to have functioned well together. Henry Squire, a medical student who was serving as an orderly, recorded in the diary he sent to his parents:

'The unit as a whole is composed of awfully nice people. I like all the orderlies and in fact all the men, and most of the sisters, though some of them are regular old hens. Lady Paget of course is simply marvellous as an organiser and she is most awfully tactful. I am sure the Unit would never have kept together without her. She smooths over all the petty squabbles which there are bound to be, and hardly ever forgets even the smallest trifles...'[16]

Although there was a good water supply to Skoplje, pumped from two artesian wells, the supply was often cut off. The drainage, was even less satisfactory and the atmosphere was unpleasant and unhealthy. There was frequent illness amongst the staff with serious attacks of septic throat and it was rare that more than eight were on duty at one time. Lady Paget attributed the problems in her later report to so much sepsis and gangrene in wards which were not properly ventilated and a serious

The Serbian Relief Fund

amount of sewer gas permeating the main building.

Henry Squire described the problems caused by ill health amongst the staff when he told his parents how difficult it was to attend a church service on Sundays:

'We are so hopelessly understaffed that every minute is occupied and as for leaving altogether for an hour it seems impossible. Even for meals we go in batches. At present we are all working 12-14 hours a day, seven days a week and it's jolly hard work...'[17]

Despite the evident problems, the British Red Cross Field Unit who were now close neighbours, were in a far worse predicament. They consisted only of six doctors and twelve orderlies and had been sent out at short notice with the intention of serving as a Field Unit at the battle front. To their disappointment, they found that their civilian status, their lack of military training and their ignorance of Serbian, meant that there was no desire amongst the Serbians to use them in a military setting. Instead, they found themselves in Skoplje, acting as a casualty clearing station for the thousands of wounded men who were now pouring in to the town. For this work, the unit was woefully under resourced. Dr J Johnston Abraham recalled the time with horror:

'There was no chloroform, we hadn't time, and the patients were afraid of it. In treatment we had gone back to the period of the Napoleonic wars.'[18]

The British Red Cross were not alone. Edward Beric Alabaster who was a dresser with the Lady Paget unit, later told a representative of the Birmingham Daily Post:

'In Uscub everything was absolutely crowded out. There were altogether about 5,000 wounded in the old Serbian capital, and all the hospitals were overcrowded and understaffed. In one of the typhus hospitals there was one doctor to 900 beds. He never went in to the wards. Serbian orderlies, who had already had typhus, did the work in the wards and the doctor came to the doors and took their reports... The hospitals were

Nursing in Serbia with Lady Paget in 1915

terribly insanitary. There were no conveniences to speak of, and patients were lying all over the place...'[19]

When the British Red Cross doctors visited the Paget Hospital, it seemed like a different world:

'How we envied them the cleanliness of the place, the smiling eyes of the sisters, the small wards of some twelve to twenty beds where no one could be overlooked, the washed faces and the clean bodies of the patients actually clad in new pyjamas, lying between real sheets which were changed whenever required. The contrast to our own place made our hearts ache.'[20]

Envy of their neighbours was compounded by irritation, when a Royal visit to the hospital by the Crown Prince of Serbia, for which they had prepared themselves with much polishing of buttons and scabbards, ended in disappointment:

'The Prince had asked for the English Hospital, been taken to the Paget Unit, said the proper polite things, assumed that this was the only English unit in Uscub, and departed.'[21]

However, despite the impressive efforts of Lady Paget and her staff, it was to be their unit which suffered the first fatality amongst the British in Skoplje. On 25 December, a nursing sister, Nellie Clark, of Bilsby in Lincolnshire, died of a septic throat and early onset of Grave's disease. She was only twenty six.

All the British in Skoplje had been invited to dine with the Paget Unit that evening, but instead of Christmas festivities, guests found events overshadowed by news of this first death.

On the following Saturday, Dr Johnston Abraham and the Russian Doctor, Dr Esther Kadisch, who had joined the British Red Cross in their unequal struggles in the Tobacco Warehouses, attended Nellie's funeral at two in the afternoon. They found the entrance gate of the Paget hospital surrounded by a crowd of curious onlookers: *'picturesque groups of*

The Serbian Relief Fund

Serbian women and children, in their most gaudy holiday attire'. In the quadrangle in front of the hospital, a military band was playing, whilst a platoon of students' corps from Belgrade stood to attention at one side of the gate. A group of high ranking Serbian officials, bedecked in gold epaulettes stood beside the empty hearse:

'Finally, out came the coffin wrapped in a Union Jack. It was put in the hearse, and the procession formed quietly. In front came the band, playing the Serbian Marche Funebre. After it came the firing party. An acolyte, swinging a silver incense burner, followed, and then four gorgeously-arrayed priests of the Greek Church, headed by the Bishop of Uskub.'[22]

The procession ended at the Cathedral where a service in Greek was performed with much chanting. At the end, the Serbian Commandant of the hospital gave a powerful funeral oration in which those who could understand Serbian, heard how *'this woman from far-off England had come to Serbia and laid down her life for the sake of the Serbian people'*. Dr Abraham noted *'many wet eyes around'*:

'When he had finished the band struck up again, and the grim procession began to wind its way through the streets, over the railway, through a sea of mud to the Christian graveyard beyond the station. There the British Consul, in full-dress uniform, read the simple, beautiful service of the English Church over the open grave, with the Greek priests, the Serbian officers, and the assembled mourners looking on. There was a pause, and quietly someone started a hymn. It was 'Lead, Kindly Light,' and all the British, standing amongst the silent Serbs, joined in.'

It was the first time that Dr Johnston Abraham had heard the Serbian Funeral March. In later years, he recalled:

'Afterwards, in the months to come it became only too familiar. I used to wonder how I could ever have liked it; for it came to be horrible, a nightmare, a dreadful thing to be pushed back in one's mind by any and every means.'[23]

Nursing in Serbia with Lady Paget in 1915

Although, in Lady Paget's official report of these events there was no room for sentiment and no account of the funeral, she later wrote of Nellie Clark:

'She was the best nurse we had, and was so very sweet and gentle that she was loved by everyone who had the honour of knowing her. As for the wounded men she nursed, they simply adored her, and it was touching to see their grief when they heard of her death.'[24]

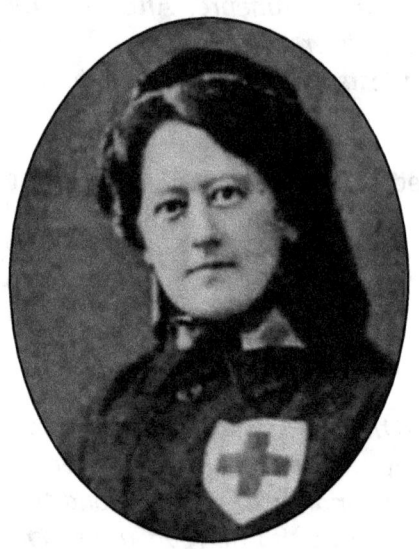

After this incident, concern at the Paget hospital about other members of staff who were sick increased substantially. In January, two orderlies and a ward maid were invalided home, leaving an exhausted unit dangerously understaffed, just as typhus and dysentery cases began to add to their worries. It was increasingly clear that help was now badly needed and at home in London, swift efforts were made to organise some relief. The sudden 'phone call to Flora Scott in Leicester was one such measure.

Chapter 3

Journey to Serbia

'Serbia was the place of all others I wished to give my services to...'

Like a surprising number of Leicester's other citizens, Flora was on holiday on the Continent in July 1914, when rumours of war first caused concern. From Switzerland, she hurried home, fortunate in catching one of the last trains for Boulogne. Back once more in her nursing home in Victoria Road, she was anxious to offer her services to the War Office but found her proprietorship of a Nursing Home a substantial problem. When she offered the Home itself to the War Office, she was disappointed to learn that whilst they welcomed the generosity of her gift, they also required it to be rent and rate free. This Flora could not afford.

It is clear that Flora remained restless, longing to serve in the war as a nurse in some capacity. She contacted the War Office once more and the Order of St John's but found that nobody would contemplate service of under twelve months and she was well aware that her financial circumstances could not permit so long a closure of her Home. Not a woman to be easily deterred, Flora now turned to the French Red Cross and found them much more sympathetic. They, it seemed, would accept her service – and apparently that of her nurses- even for as short a term as three months. Eagerly, Flora and four of her nurses filled in the requisite papers, arranged inoculations and assembled kit. Throughout December, they waited to be summoned with increasing impatience, only to be informed that as the French Red Cross was being reorganised, it would be some weeks before they would be required. One can't help wondering what it was like to be a patient in the Nursing Home at this time with all the staff intent on rushing abroad to more glamorous roles...

Meanwhile, Flora had also been following events in Serbia with great interest: *'Serbia was the place of all others I wished to give my services to. I knew the work there would be splendid, also that they were very short of Doctors, Nurses etc.'* Flora's memories of the sequence of events

Nursing with Lady Paget in Serbia in 1915

seem rather confused but she later recalled that she had contacted the Serbian Minister in London and been offered free passage and an equipped hospital if she could assemble a medical unit to serve there. She had no trouble, it seems, in finding nurses but was unable to persuade any doctors to join her venture. Reluctantly abandoning the endeavour, she now heard that a unit organised by Lady Paget was travelling out to Serbia in early November. When she wrote asking to join the unit, she was informed that the unit was already complete and it must have been then that she turned her thoughts to service in France. However, by the beginning of January 1915, France too seemed a frustrated ambition.

This then was the unsatisfactory state of affairs when at 8.35pm on Monday 11th January 1915, Flora answered the telephone to receive a trunk call from London. The message, from a Mr Bertram Christian of the Serbian Relief Fund, came as great surprise:

'Are you still willing to go to Serbia? If so, could you be ready by Friday next?'

With admirable decisiveness, Flora wired back: *'Willing to go, will write tonight.'*

Her world and indeed that of her nurses and patients was thrown in to immediate turmoil....

'Helping in the Terrible War'

Early next morning, Flora received a wire summoning her to London to meet the Committee of the Serbian Relief Fund. It was the redoubtable Miss Macqueen who interviewed nurses. Flora duly attended at 3 o'clock that afternoon and the audience must have proved satisfactory to all sides, for she left with instructions to order her kit and be ready for Friday. Her request that two of her nurses should accompany her was duly considered and when she arrived back at Leicester, she found a message agreeing to their service.

In a subsequent letter to her brother Sydney, she confessed that the

Journey to Serbia

process of persuasion had not been that easy:

'...*as you know I have always wanted Serbia much more than France, firstly because the work is much better. They have no trained nurses & very, very few Drs, so they (English) are sending only very experienced nurses out. I had to beg real hard for 2 of my nurses to come & told them I hesitated to go out alone so said I would take them as my assistant & workmaid....*'

In fact, both nurses, Ivy Pickering and Laetitia Cluley, were experienced and Laetitia had qualified at North Evington Infirmary in 1913. Perhaps, this arrangement by Flora with the Serbian Relief Fund partly explains a certain distance that grew between her and her former staff once out in Serbia. A third nurse, Nurse Turtle whom Flora had hoped to take, was now nursing at a Convalescent Home for wounded soldiers in Billesdon and could not join the party.

Before she left London, Flora called at Garrould's Nurses Department in Edgeware Road, to order her kit, explaining that her two nurses might soon require the same items. The allowance of £10 for kit was supposed to cover indoor and outdoor uniforms; wellington boots; a '*huge blue coat*'; soft large blue hat; sleeping bag or bed; buckets for washing; warm wraps and underclothes to guard against what they were warned would be the '*intense*' cold of the Balkans.

It was only on the train journey home that Flora wrote to her sisters and friends informing them of her imminent departure. Their great shock at the news can be well imagined: '*All friends asked if it was wise to go to such a terrible country & seemed to think the risk was very great*'.

Despite all dire warnings, Flora was enormously excited by the project and now had but three days in which to prepare for the great adventure, remove patients from her Home, pack and store '*this great house*' and make all other household arrangements.

Household arrangements evidently involved persuading friends and relatives to take on responsibility for a large menagerie during her

Nursing with Lady Paget in Serbia in 1915

absence. The ironically named 'Tiny'- an Irish wolfhound - was put in the care of Nurse Pickering's parents who evidently seemed to think it fair exchange for their daughter. Another hound, 'Vanity' went to Mrs Corah at Scraptoft Hall. The three parrots ('Polly Freeps','Polly Fry' and 'Mary Grey') were also a source of some concern since they were liable to fret in Flora's absence. The cat alone refused to cooperate, rejecting the loving care of 'Mrs Crosley' and insisting on remaining alone in the house where the understanding Mrs Crosley undertook to feed her with the support of 'Mrs Black'. Such domestic concerns are an endearing insight into the life which Flora was leaving behind in Leicester.

Timsons, the removal company, was employed to pack Flora's china and silver and other possessions away whilst she undertook to settle all debts and leave everything in 'apple pie order'. Amidst such preparations, the staff found themselves besieged by visitors and well wishers. 'Mr Hewitt' the local newspaper proprietor, had kindly put notices in the *Leicester Daily Post* and the *Leicester Mercury* announcing the departure of Flora and her retinue and requesting gifts for the Serbians.

The generous response of readers overwhelmed the Nursing Home. In the end three large packing cases were filled with 15lbs of tea; cocoa; chocolate; nearly 40lbs of biscuits; bottles of Bovril; Bengers Food; 30lbs of sweets; sugar; rice; candles; matches; and tinned fruits. Mrs Hewitt led the way with six dozen pairs of socks but there were also mittens, [balaclava] helmets, hot water bottles and blankets. Several Doctors in the town sent in money and the Presbyterian Church contributed 10s 10. In addition there were many personal presents of soap; tooth powder; brushes; scent and writing paper. It was heart-warming but also exhausting and Flora and her staff had little time to sleep or eat.

It was with enormous relief therefore that Flora received the message on the Thursday afternoon that departure was postponed until Tuesday. They now had three more days in which to prepare themselves

Amongst Flora's surviving papers at the Imperial War Museum is a moving collection of letters from well wishers and colleagues.[25] They afford an interesting insight into the deep affection in which Flora was

Journey to Serbia

held amongst fellow nurses and former patients. One, Ethel Alexander from Clarendon Park craved the 'kindly word and goodnight kiss which you always gave me when I was in your Home.' Another from Leire accompanied her good wishes with a New Testament and a collection of wool mendings and sewing cottons 'if you have room'. Agnes Johnson, condemned by posterity to be ever remembered as the wife of Thomas Fielding Johnson- despite many achievements in her own right- sent rubber foot warmers *'so comforting and indeed necessary in severe cases'*. Nellie Thompson, nursing wounded at Little Dalby Hall, joined in the general admiration for the courage of the departing sisters but like many was puzzled that Serbia was the destination despite all previous setbacks.

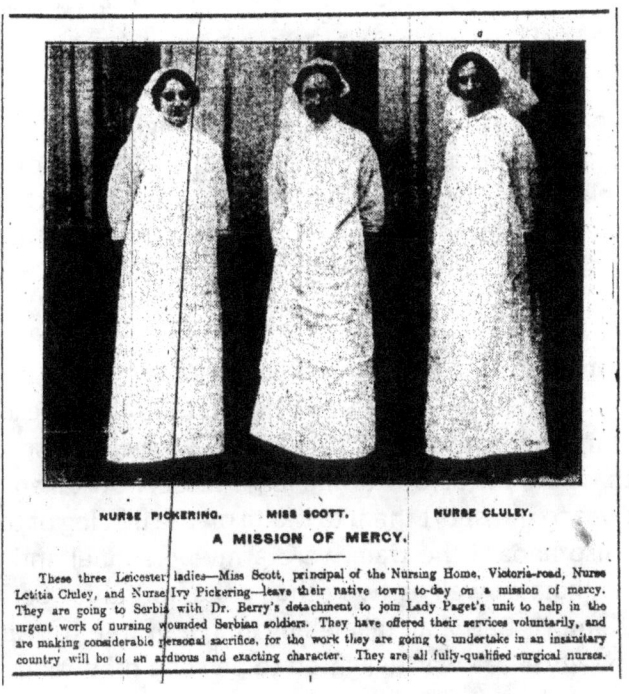

Leicester Daily Post, *18th January 1915*

Elinor Pell Smith, Flora's former employer at her Nursing Home in De Montfort Square, expressed the thoughts of many: *'It is splendid to be*

Nursing with Lady Paget in Serbia in 1915

able to help our country in her need.' and sent a pound since 'I have not a single sock etc left; no time to make anything'. In contrast, Major Goddard of the Magazine, Leicester, was more interested in Flora's nursing home. Would she be subletting and what were the arrangements for rent?

There was also a letter from the mother of one of the nurses, Frances Pickering of Humberstone Road, thanking Flora for her kindness to her daughter Ivy:

'It is good of you to take her away with you and we are both willing for her to go, as the voyage and the experience will do her a lot of good. We think it very brave of you all to go to Serbia, but, you will all have the satisfaction of knowing you have helped in this terrible war...'

'Oh how dreary everything seemed'

Preferring to sleep at home on the Monday night, Flora undertook to be at Paddington Station at 10.30 am on the morning of Tuesday 19 January. This necessitated leaving Leicester at six and the weary trio may well have had some regrets about this as they rose at 4.30 am to bathe and breakfast. *'Oh, how dreary everything seemed.'* recalled Flora in her memoirs.

Exhaustion and anxiety were forgotten however, when the party reached Paddington. The platform had been decorated and an excited crowd hustled them towards the train. They were to travel by a special train to Avonmouth where the *SS Dilwara*, a large vessel now taken over by the Admiralty, was to transport them to Malta on the first leg of their journey to Serbia. Also aboard the train were army personnel and families on their way to India as well as two other units bound for Serbia under a Dr Bennett and Dr Berry, all taking advantage of free transport offered by the Admiralty. Flora was delighted to be seen off by Lady Grogan on behalf of the Serbian Relief Fund :

'Never can we forget that platform. As the train left, flags and handkerchiefs waved, shouts of Bravo and Good Luck etc were shouted and little bunches of white heather & violets were thrown into the

Journey to Serbia

carriages...'

An immense cheer arose as the train puffed out of the station. Never adverse to having her photograph taken, Flora took note of the many photographers on the platform and excitedly advised her sisters: *'Look in picture paper carefully tomorrow'.*

'Many many people have asked me to write my experiences of nursing in Serbia. In the following, I will try to tell them, but readers, please remember I am not trying to write a book but just stating what I saw & helped to do when in Serbia in the beginning half of 1915'

In later days, Flora made several attempts to write an account of her experiences in Serbia but never seems to have concluded the task. Her literary efforts form a bundle of notes which tell us almost as much from the scribal deletions as the actual text itself. Her letters to her family provide a more intimate insight into her thoughts, fears and concerns when still nursing in Serbia, whilst her notes, written later and clearly intended for publication, tend to be less revealing. Indeed, whilst still abroad, many of Flora's letters to her family at home were published in local newspapers but in an edited form, which Flora herself did not always recognise or approve. Nevertheless, from the three sources, it is possible to piece together some impression of Flora's Serbian adventure...

One name which often appears in Flora's accounts of the voyage out but usually crossed through, is that of Dr Berry. He and his wife, were, she noted, *'very excitable'* at the station. This was James Berry (1860-1946) a surgeon at the Royal Free Hospital, London and his wife, Dr Frances May Dickinson, an anaesthetist at the same hospital. Pre-war, the adventurous pair had enjoyed long cycling holidays in south eastern Europe and were fluent in several languages including Serbian. In December 1914, they had been inspired to assemble a medical unit for Serbia after attending a talk by Mabel Grujic[26], the American wife of a Serbian minister, and would go on to establish a highly successful hospital at Vrnjatchka Banja, an elegant spa resort in Northern Serbia.

Nursing with Lady Paget in Serbia in 1915

The couple's own account of their service in Serbia *'The Story of a Red Cross Unit in Serbia'*(1916) is a lively and entertaining account of their experiences. Their hospital gained something of a reputation amongst English visitors for the dramatic and musical evenings which they hosted. One member of the unit in particular, Jan Gordon, was widely admired for his banjo playing and Flora's evident enjoyment of the music on the voyage to Salonika suggests that she too appreciated the musicality of her fellow passengers. Jan Gordon and his wife, Cora, an artist, also published an account of their experiences, dedicated to Dr Berry, under the title *'The Luck of Thirteen'*(1916) but sadly made no mention of their journey out to Serbia.

Although, James Berry or 'The Professor' as he was usually known, was born in Ontario, his father, Edward Berry, a solicitor and ship owner, had originated in Leicester.[27] It is probable that Flora was too much in awe of the Doctor to have ever discussed such matters. Whilst, Mrs Berry recorded that the Bay of Biscay was rough and those that could hold up their heads gathered daily on deck to learn the rudiments of Serbian from her husband, Flora had rather more to say about the tempestuous seas.

All had started in promising fashion. Flora found that the train had been divided up in to separate compartments for each unit. Lady Paget's unit consisted of a Doctor who is never named but was the Dr E F Eliot who is listed amongst 'Supplementary members', five nurses and two orderlies who were medical students from Cambridge. The two additional nurses were a Miss Mackintosh and Miss Moore but they seem to have made little impression upon Flora.[28]

The Doctor, Flora reported, was *'very nice, a military man, was in the Boar War & fetched ...from France to go with us...'* He was particularly concerned that Flora looked so ill after a week of feverish preparations with little sleep and prescribed *'a small bottle of champagne'* as a *'pick me up'*. Flora very much appreciated this as she tucked in to a generous luncheon of five courses. 'The Doctor' also reassured her that he would pay for everything and that they should ask for anything including tips.

Journey to Serbia

He advised that all money including *'the little gold'* which Flora carried should be sent back home, for he had been instructed to give the party everything they required to make them fit. They were well aware that they were going as a relief to a staff that *'were nearly all ill'.*

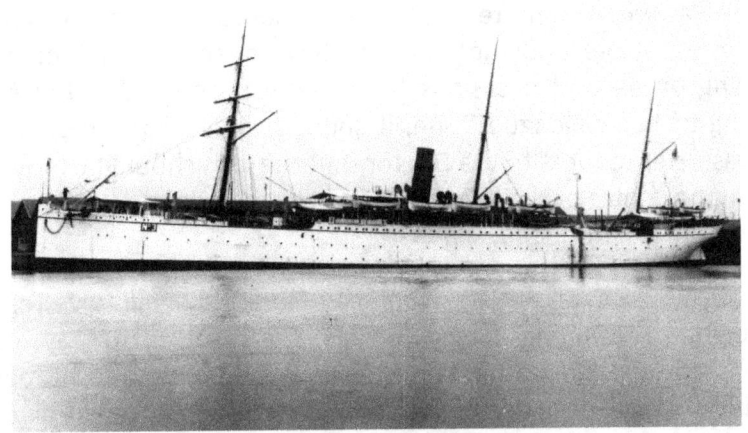

Postcard of the SS Dilwara, c. 1905

At Avonmouth, the *SS Dilwara*, a large vessel formerly owned by the British & Indian Steam Navigation Company, was awaiting the train's arrival. Flora found time to send a postcard home and then wrote a letter to her sister and sister-in-law as soon as they had settled into their cabins. The ship was due to sail at 4.30 pm but had not left the docks four hours later, when the exhausted Leicester party decided to retire for the night. By then Flora had learnt from the Chief Mate that the ship was bound for Malta on a voyage that should take seven days, calling in at Gibraltar en route. Aboard were about 120 passengers consisting of a large number of high ranking military personnel and a number of wives on their way to India. In addition to Dr Berry's unit and Flora's own group, there were two other medical units bound for Serbia: part of Dr Bennett's British Red Cross unit which, like the Berry party, eventually ended up in Vrnjatchka Banja in Northern Serbia and a group bound for Montenegro which was probably the unit led by Dr Clemow *'late of the*

Nursing with Lady Paget in Serbia in 1915

Constantinople Embassy'.[29]

At seven the next morning, when the steward brought tea and biscuits, all seemed calm and quiet and there was some debate amongst the nurses as to whether they were at sea. All doubt was cast asunder, however, as within minutes, both nurses succumbed to overpowering sea sickness. Flora does not seem to have been awfully sympathetic, recording on several occasions her great amusement at the evident suffering of her colleagues. She, it seems, went off to enjoy a hearty breakfast. Her request to the Doctor that the girls should be moved to a cabin in the centre of the ship for their own good does not seem to have been totally disinterested.

However, when a gale arose at midday Flora may well have regretted her laughter. Wrapping herself in rugs, she resolved to stay on deck but was advised by the Captain that it was not safe and instead was permitted to sleep in the music room. The gale worsened and Flora, bravely attempting to take a bath found herself almost tossed out on to the floor. Her troubles were compounded when the bathroom door slammed on her left hand, trapping a finger. She ruefully recalled that she became the ship's doctor's first patient and fainted several times before being carried to the music room where she remained for the next three days. Even here, the 'windows' had to be boarded and shuttered but Flora still preferred it to the cabin. Meanwhile, her nurses were also very ill and could take only a little champagne - apparently the main cure prescribed for all ills.

It was difficult, however, to repress the high spirits of the Berry party and on Friday evening, Flora found her temporary cabin in the music room disturbed by several gentlemen, intent on a musical evening:

'I don't think I have ever laughed so much. One started to play, another to sing. Several sat around listening. Over went the stool and everyone rolled on the floor & went together first to one side of the ship, then to the other [and] could not keep their seats even on the floor...'

Dr Berry strapped himself to a seat and more hilarity ensued when the

Journey to Serbia

strap gave way and he was hurled across the room, sustaining, amidst rather unsympathetic laughter, an injury to his eye. Dr Berry may not have told his wife about these high jinks, and she was probably 'hors de combat' for she made no mention of the incident in her account and recalled first encountering the banjo and inimitable songs of Mr Jan Gordon *'which during so many months were to be such an antidote to depression and influence of sociability in the Unit, as well as such an unfailing attraction to lay before our Serbian visitors...'* only when the party left Malta.[30] Flora certainly seems to have enjoyed herself in their company.

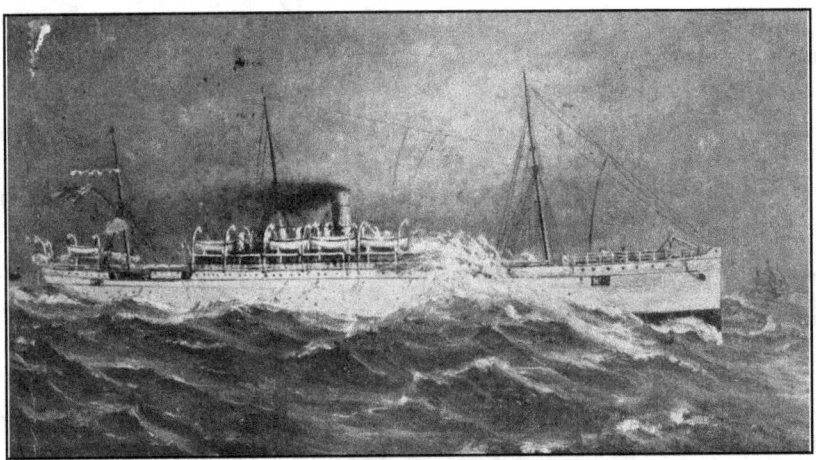

Postcard of HM Transport Dilwara in stormy seas, c. 1915

The storm appears to have been particularly bad, even for the notorious Bay of Biscay and it was not until noon on the Saturday that the gale finally ceased. The Captain's bridge had been blown away, large quantities of crockery had been broken and more than half of the crew had been ill. It was not a good introduction to sea travel for Nurses Pickering and Cluley. Now, the fiddles [rails or battens to prevent things falling off] were removed from the tables, plants and flowers decorated the dining room once more and life seemed a little brighter.

In Flora's letters to her sisters, written when the horror of the experience was still fresh, the storm and her own affliction with headaches are

Nursing with Lady Paget in Serbia in 1915

described rather more graphically:

'This is the first morning I have wished to be alive. Oh, we have had an awful time. It has not been sea sickness that has troubled me, more my head & a feeling of general helplessness & so tired. I have scarcely felt able to keep awake even for food but today I feel quite different although my head feels so tender & strange (not able to touch)....I have realised little except when the ship has thrown me out of bed, or used me as a shuttlecock. Oh it has been terrible. Am told that out of 120 passengers only 5 were at meals for 2 days...I told Dr from the first, I really thought if I had to sleep in cabin with shut port hole, I should just die, so they have let me have my sleeping bag in the music room... The cold has been intense & oh dear, never never do I wish to see or feel the Bay of Biscay again...'

Flora concluded the letter with anxious worries about her various pets distributed around Leicester and concerns about packing up her house. She felt as if she had been away weeks already and was alarmed to hear how bad the postal service was to Serbia:

'How about my house...? Did you manage to get it all packed up & straight? Am afraid there was a lot to do. I could never never go through that last week at home again. No wonder my head has been bad. It was terrible & oh, I do wonder when I shall see it again. All seem to have come for three months, says it is as long as anyone can stand. We say we shall strike & refuse to cross the Bay again, come overland if we can.'

Flora's misgivings about the coming adventure were understandable, especially since she seems to have had little idea about what awaited her in Serbia. She was unaware of what was planned once the party reached Malta and surprisingly ill informed about Lady Paget herself:

'We are not going with Dr Berry's party but straight to Lady Paget. She is the wife of our English Embassador in Servia, so of course partly lives there. She is said to be very charming, an American, I believe...'

In addition to her troubles, Flora was being pressurised by the remarkable

Journey to Serbia

Doctor to take up smoking:

'Dr insists upon me smoking. I certainly don't like the idea & yet cannot bring myself to it but he says if I am out & about [in]fields etc, it would certainly be wise for me to smoke. However, I will see later. I am not up to it at present...'

By Sunday morning, even Flora' s nurses appeared on deck once more, looking ill and weak. Flora teased them about their diet of champagne and fruit. As the coast of Portugal and Spain came in to view, they were assured that they would soon be entering the Mediterranean. All began to feel more optimistic. Flora noted that the other nurses *'seem nice'* and the orderlies *'quite gentlemen, Cambridge men...'*

One of the intriguing aspects of the British missions to Serbia during the First World War was the complete mix of those whom class distinctions would previously have kept apart. Mabel Dearmer, a well known artist and children's writer, was an orderly at Mrs Stobart's Field Hospital in Serbia and wrote in her *'Letters from a Field Hospital'*, published posthumously in 1915:

'The sets here are curious. Everything is reversed. The orderlies are ladies – the poor useless ladies who have been trained to nothing – we have to take our orders from the nurses...'[31] Flora makes no comment on this aspect of life in Serbia, but evidently gloried in her contact with the titled and upper class figures she encountered both now and later in her nursing career.

At Gibraltar, the ship called for four or five hours and Flora enjoyed viewing the rock and harbour in brilliant sunshine whilst a Colonel and former resident pointed out the highlights. She wrote with the first signs of enthusiasm to her brother Sydney:

'What a lovely place. Well worth seeing. Sunday and yesterday were lovely days, brilliant sunshine, light blue sky & water & quite smooth.'

High spirits were short lived:

Nursing with Lady Paget in Serbia in 1915

'*Today is terrible: rain simply pouring, so dark & grey, cold & rough. The boat is rolling terribly. We get to Malta on Thursday & stay there until the 6th when we get another boat to take us to Salonika. It will be a grand voyage if we can only have good weather, all through Islands of Greece etc 4 days voyage...*'

She was to be disappointed.

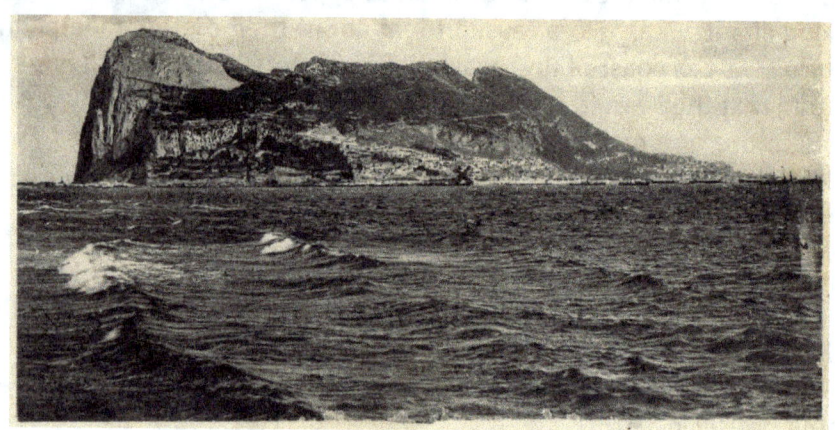

Postcard of Gibraltar, c. 1910

'It is impossible to tell you how lovely Malta is'

Despite the bad weather on Monday morning, Flora recalled '*a jolly time*' and particularly relished the '*delicious meals*'. She obviously enjoyed the company of the officers, and in particular listened with interest to the 'weird and heartening' tales of a Colonel Cunliffe Owen, who was on his way from the trenches of France to Egypt. She reported seeing 'water spouts' all day and found the only other interest was the sight of the coast of Africa. Amongst several islands, she took especial note of the Isle of Pantelleria where the Italians kept convicts, closely guarded by 'Men of War'. The ship reached Malta about 9am on the Thursday morning:

Journey to Serbia

'What a lovely picturesque place it looked in brilliant sunshine, standing very high on immence [sic] white rocks with oriental buildings & large palms. The entrance to the Grand Harbour is very magnificent...'

Although mightily relieved to be on land once more, Flora was sorry to leave her fellow passengers, now bound for India. She was enchanted by all that she beheld as she was rowed ashore in a *'pretty little boat'* and saluted by a detachment of Maltese soldiers. Amidst pomp which clearly delighted Flora, Lady Paget's unit were met by the English and Russian Consuls and escorted through customs to the perpendicular lift which raised them to the town of Valetta, *'the beautiful capital of Malta'*. Here carriages awaited them to convey them to the The Royal – the *'best hotel'*.

At the hotel, even an altercation with a very irate manager failed to dampen spirits. General embarrassment had ensued when the Doctor discovered that only four rooms had been reserved for their party of five ladies and three gentlemen, despite his having telephoned from Gibraltar to request a room for each member of the party. The manager, claiming that he did not have eight rooms available, was mollified- rather suspiciously- by the Doctor agreeing to pay double.

Flora rejoiced in the large comfortable bedrooms, marvelling at the canopy of the bed from which hung *'an immense piece of thin white muslin which entirely envelopes the bed from top to bottom'* [mosquito net]. She found the food delicious and well served with abundant fruit. Fresh from the delights of Leicester in January, she gloried in the warm weather and scenes of palm trees, orange and lemon groves and parks already displaying the colour of geraniums. Like many of the nurses who would pass through Malta on their way to Serbia, Flora was astonished at this *'land of bells'* noting that the churches seemed to hold services every hour.

Margaret Munro Kerr who served as a cook with a unit of the Scottish Women's Hospital when they called at Malta in April 1915, was equally impressed with the noise:

Nursing with Lady Paget in Serbia in 1915

'Valetta never sleeps, nor allows a visitor to do so. From 12pm to 4am there is a slight lull; but at 4am the church bells burst in to song and continue until midnight, whilst between their lusty clanging the goat bells tinkle a running comment...'[32]

The ubiquitous goats were a constant concern to an animal lover like Flora. As she climbed the steep narrow streets, fascinated by the oriental bazaars she noted *'a miserable looking goat'* beside many of the doors:

'Thirsty people pay their coin, take a mug, milk the goat & drink'

She worried very much as to when these hapless animals were fed. But a few months later, concern for hygiene and fear of fever would lead the authorities to instruct all 'troops of His Majesty' to refrain from goat's milk and to boil all water, fruit and vegetables, whilst always washing hands before a meal in a solution of potassium permanganate.[33] At this stage, however, rules were still relaxed.

Notwithstanding her concern for animal welfare in Malta, Flora evidently enjoyed exploring the tourist sites in the company of government officials. She noted that wherever they went, the Red Cross of their dress aroused much curiosity and crowds of interested onlookers followed them.

Amongst the tourist sites which it was, apparently, obligatory for all English visitors to admire was the ' Chapel of Bones', a bizarre chapel, built initially in 1619 but remodelled in Baroque style in 1731. The chapel lay close to a cemetery where deceased patients from an adjacent infirmary were laid and in 1852, the questionable decision was made to decorate the chapel's crypt with skeletal remains from the cemetery. Flora found the *'wall and ceiling thickly covered & decorated with human bones , rather gruesome but wonderful'*. Mercifully, perhaps, the chapel was badly damaged by bombs in 1941 and demolished in the 1970s.

She marvelled too at the *'finest armoury'* in the world, a collection of arms and armour housed in the Grandmaster's Palace which had been opened as Malta's first public museum in 1860. This remains even today one of the largest collections of armour still housed in its original

Journey to Serbia

building. Flora refers too to an underground village guarded by a soldier although it is more difficult to identify this particular attraction.

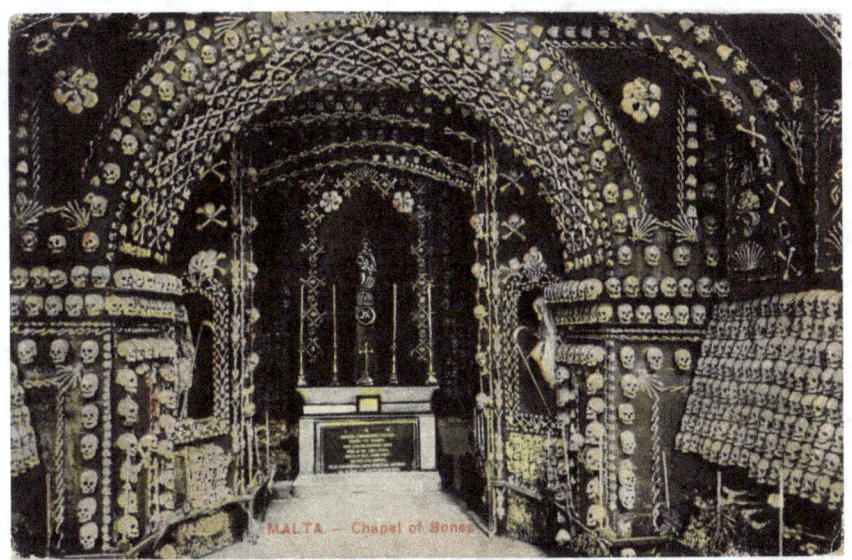

Postcard of Chapel of Bones, c. 1915

Rather more of interest, presumably, was the old hospital used by the hospitallers of St John of Jerusalem and now adapted for use as a modern hospital. Only a few months later, nurses of a Scottish Women's Hospital unit, on their way to Serbia would be commandeered by the Governor of Malta to assist with the reception of wounded from the Dardanelles in this hospital: a point of great satisfaction to the women since only a few months previously the War Office had rudely dismissed any idea of accepting help from a unit staffed entirely by women.

> **'What their other vessels are like, I cannot think , if this was their best...'**

Lady Paget's party spent from Thursday until the Saturday enjoying the hospitality and kindness of Malta but, all too soon, Flora was disappointed to learn that it was time to continue the journey. The *Caledonien,* a French vessel owned by the Messagerie Line, plied regularly between Marseilles

Nursing with Lady Paget in Serbia in 1915

and Turkey calling at Malta, Athens, Salonika and Constantinople and would be calling in four days time. If this ship was missed, there would not be another until 6th February. Flora was advised that they were lucky in securing the largest and finest vessel of the line but she remained unimpressed.

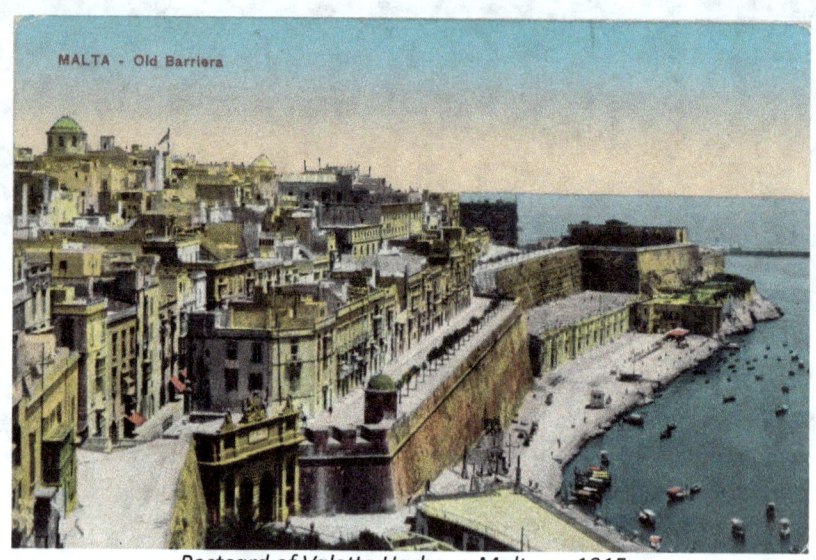

Postcard of Valetta Harbour, Malta, c. 1915

Although, vessels were not normally permitted to enter or leave the harbour after sunset – about 5 o'clock in January - the Captain of the *Caledonien* obtained special permission to leave at about 7pm. Flora was keen to see the barriers open and very untypically elected to forgo dinner in order to remain on deck. She did not regret her decision as the vessel slipped out under a large clear moon:

'It certainly was one of the finest sights I have ever witnessed. The gun from high watch tower fired 3 times, then the gates slowly opened & we passed through. I fetched all friends from dinner to see lovely sight: Malta brilliantly lighted standing high in the sea, a brilliant moon & seven immence [sic] search lights flashing all around the island. These we saw many miles right up until we went to bed about 10pm...'

Journey to Serbia

Dr F May Dickinson Berry also recalled that *'beautiful evening...sitting on deck watching the moonlit sea and sky'* and listening to Jan Gordon - or Herr Ingenieur' as he was known in his unit- singing to his famous banjo.[34] Her only other comment on the voyage was to observe bitterly that the *Caledonien 'soon showed that she could roll as well as the Dilwara'*.

Flora too had nothing but bad memories of the *Caledonien*. She found the food *'very poor'* and took particular exception to the *'luke warm'* nature of the offerings- *'all French'* she lamented:

'We never got a hot meal. Warm meats etc served on cold plates. Breakfast 6.30 until 8 coffee, black bread and jam. Lunch supposed to be hot, 4 courses, tea & biscuits. At 4pm Dinner 5 courses always luke warm. We all were hungry, yet no one could fancy or eat food. Lived principally on fruit.'

She found the boat *'dingy and dirty'* and *'First Class little better than our 3rd'*.

When the unhappy vessel reached Piraeus around midday on Monday 1 February, Flora and her party were quick to seize an opportunity of escape since the ship was due to remain there for nine hours whilst stores were loaded.

Athens was only an hour away *'by a funny little train'* and like most parties of English en route for Salonika, the group made haste to seek out the Offices of Thomas Cook the tour operators, strategically located opposite the Tramway station. Here they requested details of the nearest 'nice English hotel' and made arrangements for a guide and carriage to show them all the wonders of the city once they had eaten *'a good lunch'*:

'Oh it is past description, so beautiful; those ancient temples of white stone are grand & so enormous. Again brilliant sunshine favoured us. We had another meal before going on the boat and bought a little food...'

After a tour of five or six hours, during which the excited nurses

Nursing with Lady Paget in Serbia in 1915

admired the King's Palace with his special guard *'in their funny kilts'* and fascinating shops, the party descended with evident glee upon an English Tea Shop and Flora delighted in the unlikely feast *of 'white bread, butter, cream and scones'* as well as *'well made tea'*.

Flora was impressed by the beauty of Athens and in a reminder of the insecurity of the times, reflected sadly: *'...how terrible it seems to think it may be destroyed by warfare...'*

'Why did I leave my dim fireside?'

The party returned in good time for the promised departure of 10pm but found that the loading had not progressed well and that the ship would not now sail until seven the next morning. Flora ruefully recalled later that they were advised that the voyage would only take three more days. All retired to bed, grateful at least that they would have a quiet night. Sadly, this was not to be...

At around 2am, a terrific gale arose and it became clear that it would not be safe to leave harbour. Unable to go ashore, the hapless passengers remained on board as the ship rolled and rocked for the next twenty four hours. Flora spent the time watching *'poor wretched refugees'* from Constantinople struggling ashore with their worldly possessions: *'a very pitiful sight'*. These were ethnic Greeks displaced from Asia Minor by a Turkish government intent, now that they had joined the war against the Allies, upon a ruthless policy of ethnic cleansing.

 During the night of 2 February, the gale appeared to abate and at seven the next morning, the ship ventured out of the harbour. For a few hours, the decision of the Captain seemed justified but as the ship turned into the Aegean Sea, a gale of even greater force confronted the vessel. Flora who was not well versed in nautical matters described the ordeal in graphic terms:

'The Captain tried to turn & go back to harbour, was unable to do so & after struggling some time, took the vessel into islands & for 8 or 10 hours we went round & round these islands at almost 2 miles an hour,

Journey to Serbia

water too deep to anchor, then put to sea again and no one on that boat can ever forget the next 48 hours, could not hear yourself speak, tossed out of bed, every one had cushions on their floor, only 5 on the vessel (I was one of the lucky 5) not sick, the Captain & crew got all boats ready & we were prepared to get into them at a few minutes notice. It was a terrible experience. Women screamed (several French ladies on board) & fainted & oh, the noise of storm etc was deafening...'

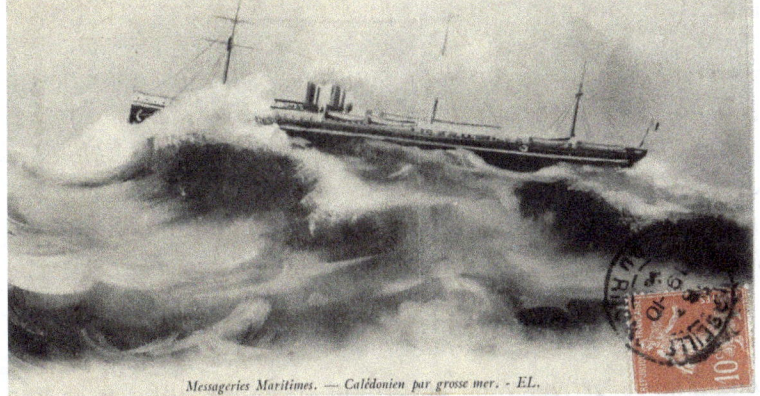

Postcard of SS Caledonien in heavy seas

The poor Leicester nurses were once more prostrate and Nurse Pickering declared herself quite willing to go to the bottom of the sea if only peace and quiet was granted: *'I feel too ill to care if we drown or not.'* Flora, with lamentable lack of sense - and supervision - determined upon tucking herself up *'quite snug'* under a rug on deck:

'when the ship gave a tremendous lurch, sent chair & myself with a bang to side of ship then the other side. I was quite insensible for a short time. The sailors carried me to the ladies cabin. I fainted. Dr Berry came & he thought I had broken my femur. I was left there with a nurse, hot bottles etc for several hours...'

Fortunately, Flora's leg was not broken but only badly bruised and the injury does not seem to have caused any long term damage. The foul weather continued for days and the height of anxiety seems to have

Nursing with Lady Paget in Serbia in 1915

been reached on Wednesday night when the ship's boats were lowered and made ready. Even the crew were now, apparently, expecting the worst and several French and Russian ladies were quite understandably reduced to hysterics. According to Flora, a gun boat was sent out from Salonika to aid the stricken vessel but around mid day on the Thursday, the storm abated just as suddenly as it had arisen. Now under military escort, the *Caledonien* sailed into Salonika next morning in beautiful sunshine:

'It looked very lovely in brilliant sunshine, such a magnificent bay, scattered all over with picturesque boat & boatmen, large oriental building on the seafront, with towering snow mountains behind. Oh, it is impossible to say how thankful we were to get on land & feel we were safe once more. One did not dare to think we might have again to face such dangers on our way home...'

All resolved to return to England overland when the time came.

The *Caledonien's* arrival was, according to Flora, three days late and there had been great concern about the fate of the vessel. Dr Dickinson recorded the voyage more laconically but less vividly:

'...in the narrow channel of the Doro such bad weather was encountered that the boat actually turned back and spent several hours steaming up and down in a more or less sheltered bay, thus prolonging by another twenty-four hours the pleasures of the voyage...'[35]

There were certainly no screaming women amongst the Berry party...

At Salonika, the Paget party was met by the Honourable Richard Chichester, Lady Paget's cousin and secretary who gave them a 'great welcome', having already reported to Lady Paget that the ship had been wrecked. He escorted the somewhat shaken party to the Olympus Palace Hotel, where rooms had been reserved. Flora delighted in the magnificence of the hotel, thrilled to find herself in a beautifully furnished bed room with bathroom attached. The view from the verandah was breathtaking:

Journey to Serbia

'It looked right across the harbour on to the Mount Olympus, the highest in Greece. Oh if only I could just describe this picture, a brilliant sunshine on very blue silent water, picturesque boats, barges, men etc moving about & all around those lovely mountains covered in snow. The sunset over the sea & mountain that evening was most wonderful...'

Flora scribbled a hasty letter to her sisters, keen to describe her 'terrible experience' assuring them that they would laugh to see how terribly thin she had become since last Saturday, after all the bad food and anxiety. She recognised that the party had already 'had some great experiences and seen some wonderful sights' but also admitted to that feeling of regret which many a traveller will recognise:

'Still, I have said once or twice lately 'why did I leave my 'dim fireside' & oh what would I give for a cup of tea & piece of bread and butter.'

'Oh, the dirt & wickedness'

After a bath and good meal, the party spent the rest of the day exploring the town of Salonika. Flora found the Eastern dress and ancient buildings fascinating, delighting in the bazaars and narrow streets but like many English visitors at the time was shocked by the dirt and flies:

'Oh, the dirt & wickedness. We were not allowed to go out alone, only in parties of 3 & 4. They are great thieves & their appearance rather strikes fear into one...'

Flora had little understanding of the problems arising from severe overcrowding. Salonika like Athens, was filled with Greek refugees from the Turkish coast of Asia Minor, not to mention military personnel of almost every nationality. A few months later, nurses bound for Serbia would assist in soup kitchens for the refugees, horrified at the numbers of destitute families they found crammed in to churches. Mabel Dearmer shared Flora's distaste for the city:

'This is a curious place – it seems to be crowded with the sickness and deformity of the world. Everybody is marked with small pox – some

Nursing with Lady Paget in Serbia in 1915

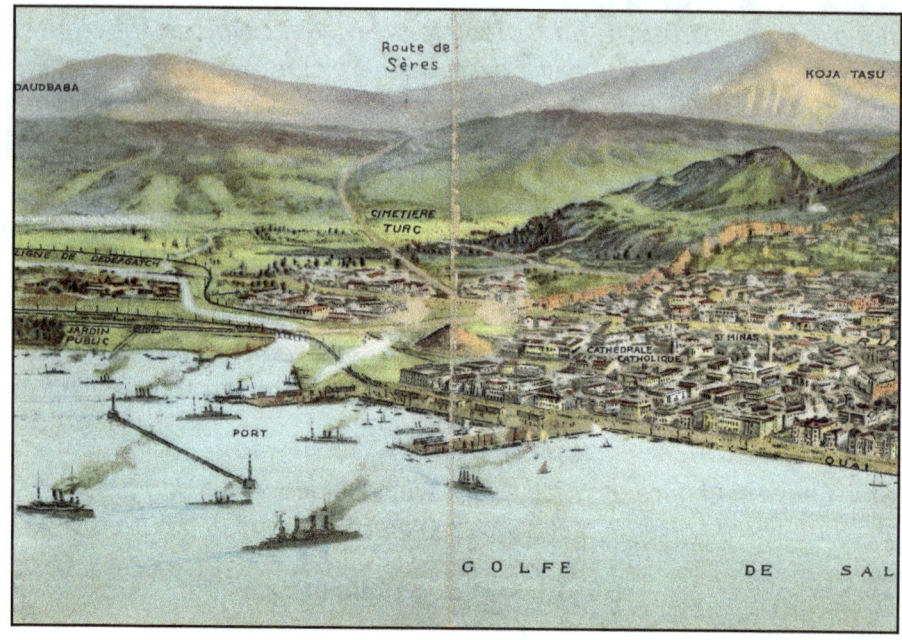

people without noses or ears. There are great crowds everywhere- we are not very much stared at, for the place is full of Red Cross – doctors and nurses, French, English, American. We heard there was a strong Anti-Allies feeling but we have not met it. The place wants cleansing – washing out with disinfectant or burning down – burning down would be best...'[36]

Mrs Dearmer might well have regretted her unsympathetic observations when, in August 1917, a terrible fire destroyed two thirds of the city leaving some 70,000 homeless. However, by then she was already dead, having died of typhus at Kragujevatz in July 1915.

Amongst the reception committee of four gentlemen, Flora was particularly impressed by the Honourable Mr Chichester, son of Lord Templemore, calling him *'very charming & so beautifully dressed'*. When he found that Flora and her companions had brought with them no bed

Journey to Serbia

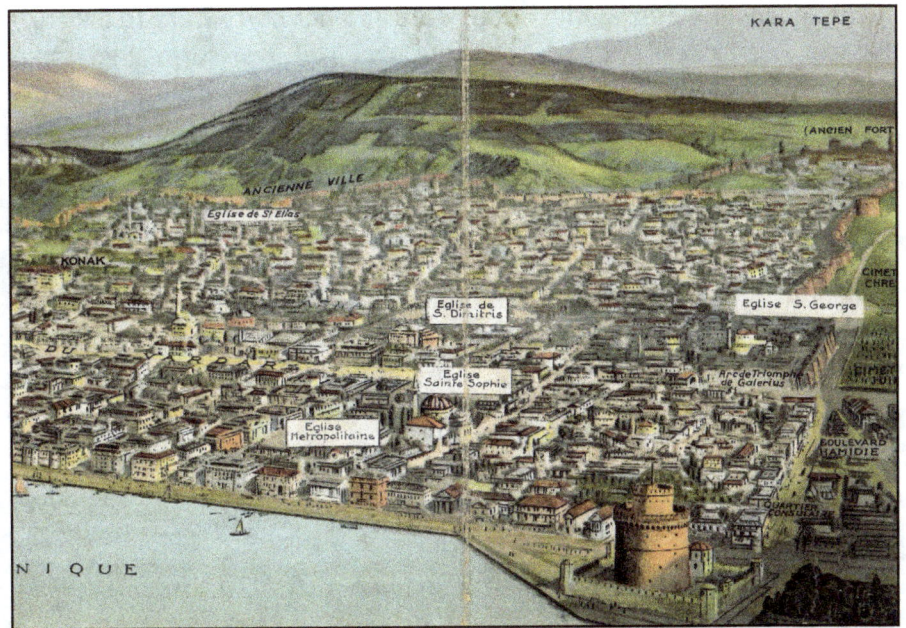

Panoramic view of Salonika, sold as a postcard, c. 1915

or bath, he hurried off to buy them, explaining that nothing could be purchased in Serbia. Understandably, he was keen to return to Lady Paget's hospital as soon as possible and he told the party that a train had been chartered for them on the following day.

Meanwhile, Dr Berry's party would stay a few days longer to supervise the unloading of supplies for their own unit as well as several other medical missions to Serbia. These included packing cases for the British Red Cross Mission under Captain Bennett, as well as Lady Paget's Hospital and a Serbian Red Cross unit at Nish. Although some of Captain Bennett's staff had arrived with Flora, others had travelled overland and been privileged to cross the Mediterranean on Sir Thomas Lipton's yacht. At one stage, Flora had thought that she too might be a guest on this yacht but was disappointed.

Nursing with Lady Paget in Serbia in 1915

After an evening meal in the hotel, Flora and her party went to a Picture Palace *'just to see what a Greek one was like'*. Not surprisingly, they were able to appreciate only the pictures. With the peculiar arrogance which the English often exhibit abroad, they seemed surprised that they could not understand the language...

The next morning, the party rose early at 4.30 in time to see the sun rise over the sea before a hurried breakfast of poached eggs, rolls and goat's milk butter. The train was due to depart at six, and the 'old Arab driver' thrashed the horses into a haphazard gallop as the carriages bumped over huge pot-holes and stones. At the station, passports were carefully examined for the first time on the journey. Hotel staff dealt with the luggage, as the somewhat shaken passengers located the reserved compartments and climbed with difficulty into the high train. There was no platform and the train seemed much higher than those at home:

'The carriage (1st class) was fairly clean, very very hard cushions on seat & back covered with a shiny cloth, so narrow our knee met those on the opposite side...'

The train finally departed an hour and ten minutes late: *'quite the usual thing we were told'.* Flora now gazed in wonder as the landscape unfolded before her:

'Every minute one seemed to see different strange sights, the whole time being reminded of bible stories & bible pictures we learnt as children, large wastes of sandy ground, huge mountains (snow covered) in the distance, men riding on donkeys, arab dress, shepherds minding their flocks, mules, buffalo, oxen, strange large beautiful coloured birds & quite wonderful sights...'

After travelling for around four hours, the train stopped at Ghevgeli beside a train packed with goats and cattle. All were ordered to get out and take their luggage about a quarter of a mile to the Serbian frontier where another train awaited. With no porters and no platform, the party struggled to transfer the luggage but were assured that there was no hurry: *'the train would wait any length of time'*. Flora noted the chivalry

Journey to Serbia

of the Doctors with a certain relish:

'The D[octo]rs had to carry all our luggage along the line to another train some good distance away... It was such a funny sight'

Near the station here, were the buildings of an American Mission which was already overwhelmed with typhus cases. Flora and the other nurses talked to American nurses at the station and heard with concern that they had already lost two or three of their staff to typhus. A few days later, Dr Berry and his staff on the same route, would also meet some of the American staff of the hospital *'which was waging a terrible fight against typhus'*. Dr Dickinson recalled:

'The enormous numbers they had to deal with made it impossible to secure proper conditions for the satisfactory treatment of the sick or the safety of the staff...they had already two members of their staff down with typhus and seemed very depressed and overworked...'[37]

The situation was about to get far worse. Dr Johnston Abraham of the British Red Cross, recalled the situation at the height of the epidemic:

'We had asked questions about the American Hospital at Ghevgeli on several occasions, and always met with evasive answers. Now we knew why. All the doctors were down with typhus, and most of the nurses. Donnolly, the head doctor, was dead...'[38]

In fact, James Donnolly had fallen ill with typhus and in his delirium, had seized an old musket from a Serbian sentry and shot himself.[39]

Flora seemed, at this point, oblivious to the dangers she was about to encounter. Her main preoccupation was the unreliability of the Serbian postal service... and the state of the trains.

She found the compartment in the Serbian train an improvement on the Greek one but *'one did not really fancy it'*. She was fortunate not to be a travelling a month or so later when the typhus scare led to train carriages being disinfected with formalin and passengers coating themselves in paraffin which combined to emit a particularly nauseous smell.

Nursing with Lady Paget in Serbia in 1915

In her letter to Syd and the girls, written upon arrival at Skoplje, Flora was less guarded in her description of the train:

'Trains here are rotten. Although reserved compartment had been put on for us by the Servian Government, they were little better than 3rd class carriages of the L & N W Railway...'

The journey to Skoplje was expected to take around eighteen hours and food for the journey as well as candles and matches had been purchased in Salonika in anticipation of the discomforts to come. Now the party of four men and five nurses fell upon the lunch boxes. Provision had been generous and Flora greatly enjoyed the lunch which consisted of six cooked chickens, two dozen hard boiled eggs, goat's milk butter, rolls of bread and an unspecified number of bottles of wine and lemonade. Since no one had thought to provide cutlery, the party relied upon pen knives and teeth and Flora found the meal 'great fun'.

'All along the mountains & roads you saw men on mules in such funny dresses riding or walking, shepherds watching their flocks of sheep, goats or pigs, all mud houses, no clean or tidy looking place & so often wooden crosses on lonely parts or mountain sides to mark soldiers' graves....'

The railway followed the valley of the river Vardar, crossing rickety bridges of planks, only just repaired after recent raids from nearby Bulgaria. It was a mystery to Flora as to how the planks were able to support the train as it crawled slowly over them: 'we expected every minute to be thrown into the deep and rapid torrent.'

The river ran swift and clear through *'high rocks and glorious sunny mountains'*. Like many of the English visitors Flora admired the beauty of the landscape. The whole line was guarded closely by Serbian soldiers:

'What poor creatures they looked, standing beside their funny little whattle huts, part Serb uniform & any extra clothes they could get. One had a coat of khaki evidently given by one of the English... we amused ourselves throwing cigarettes to them as we slowly passed for many

Journey to Serbia

miles up the line.'

There was other evidence of the recent conflict too. On the mountain sides there were little wooden crosses marking graves where battles had recently been fought *'showing and speaking of brave deaths in that desolate and lonely part'*. Every three or four hours the train shuddered to a halt and passengers were allowed to get out and wander about until a bell summoned the passengers to return. Flora told her family nonchalantly that one then ran after the train and climbed in *'as best you can while it is on the move'*.

By tea time, the party had obviously adapted to the relaxed regime on the train and the Doctor 'ordered' the train to be halted so that the group could fill their kettles from a well. As the train rocked and rolled, it was found to be impossible to fix a stove on the floor so the party resorted to holding their spirit lamps on their laps and holding the kettles over them until they boiled, in what sounds a highly hazardous operation. With admirable ingenuity, the intrepid travellers put tea into the kettles and used them as tea pots with the cups from their thermos flasks:

'It was all very funny & we said if only our friends could see us there how sorry they would be for us but we were quite happy.'

The cold however, was intense and Flora found the journey *'a weird and strange travelling experience'*. As dusk fell, the nurses lit their candles and kept them in their hands since the train's motion was too violent to fix them anywhere. Rolled up in their sleeping bags and rugs they tried to sleep or read until finally at around eleven in the evening, the train reached Skoplje where an anxious Lady Paget awaited them.

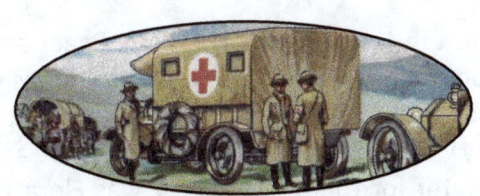

Chapter 4

Lady Paget's Hospital

'I think I shall love being here but the work will be terribly hard...'

Flora and her colleagues were conveyed *'through pitch black streets'* on *'funny little donkeys'* to a local school where the nurses were lodged. A room had been prepared for the new nurses and temporary beds erected:

'It was a strange looking home, furniture consisting of packing cases but the most welcome sight, was an old fashioned stove, with a huge fire in & heaps of wood beside it to keep it alight... Our room really was a funny sight, 4 little camp beds in a great school room, tables, chairs etc made of packing cases...'

The room was divided by curtains which separated each bed and beside each bed was an enamelled wash basin and a large *'lard tin'* evidently intended for use as a bath. A map of Serbia on the plaster wall afforded the only decoration.

After a brief meal, the nurses gratefully retired to bed, anticipating a good night's rest. They had reckoned without the intense cold, the antiquated beds and the local mice population....Unable to settle, Flora lit a candle to examine her bed more closely and found to her discomfort that her temporary bed consisted merely of a bag of straw resting upon hard planks: *'Tired as we were, none of us got much sleep.'* All were glad when morning finally arrived.

From the start, back in November 1914, Lady Paget and her staff had relied heavily upon Austrian prisoners of war to act as orderlies in the hospital. Now, the startled nurses were greeted at six by an Austrian orderly who calmly walked into their room, lit a candle and the stove and brought pails of water for them to wash. It was Flora's first encounter with a group of workers for whom she would develop a great affection

Lady Paget's Hospital

in the difficult days to come.

After dressing, the nurses made their way to the hospital for breakfast. It was Sunday 9th February and they wondered whether they should have a service or go to church. Lady Paget, however, reassured them that nothing was expected of them that day. They were to unpack and arrange their rooms and acclimatise to their new surroundings.

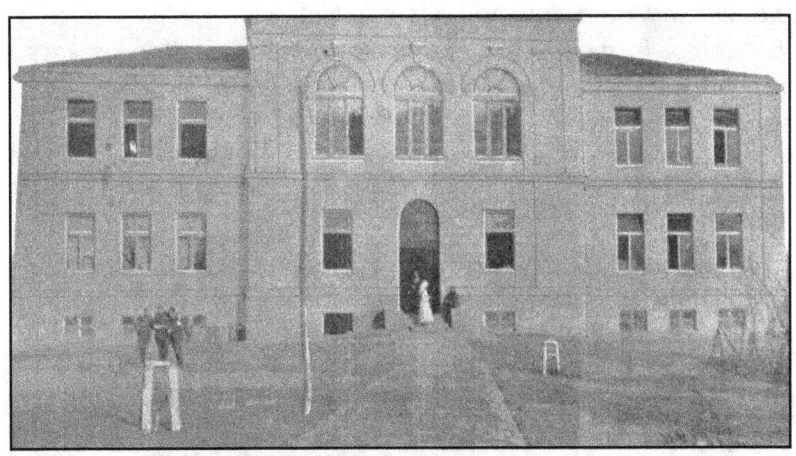

Lady Paget's Hospital (from Experiences in Serbia *by J T J Morrison, 1915)*

Having located their luggage, the nurses settled their room as best they could. They had found dressing in the poor light tedious and resolved to purchase a mirror and some hooks for clothes as soon as they could, as well as some mouse traps. The mice were to be a constant irritant, often keeping poor Flora and her companions awake by running across the beds and even, on occasion, across their faces. Flora was used to the problem of mice in Victoria Road and in her letters had warned her sisters to keep them away from her office and its papers but even so, she did not find them welcome bedfellows.

After lunch, the nurses went for a long walk, marvelling at the strange sights around them. It was a beautiful day of sunshine and all longed to climb the distant snow covered mountains. Flora's letter home to her

Nursing in Serbia with Lady Paget in 1915

sisters conveyed some sense of the culture shock:

'This place is most interesting & quaint. It is really in Macedonia & belonged to Turkey until the last war. There are people of nearly every race, especially lots of Turks. Their part is very funny to see. They sit in their bazaar making rugs, eider downs, nails, hammering those beautiful brass trays & ornaments etc. It is wonderful to see the things & places around. All the time you are reminded of Bible pictures. One of the funniest things is to see great Arab men riding sweet little donkeys & the women walking behind carrying loads or children. Never do you see a woman riding...'

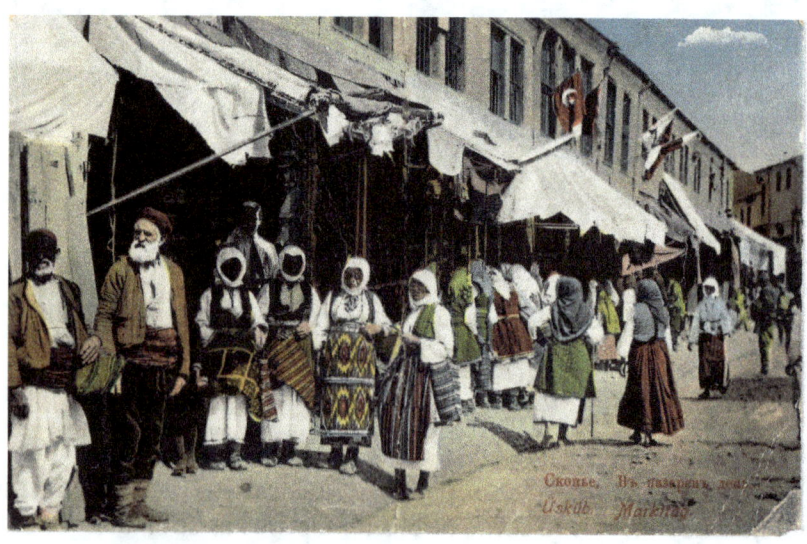

Postcard of market day at Skoplje (Uskub) c. 1916

'Skoplje is a town of great antiquity and interest, though it contains today but few really ancient buildings'[40]

The chief town in northern Macedonia, Skoplje, had always fulfilled a vital strategic and commercial role within the area. As early as the Second Century, Roman 'Skupi' was established as an important city within the Byzantine Empire, favoured by Constantine the Great. After a great earthquake in 518, the town had been rebuilt by the Emperor

Lady Paget's Hospital

Justinian and it is thought that the great fortress that dominated the town had been first built at this stage. The Serbs had seized the city from the Byzantines in 1282 and for a brief period the city played an important role as capital of the Serbian Kingdom. From 1389, when the kingdom fell to the Turks, until 1912, the district of Skoplje had remained part of the wide flung Ottoman Empire. Under the Turks, the city remained an important city, now known as Uscub, flourishing in the trade of hides. However, in the seventeenth century, the city was destroyed once more - this time by fire on the orders of an Austrian general. Most of the buildings which survived in 1915, dated from the rebuilding at this time.

During the city's turbulent history, the ancient fortress - known as 'the Grad' - had been rebuilt and remodelled by successive conquerors and its remains, perched on the hill which rose from the old part of the town, still dominated the skyline. Dr Johnston Abraham of the British Red Cross unit in Skoplje described the scene well:

'In Uscub the Grad dominates everything. The town itself lies in the middle of a triangular plain, with mountains all around. In this plain, overhanging the river, there rises a solitary precipitous high hill; and on this hill is the Grad...Always from any part of the old city, its battlemented white walls could be seen, and often, when we had got hopelessly lost in the Turkish quarter, we used to steer by it to known country again...'[41]

The Serbs had finally recaptured this prize from the Turks at the end of the First Balkan War just three years earlier and the town still retained much of the Turkish influence as well as a sizable population of Turks. Now as the capital of 'New Serbia', her population consisted of some 35,000 Serbs, Turks and Albanians. The town was part of a territory upon which the Bulgarians looked with great envy and resentment, having failed to secure their share in the recent conflict.

Reactions to the town from British visitors seem to have been mixed. Jan and Clara Gordon, the adventurous banjo player and his artist wife, taking time off from Dr Berry's unit, visited the town after Flora had left and described it in vivid terms:

Nursing in Serbia with Lady Paget in 1915

'Uscub is a Smell on one side of which is built a prim little French town finished off with conventionally placed poplars in true Latin style; and on the other side lies a disreputable, rambling Turkish village culminating in a cone of rock upon which is the old fortress called the Grad[Slavic word for castle]... Strange old streets there are in Uscub. One comes suddenly upon half-buried mosques with grass growing from their dilapidated domes, a refuge only for chickens...'[42]

Other, less critical visitors simply delighted in the Turkish character of the town. Monica Stanley, a cook from Mrs Stobart's Field Hospital, which was stationed further North, visited Skoplje whilst convalescing from a fever:

'I have thoroughly enjoyed being here, and am quite in love with this place. It is so Eastern.... This is the most ideal place in Serbia; it is like an Eastern village, and it is full of Turks, and the costumes are most picturesque...'[43]

It an interesting reflection of the mixture of cultures and races represented in the town that it was the birth place in 1910 of the future Mother Theresa, whose ethnic origins were actually Albanian. She spent the first eighteen years of her life there and it is a curious thought that she may well have remembered the sudden influx of foreign visitors who were drawn to Lady Paget's Hospital. Perhaps, she even first learnt the value of nursing from their example?

It must have seemed strange indeed to Flora and her nurses as they wandered round on that first afternoon but first impressions seem to have been favourable:

'I am charmed with this town. I never go out without finding something fresh & very interesting. The people are wonderful. Never two dressed alike & all in such bright colours. Since leaving England we must of seen [sic] quite a thousand different dresses & costumes.'

'A fairly decent lot...'

Lady Paget's Hospital

After tea, in the evening, Lady Paget visited their room and gave them directions about work. She impressed upon them that they should ask for anything needed and obviously tried to make them feel as welcome as possible. Flora and the nurses retired to bed, certain this time that they would be able to sleep soundly. However, this was not to be:

'Again we were doomed to disappointment. First a cockerel started to crow (he did every night about 10) & his noise was great. Then we all complained of cold coming through the bottom of our beds. & even our faces. Sleep left us...'

True to her word, Lady Paget listened to the complaints from her new arrivals and provided woollen mattresses which greatly improved the situation. If she had any misgivings about Flora and her sensitive nurses, she did not betray them. On one member of staff at least, they had made a good impression:

Henry Fremlin Squire who served as an orderly at Lady Paget's hospital from November 1914 until he was invalided home in February noted the arrival of Flora's relief party in his papers, preserved at the Imperial War Museum:

'Some of the party have been down to Salonica to collect stray bales & to welcome new arrivals. There are 8 new ones altogether, another doctor apparently a keen humourous [sic] man with a physiognomy like a prize fighter. Two orderlies, one of whom has had absolutely no previous experience of hospitals or medical work at all & doesn't like smells & the 2nd one I don't know anything about. The sisters seem a fairly decent lot as far as I can judge, quite competent at any rate...'[44]

The 3rd Reserve Hospital, Skoplje

The hospital which Lady Paget and her party had selected was a former high school or gymnasium which had been built only a few years ago and 'was not quite finished'. Although the building had been taken over as a Serbian hospital at the beginning of the war, the Headmaster of the school and his family still occupied the ground floor. The main

Nursing in Serbia with Lady Paget in 1915

block, facing the entrance gate was a large two storeyed building with outhouses and a pavilion occupying three sides of a large courtyard. The fourth side was a wall with a strip of garden beneath it. A Serbian sentry guarded the entrance.

Inside the main building, was a central stairway of stone, lit by tall windows and flanked by corridors giving access to twenty one large rooms, eighteen of them equipped as wards. Halfway up the stairs, a landing gave access to the recreation room which by day was used as a dining room for the staff. By night it was used as a drying room. Here was a stage, used as a granary – mainly for bags of rice - and a gallery where all the school furniture had been stacked. It was here that Sir Ralph and Lady Paget, the Doctors, Sisters and orderlies all ate together. Flora, to whom food was always a subject of great interest, was not altogether impressed:

'The tables were covered with white oilcloths, knives, forks, spoons were same as we get in our funny bazaars & we used emamelled mugs. The food was not very appetising, cooked in a strange way to us, but we had just to eat or go without...'

The buildings were lit by oil lamp although an unreliable electric light was sometimes available in the operating theatre. When the electricity failed, a large oil pressure lamp, purchased in Malta, was swiftly brought into service. Whilst there was an intermittent water supply to the main building – when the pumps were working- there was no supply to the pavilion and outhouses. Drainage was in a 'hopeless condition' and frequent protests to the Serbian authorities had so far led to no improvement...

A reminder of the former educational nature of the building emerges from 'My Balkan Log', the memoirs of Dr Johnston Abraham who served with the British Red Cross in Skoplje. When one of his colleagues, Dr Stretton, fell ill from what they called 'relapsing fever', it was felt that only good nursing could save him. Since their unit lacked nurses, he was sent to the Paget hospital, with whom the unit maintained a close relationship:

Lady Paget's Hospital

'... *four stolid Austrians carried him to his sick room. It was a little chamber, formerly used as a natural history class-room, containing large jars of snakes, skeletons of various ganoids, a huge stuffed eagle hanging from the roof, botanical charts on the walls, glass cases of small stuffed birds around. Stretton stared at these uncomprehendingly... The nursing saved him.'*[45]

'**How I longed for an English ward with its space, air, cleanliness & every convenience & comfort...**'

On 11 February, two days after arrival, Flora wrote a swift letter home, hastening to finish it so that Sir Ralph Paget could take it with him to England, thus evading the strict censorship of outgoing letters. The dates of her letters are confusing because of the discrepancy between the Gregorian calendar in use in Western Europe and the Julian calendar favoured by the Eastern Orthodox Church of Serbia. Dates were some thirteen days behind those in England and it is not always clear by which calendar Flora was working.

She reported that she had taken charge of two wards containing thirty eight beds:

'The poor fellows look terrible, just lie on planks with bags of straw, so close together, one cannot get between only side ways & often one finds another man lying beneath just on a blanket. It is too terrible, but they do seem nice & sweet & oh how they love you... I think I shall love being here but the work will be terrible hard. So many nurses & orderlies are ill & things are very very serious. They say there will be no more fighting for a very long time but cholera is terrible bad all over Serbia & Austria. All the soldiers have it & they are dying in thousands. Also the floods are very bad in the north...'

In her memoirs, Flora described commencing work at nine in the morning on the second day of her stay. She was put in charge of two wards under Professor Morrison. In something of an understatement, she described the state of the hospital as *'topsy turvy'* since so many staff were ill and off duty. The sister in charge of her wards had been off

Nursing in Serbia with Lady Paget in 1915

sick for more than a week and all duties had fallen upon a single orderly. The fact that the hospital was still able to function was due entirely to the Austrian prisoners of war who acted as ward maids, sweeping, scrubbing, serving meals and waiting on the Serbian patients. Flora marvelled at the kindness and patience of these men as they ministered to their erstwhile enemies:

'Never can I speak too highly of those Austrian prisoners. They were beyond praise. Nothing was too much trouble for them to do either for the Serbs or the English. Their beds were on the ward folded under patients' beds so they often were at work at night & day, without any comfort or rest...'

With characteristic determination, Flora set about taking temperatures and opening windows although she noted that they were quickly closed as soon as her back was turned: *'Serbians (like many of the English) do not like fresh air in the room.'*

Then she set about the dressings. It was all a far cry from her comfortable nursing in Leicester:

'Needless to say, nothing was sterilized. Water was boiled in paraffin tins (these tins were used for everything out there). I dare not tell you about the urinals. They were too dreadful. Nothing clean. Every[thing] swamped in pus, in addition to their wounds. Most of the men had gangrene feet and hands. Lots had lost toes, heels, part of foot & some a whole foot. I thought I should never get done....'

With rare sarcasm, Flora noted that the orderly left in charge had had two months's training at St George's [Hospital] in London before leaving England *'and knew better than even the professor how things should be done'*. The orderly, it seems, had been in the habit of using the same bowl of cotton and instruments for all the dressings until Flora, horrified, insisted that he used different instruments and washed hands between each dressing. The orderly was equally shocked when Flora proceeded to introduce her own regime for hygiene and he saw her disinfecting wounds with hydrogen peroxide:

Lady Paget's Hospital

'*In fact he started to criticise the Professor's fads to me & I really think he thought I was absolutely daft when I dry shaved a man to prepare for [an] operation; also when I started to use Hyde peroxide to syringe out wounds.*'

'*Those first weeks were difficult work*' she recalled.

Flora did not condemn her fellow nurses for the sorry state of affairs. She understood that the hospital had been established under difficult circumstances:

'*You see there had been no chance for our English sisters to get the wards to work in anything like order. They poor things had the school to thoroughly scour & clean, put up beds, unpack stores. Before they were nearly ready, wounded started to arrive, kept coming in so quickly they could not keep pace. Also the weather was very terrible, intense cold, deep snow, food scarce & bad, no off duty time etc. First one got ill then another. They began to get low spirited & disheartened. This accounted for the state of wards & dressings.*'

Flora set to work with a will. She asked Professor Morrison, '*The Chief*', for permission to have her patients put into a corridor on stretchers whilst she and fifteen Austrian prisoners scrubbed the ward, disposed of the old straw in the bedding and brought in clean linen: '*After that I was able to get things better*'.

Flora loyally makes no comment about Professor Morrison although his own account of his experiences working with Lady Paget, published in 'The Lancet' in November 1915, suggests that he was not an easy man to work with.

Professor J T J Morrison had taken three month's leave from his post as Senior Surgeon of Queen's Hospital in Birmingham, although it was later extended to five months. The opening paragraph of his report made it clear that he had expected to take sole charge of a Serbian Hospital expedition proposed by the Order of St John of Jerusalem. However, since the aims of the project overlapped so closely with the objectives of

Nursing in Serbia with Lady Paget in 1915

the Serbian Relief Fund, it had been resolved to form a joint unit under the auspices of both bodies. Since the Serbian Relief Fund was providing most of the funding, Lady Paget was appointed as Superintendent with her cousin the Hon R F C Chichester as Secretary. The direction of the Hospital was assigned to Morrison as Surgeon in Chief. It was not a natural alliance, as Morrison made clear:

'It was not to be supposed that an ideal scheme for the purpose in hand would be produced within the available limits of time and resources.... No formal regulations were prescribed for the party, who were for the most part, strangers drawn from all quarters. Difficulties, domestic and external, inseparable from such an enterprise cropped up, and mistakes were made; these afforded scope for forbearance and some measure of give-and-take and were surmounted by keeping steadily in view the common purpose...'[46]

Whilst the other Doctors had rooms in the hospital, the nurses occupied a nearby school and the orderlies another school, Morrison and Mr J W Wiles, who acted as his *'secretary – interpreter'*, were accommodated with the four dressers in a villa put at his disposal by the Italian Consul. The four dressers, Mr E B Alabaster, Mr H W Hall, Mr Frank Newey and Mr Cloudesley Smith were all medical students firmly under Morrison's patronage. Professor Wiles *'...a large, blond man, loosely built, carefully dressed and full of enthusiasm'*[47] had formerly been the lecturer in English at Belgrade University and was an old friend. Meanwhile, Lady Paget and her secretary lodged with Major Suskalovitch, the head of the Serbian Red Cross and former Medical Officer of Health in Skoplje. It seems likely that there was little warmth in the relationship between the different parties.

Perhaps more eloquent still was the final appreciation in Morrison's report of the medical personnel of the unit, which mentioned by name only the Doctors and the medical students who served him as dressers and orderlies. There is no mention of the nursing staff or Lady Paget by name.

An insight into the degree of friction between Lady Paget and her

Lady Paget's Hospital

surgeon in chief might be discerned in their respective reports of the death of Sister Clark on Christmas Day. Whilst Lady Paget attributed her death to the early onset of Grave's disease and a septic throat, Morrison explained it as *'a fever, presumably scarlet fever, supervening on acute tonsilitis'.*[48] There seems to have been a great deal of confusion about the nature of the fever which overcame so many members of staff but the slight discrepancy in the diagnosis is perhaps indicative of a deeper rift. Down the road at the British Red Cross hospital, Dr Johnston Abraham noted that this recurrent fever or 'Relapsing Fever' as he termed it, was a comparatively new disease to the British but was endemic in Serbia: *'Amongst ourselves, at first, we labelled it 'Uskubitis'...'*[49]

Morrison certainly does not appear to have been a particularly sympathetic man. He seems, in fact, to have represented a fairly typical example of the class prejudice and misogyny of the period. His arrogant and chauvinistic analysis of the Serbian nation leaves several points with which one might wish to take issue:

'The characteristic mental attitude of the native official in Macedonia is the product of centuries of Ottoman influence, and he himself belongs as yet to the East rather than the West. This attitude finds expression in three words, which were constantly and unforgettably dinned into our ears- 'sutra' (tomorrow) 'polaka' (go slowly) and némojé (impossible).... Another point worth noting is the fewness of educated men trained to bear responsibility. A nation of peasant proprietors, intensely democratic, with no aristocracy and no titled persons beyond the Royal Family, is not likely to produce numerous men of marked capacity.'[50]

Surprisingly, Henry Squire was not one of the medical men under Morrison's spell. In November 1914, he confided in his diary: *'Morrison is not such a skilful surgeon as I had expected, very slow and rather clumsy. Also very vain...'*[51] By January, he was even less impressed and reported to his parents:

'There have been great rows here, unfortunately, between Morrison and Lady P. as Morrison had got into his head that he was the head of the expedition and has acted accordingly. Of course, Lady P had to explain

Nursing in Serbia with Lady Paget in 1915

matters and consequently there have been ructions. Morrison has shown himself utterly incompetent to manage things, or else Lady P would have let him imagine himself the boss, besides being very bombastic and tactless. I suppose the real fault is that he is too old and a Plymouth Brother...'[52]

No doubt, Flora had encountered worse examples. In any case, she had more important problems:

'...dressing equipment was not like that we had been used to & there were no conveniences. Water had to be fetched & boiled on primus stoves. Bowls, trays etc were very primitive, paraffin oil tins served as cans to carry & boil water in , as foot & arm baths, soiled dressing receiver etc & I have even had to use them for making large quantities of cocoa, Bengers etc in. There was no sterilizer in the ward so I used a cigarette tin & boiled it on my spirit stove. Often it seemed like playing at makeshift. One was so short of everything & used all kind of odd things unheard of before to do dressings...'

'How one longed to take them to England & have them in delightful English wards where there was plenty of everything necessary & all the comforts.'

Flora found it hard to acclimatise to conditions where instruments were in short supply and precious and dressing appliances made of *'all manner of things'*. She learnt to admire greatly the skills of the storeman *'a splendid man, most handy & very clever',* who with his team of Austrian prisoners, undertook to turn paraffin tins and packing cases into stools, tables, shelves, trays and buckets:

'It was so funny & laughable but really very clever. One had only to ask for a thing, make a suggestion as to shape etc & very soon you would get a remarkable thing to make use of. Life there was a whole world of make belief...'

Lady Paget herself, had observed that the bedsteads supplied by the Serbs were *'somewhat primitive',*[53] consisting of wooden planks resting

Lady Paget's Hospital

upon iron frames and mattresses filled with straw. As Flora soon discovered, they were hard to move and tidy. On each bed was placed a brush, flannel, soap, towels, slippers, stockings, nightshirts or pyjamas brought from England.

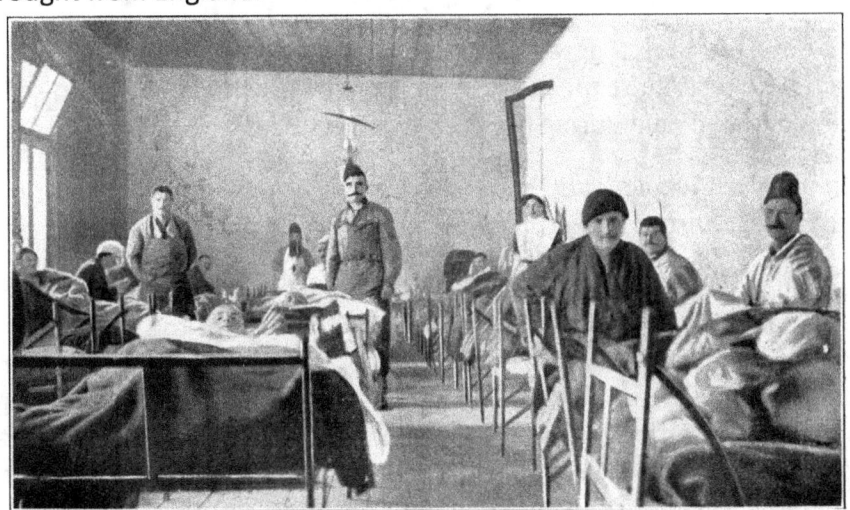

Interior of a ward at Lady Paget's Hospital (from Experiences in Serbia by J T J Morrison, 1915)

Most of the men had come straight from the battlefield and had arrived at the hospital after travelling long days and nights in cattle trucks without medical attention. As a result many had suffered from frost bite and lost toes and fingers. Many had bed sores in addition to their shocking wounds:

'One of my patients had lost both eyes. Shrapnel had gone right through his body, also his thigh & in addition to these [he] had gangrenous feet, another had lost right arm & leg another both legs... One had a large piece of skull blown off, his ear & eye also & one leg injured & so not one man had less than two wounds. They watch carefully everything you do & English always do the right thing. They have implicit faith in the English. All fractures were in bad condition & really their wounds were gruesome & not one bit English. Pus poured from everything. The wards reaked with smells of septic wounds, gangrene and iodoform...'

Nursing in Serbia with Lady Paget in 1915

Despite all, Flora found the men to be *'brave & plucky'* and *'all were most anxious to get quickly well & would often ask how long it would be before they could fight again'.* Astonishingly she found the soldiers *'always able to see the funny side of things.'*

The Serbians took a great interest in each other's wounds and would follow Flora around the ward, mocking those who made a noise or complained of pain during the dressing:

'... the others would laugh and make fun & call him a donkey that is one of the most hurtful things in the East to be called out there...'

Serbian and Austrians lay side by side and Flora relied upon the patients to explain their identity. Each nationality would point to the other and pretend to shoot and kill the other *'but they were always so happy & kind together, how sweetly they sang & were always in mischief.'* Although many of the men looked middle-aged, most were only between eighteen and twenty five and were the veterans of several battles. Besides their courage and love of fun, Flora found their most notable feature to be their strong white teeth, remarking that she never found anyone with bad teeth. Like many, she commented that the men were almost child-like in their demeanour.

The Serbians delighted in music, singing patriotic songs *'in a weird sing song style'* to the accompaniment of an instrument known as a 'guslar' which rather resembled a mandolin. Observers, less kind than Flora, often referred to this instrument in unappreciative terms, one in particular describing it as making a sound like a *'hive of bees'.*[54] Also, Flora recalled, the men greatly appreciated the wild flowers and wonderful blossom of the orange, lemon and cherry trees which first appeared in late February.

Nonetheless, the greatest pleasure for the men was an English cigarette and soon Flora was begging her sisters to arrange shipments of cigarettes for her to give to her patients. One story which she was fond of recounting was that of young soldier who lay dying in her ward. It was the custom for Serbians an hour or so before death to hold a

Lady Paget's Hospital

lighted taper on their chest, presumably to light their way in to the next world. On this occasion, English cigarettes were being handed round the ward and when a moribund patient nursing a candle on his chest, looked pleadingly for a cigarette, one was placed on his hand. The poor man managed to light the cigarette from his candle and smoke it just before death took him. Flora longed for cigarettes to arrive from England since they were unobtainable in Serbia although she herself still resisted the 'pleasure': *'I am real proud Con, to say I do not yet smoke. I am the only nurse here who does not.'*

Although she found the language very difficult, Flora was amazed at how much could be conveyed through signs and gestures. Great misunderstandings did of course occur and she was particularly fond of recounting the disaster which ensued when a king's messenger with a dispatch for the General of Skoplje unluckily arrived at the same time as a convoy of wounded from the battlefield. The confused and rather indignant man was received with all the other patients and despite his protests was forcibly undressed, bathed and put to bed where he was watched closely until the interpreter arrived to sort out his troubles. Flora's main regret was that a bath and much energy had been expended to no purpose. The story was a popular one amongst other English missions in Serbia at the time.

'Oh what I would give for a piece of thin white bread'

Flora wrote little in her letters home about the actual conditions but described an exhausting work routine:

'We have breakfast at 8.30 & go on duty at 9. We come off at 9pm very very tired. We are standing or rather running round all day, never sit except for meals...Work is very very different to England'

Breakfast consisted of porridge, eggs or omelette and bacon *'or what they call bacon'*, honey and sour black bread accompanied by *'wish wash tea or coffee.'* Food was *'fairly good'* but cooked rather strangely as there were no ovens. The diet included plenty of chicken, turkey and pork but it was rather disconcertingly difficult to identify the meat because of

Nursing in Serbia with Lady Paget in 1915

the nature of the preparation. There were lots of omelettes, vegetables and copious amounts of rice and macaroni. Sir Ralph Paget, had been recently presented with a gift of three hundred sacks of rice but the appeal was already beginning to decline since puddings were made with water instead of milk. Flora hugely resented the coarse brown bread and longed for the white bread at home: *'You cannot think how I long for some bread & butter.'* She did not like the strongly tasting butter which *'came in tins from France'* and was not at all impressed with bullock's milk, preferring now to take her tea as the Russians with a little sugar and lemon. *'More often than not'* she recalled *'it was impossible to eat the food, it was so badly cooked and served.'*

Each afternoon at 4.30, all the nursing staff sat down for a cup of tea and a strict ration of three biscuits each. No extra helping was permissible whatever your rank and the nurses thought longingly of the cake awaiting them in the luggage which was still in shipment. All would soon come to rely upon their own private food stores, shared regularly at picnics in their rooms and Flora quickly became resigned to the new diet: *'Still, there is no need to grumble. I can eat anything now, am always hungry...'*

The patients had a different diet and the feeding was left entirely to the Austrian orderlies. Lunch at midday, Flora reported, was a very coarse meat in some sort of stew followed by the inevitable rice pudding, served in enamelled basins or mugs *'not washed between the courses'*. At four, there was *'chi'* or what the Serbians called tea: *'What terrible stuff, just like dish water, no milk & dry bread'*. Each patient was allowed a loaf of bread per day and bread was served again about half past six accompanying an evening meal of haricot beans in gravy. Flora knew nothing of breakfast since she never did night duty but she recorded that it was usually coffee and bread unless there were eggs which were boiled hard, kept a day or two and then eaten cold with fingers. The greatest delicacy which could be found for the men was a Bulgarian dish known as 'kaimak' which consisted of sour milk *'rather like our cream cheese'*.

The egg supply was rather erratic: *'Lots of patient able to crawl almost would get themselves eggs. Where they really came from was a mystery.*

Lady Paget's Hospital

One poor soul, with gangrene feet, unable to get out of bed, handed us a warm new laid egg each morning.' When a puzzled doctor turned back his bed clothes, there lay the hen beside the patient. This story, which was also often repeated amongst the British community, does seem to raise certain questions about the hygiene of a ward where hens were permitted to wander in and out but Flora chose not to provide further details. The story is repeated by Monica Stanley, a cook with Mrs Stobart, although ascribed to a different hospital.[55]

'All we English people seem lame & hobbling'.

Laundry washing did not meet Flora's high standards either:

'The clothes here are terribly washed. White things are a great novelty. The women never boil clothes, so can scarcely tell if they have been washed or not. No mangles either & everything done by hand. We cannot get half the clean clothes necessary for patients. As regards our clothes, I wash my own combos, n[ight] dresses, handkerchiefs, stockings, camisoles etc but dresses & aprons etc I have not attempted...'

In an apparent attempt to combat the problem of washing such a cumbersome uniform, 'the Turkish dress' of blouses and trousers was now being made for all the nurses. Flora looked forward to sending a photograph of herself modelling the new style.

Another difficulty about which Flora complained, was her feet. Roads in Skoplje and Serbia generally were terrible with no paving and huge stones. On drives, one clung to the sides of the carriage for fear of being thrown out as the conveyance lurched over stones and potholes, and Flora reported roaring with laughter with her colleagues as they suffered this indignity. Walking was equally difficult and strong foot wear was demanded. However, in the wards, the high rubber boots which the nurses were required to wear made their feet hot and tender and few could cope : *'All we English people seem lame & hobbling'.*

Flora asked her sister Connie to send out a coat and mackintosh as well as some rubber half shoes or galoshes, warning her to send them in

Nursing in Serbia with Lady Paget in 1915

wooden box via Mr Christian at the Serbian Relief Fund since he would be sending more nurses out at the end of March. The parcel service, she explained was very unreliable, taking nine or ten weeks. Flora was now mightily relieved having received her first letter from home. It had been posted in Leicester on 3 February and taken fifteen days which was regarded as unusually efficient.

'The donkeys are really sweet. Such dainty pretty little things & carry such large loads, but they will walk where they think best. Cannot be made to go where the men want. People here are not really kind to dumb animals...'

Although other British visitors frequently commented on the tameness of domestic animals in Serbia, Flora was not so impressed with animal welfare in Skoplje. Her letters home were still full of enquiries about her many pets, but now she had a new worry:

'There is a big vulture here & I am terrible sorry for it. [It] is in such a small space and cannot open its wings. I declare I shall let it out some day but of course it might carry me with it so I shall have to be careful...'

This unhappy creature is mentioned too in the writings of Alice and Claude Askew. This rather supercilious couple travelled out to Serbia in April 1915, *'essentially as writers'*[56] attached to a unit led by Dr J Hartnell Beavis and serving as special correspondents for the *Daily Express*. They spent six weeks at Skoplje with Lady Paget's hospital and must have coincided with Flora although by then she was probably at a different hospital and preoccupied with far greater problems. The *'vulture'*, it seems, was actually an eagle:

'I cannot refrain from mentioning another queer 'pet' we had. This was an eagle, and we found it at Skoplje, shut up in a wooden case ever so much too small for it. Someone had caught it, intending, I believe, to take it out of the country, and had then gone away, forgetting all about it. We decided that the kindest thing would be to let it free.'

We thought it would fly away, but it could not – at any rate, it did not.

Lady Paget's Hospital

It elected to take up its residence in the hospital yard – much to Soona's [their dog's] indignation, and occasionally to the alarm of our visitors. Now and then, in a spirit of curiosity, it would invade the hospital itself, hopping solemnly up the broad stair case, and rather disposed to resent ejectment. Curiosity was certainly a conspicuous trait in that bird's character; we were lucky enough to get a snapshot at it one day while it was inspecting a bottle of Perrier Water with the greatest apparent interest and with all the aspect of a connoisseur.'[57]

'I seem to have been here years, yet it is only 4 weeks today we really arrived here in Skoplje.'

In rare *'off duty time'*, Flora would escape the town and climb the surrounding hills to write her letters, perched on high rocks. Although reticent about her actual work, she wrote enthusiastically about the scenery:

'How I wish you could see it. It is really magnificent & picturesque. The town is so quaint, white or yellow houses built so funny, with bright red roofs... As I sit, I can count 14 mosques. I have not yet been into one but will go some day & see what they are like. The mountains near have no snow on now but those in the distance are still covered and very very lovely they look...'

There were sober reminders of the recent conflict:

'On one mountain, to my left, the whole side, is covered with tiny white crosses, thousand & thousands of them. I am told it is where one battle was fought & the dead are buried there. On the mountain right hand side, there is another good sized cemetery where the Turks buried their dead. The tomb stones to theirs are flat...'

At the beginning of March, Flora reported heavy rain and mud in the streets which came *'well over the shoe tops'*. Despite the weather, she gloried in the burgeoning green and the lovely orange and lemon blossom. She was enjoying shopping too and had apparently recovered from the disappointment of their newly acquired mirror cracking on first

Nursing in Serbia with Lady Paget in 1915

use: *'So much for Serbian mirrors'*

'Shopping is great fun here. You go into a shop, make sign what you want. Oh we are fearfully clever now in making dumb signs & shrugging our shoulders. Well, this is what happens. I went for a reel of cotton the other day. I said 'Bovly cottoro'. Man shrugged his shoulders & said 'Nay Nista' meaning 'Nay' & then made signs of stitching. Still, no, so I walked behind , fetched boxes down etc & hunted myself. After a lot of searching, found it. They will let us do just what we like & never seem to mind how we search, but every one is the same. All the sentries let us pass anywhere. How we shall miss the salutes & attention when we leave them...'

'One cannot help but love them'

Whilst life clearly had its lighter side, Flora was now very busy in the hospital with responsibility for four wards of fifty five beds. The Serbs were grateful to their new 'Englisher Sistra' and Flora quickly learnt to love them, marvelling at their good relations with their former enemies. The other Leicester nurses had also acclimatised well. Letitia Clully wrote enthusiastically to her mother, home in Lansdowne Road, that the men in her ward were teaching her Serbian in return for English lessons:

'Imagine me in a ward with thirty foreigners of three or four nationalities. They are all so good and considerate. Nothing is too much trouble for them to do if they are able to do it. My orderly (an Austrian prisoner) speaks five languages...'[58]

Flora too was struggling with the Serbian language but she found the Serbians and Austrians *'picked up our language much quicker than we theirs'*. Few of her patients could read or write but those who could, would buy newspapers and read the news to the ward amidst great excitement and interest. There was similar delight exhibited when Flora was able to bring in one the English picture papers:

'There was always a great scramble if I took my Daily Mirror or Sketch, the Sphere etc for them to see & they were so interested in pictures of

Lady Paget's Hospital

guns etc & would ask many questions. Such little things pleased them. They are always as happy & child like, full of fun, always teasing each other...'

'How one's heart ached for these poor brave fellows.'

When the soldiers were discharged, Flora was shocked to find that their clothes were returned to them still caked in mud and blood stained. Although, Lady Paget was able to supply a couple of pairs of good stockings and a pair of Serbian shoes, it was impossible to provide new suits. Most left at seven in the evening, catching one of the two trains which passed through Skoplje each day, one going north and the other south:

'How one's heart ached for these poor brave fellows. I used to think of our soldiers with all their great comforts, clean, cosy clothes, being sent to a convalescent home, travelling comfortably, being met, well fed etc & see these poor souls travelling alone in open trucks through the cold nights, just getting bits of food as best they could on the journey but they went so cheerfully & happily & were so grateful to we English...'

Flora was quite overwhelmed on the first occasion when a patient left her ward:

'... he took my hand, knelt down, kissed it, put it to his heart, then to his head, kissed it again, got up off his knee, shook it. Although quite a poor man it was done so reverently & beautifully. They were so delighted with our nursing. I never heard a grumble...'

Only one complaint was recalled by Flora and that from a disgruntled former patient who had been given a glass eye and returned after two or three days, to report that he could see nothing through it.

'Oh it made me cry more than once'

Despite her admiration for the Serbians, it was the Austrian prisoners of war who most impressed Flora: *'What we should do without the Austrian prisoners I cannot think. They are such workers & really clean*

Nursing in Serbia with Lady Paget in 1915

clever men. In every ward there are 2 or 3 . They do ward maids' work , serve foods & wait on the patients hand & foot, it seems impossible they can be enemies & oh they are good to us English.'

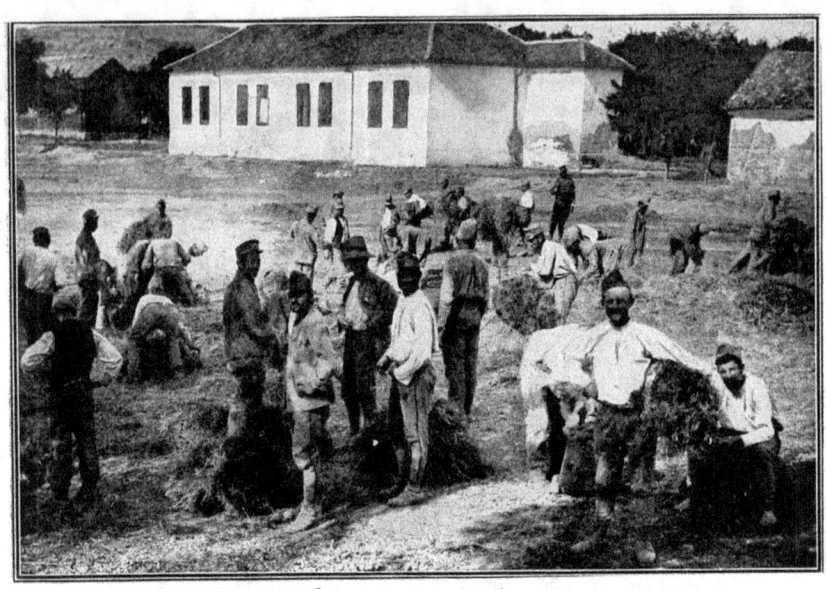

Austrian prisoners-of-war engaged in farm work at Skoplje
(from The Great War III, *1915)*

Around Skoplje, there were around 8000 such prisoners of war who were put to work mending the local roads. The men were ill fed and neglected, with little or no provision made for their accommodation let alone their medical needs. Flora wrote home to her family that she was moved to tears on several occasions when she encountered groups of eighty or a hundred former citizens of the Austro-Hungarian empire, as they finished work for the day: '*their faces white & drawn, too weary to drag one leg after another.... It is too awful, for there is not food enough to feed them & lots & lots of them are dying from fever & loads dying of home sickness. I have never so much longed for money or rather to be rich as I have longed here. Today, I put my hand in my pocket to give a wretched looking Austrian money ,then thought most likely he was a gentleman & would be hurt if I offered him a para. I had no more with me.'*

Lady Paget's Hospital

It was to be amongst the wretched Austrian prisoners, that the dreaded typhus would first take hold. Lady Paget and her staff were about to be overwhelmed by the consequences...

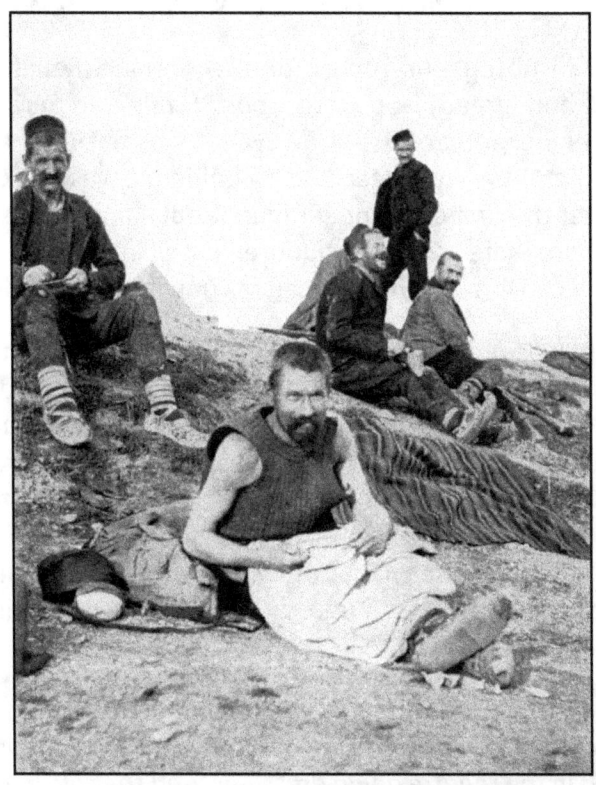

Serbian soldiers hunting for lice (from My Balkan Log *by J Johnston Abraham)*

Nursing in Serbia with Lady Paget in 1915

Chapter 5

The Typhus Epidemic

The Typhus Hospital, 6th Military Reserve

Lady Paget's subsequent report to the Serbian Relief Fund stated that typhus had already appeared *'sporadically'*[59] in Serbia as early as November or December 1914. However, it was not until the latter half of January that it became clear that an epidemic was fast developing. It was then that the first case appeared in Skoplje and by the first week in February, there were over four hundred cases in the town. It was into this crisis which Flora and her colleagues unwittingly wandered.

The problem was not confined to Skoplje. Further north at Kragujevatz, the staff of Dr Eleanor Soltau's unit of the Scottish Women's Hospitals were also struggling. Dr Elizabeth Ross, a Scottish woman who was working independently at the Serbian Fever Hospital there, fell ill with typhus and was nursed by her fellow countrymen. Her death was swiftly followed by the death of the two nurses who had cared for her: Sister Louisa Jordan and Nurse Margaret 'Madge' Neill-Fraser and then by a further death, that of Sister Augusta Minishull. Dr Katherine MacPhail, one of the doctors recalled:

'Those were the darkest days for us all, and the unit was never the same again...I remember Dr Campbell, who was the other junior doctor with me, working in the theatre doing dressings, and she said to me: 'I wonder who we will bury next Sunday?' It was four consecutive Sundays we had buried four people.'[60]

Flora herself did not recognise the scale of the crisis until she had been at the hospital for a couple weeks:

'Towards the end of February, we all realized Typhus Fever was raging everywhere throughout Serbia & especially in Skoplje. Often when out, oxen wagons loaded with coffins would pass. I have seen as many as 20 to 40 at a time . These coffins made of white wood, slatted bottoms

The Typhus Epidemic

& red cross painted on top were never screwed down & it was not an unusual thing to see an arm or leg hanging out of coffin. The cemetery was right out of the town at the foot of a mountain, but you could see 50 or 60 coffins lying waiting for burial. Graves could not be got ready quick enough. No attempt was made to isolate this terrible fever until the English felt something must be done.'

When Letitia Cluley's letter was published in the *Leicester Daily Post* on 8 April 1915, the editor highlighted her comments about the same scenes:

'The horrible effects of war are shown in one sentence in which the writer tells how she often sees coffins like 'sheep troughs with lids on' borne along in bullock carts. The coffins look as if they are made of matchwood, and have no furnishings whatsoever'

Letitia too warned of the imminent crisis:

'The number of deaths in the different fever hospitals has been terrible. Lady Paget is going to leave us to ourselves, or rather in charge of the doctor, and is going to help with the fever patients. She does work hard: she is always on.'[61]

Flora wrote of the other hospitals in the town with many deletions and had clearly struggled to describe the appalling situation:

'The other hospitals in the place, a Greek, American, Russian, Serbian etc were all crowded out with typhus. The Isolation Hospital was very overcrowded. Patients were lying 3 in 2 beds or 5 in 3 beds, men, women and children together, also they were lying on the floor & around, scarcely a soul to look after them, not Austrian prisoners many of whom were already sickening with the terrible disease. The Serbians did not seem to realise how grave the situation was...'

The Isolation Hospital, set aside for contagious diseases, was called the 'Polymesis' [half moon] and lay on the outskirts of Skoplje on the far side of the river. During the first Balkan war, the fine building had served as the British Red Cross Hospital. When Dr Johnston Abraham visited the hospital, shortly after his arrival in November 1914, he found it full of

Nursing in Serbia with Lady Paget in 1915

'*relapsing fever, with a few typhoids and diphtherias*' staffed by a Greek doctor and Austrian prisoners.[62] Whenever an infectious disease was detected at his own hospital, a notice was sent to Major Suskalovitch, the Commandant of the Serbian Red Cross and former Medical Officer of Health in Skoplje, and a horse ambulance was eventually sent to collect the patient and deliver him to the Isolation Hospital.

There was little confidence in the nursing available at the Hospital and when British Red Cross staff themselves started falling ill, the idea of sending them to the Isolation Hospital was not entertained. It was at the Isolation Hospital that the first cases of typhus in Skoplje were reported. Dr Johnston Abraham who was one of the few doctors to have experience of the disease, having encountered it in Ireland, was horrified and warned his curious colleagues to keep away. His fears were well founded. When at the height of the epidemic, he passed the Isolation Hospital, he noted :

'*On the way we passed the Polymesis, now a veritable pest house, crammed to overflowing with untreated cases. The Greek doctor had died, and it was being run by a Serbian helped by Austrian prisoners...*'[63]

At first, there had been no system at the Paget Hospital for isolation of typhus cases. Two large tents had been erected for new arrivals but these had received all new patients regardless of their symptoms. Overcrowding often led to two patients sharing one bed and under these conditions the typhus fever understandably spread 'like wildfire'. All too often, those that tended them were Austrian prisoners who were already sickening themselves.

Flora was only too well aware of the wider crisis in the town:

'*The death rate was enormous. One of the sisters in our hospital caught it & several patients. Our isolation tent was put up & all high temperature suspected & taken there. ...*'

It had only been relatively recently, in 1909, that a French medical team had discovered that lice transmitted typhus. Although the Serbs liked to

The Typhus Epidemic

blame the Austrians for bringing the disease with them, most medical authorities agreed that it was already present within the population. Typhus – or Typhus Exanthematicus (Black Typhus) to give its correct name and distinguish it from Typhus Abdominalis (typhoid or enteric fever)[64] - often surfaces in times of war, since it thrives in conditions of bad sanitation and overcrowding. It also spreads most successfully in cold conditions since this is when dirty, neglected groups such as soldiers, refugees or prisoners of war draw together seeking warmth and shelter. Whilst a healthy well nourished patient could hope to survive the debilitating fever, those weakened by deprivation and wounds often succumbed to secondary problems of severe pneumonia and gangrene. The one defence against this virulent disease was the eradication of the lice and to this purpose the British staff committed themselves to shaving every patient of all body hair before any other attention, however callous this treatment might appear.

Realising the enormous humanitarian disaster which was threatening to engulf them, Lady Paget with Doctors Knobel and Maitland met with Doctors Barrie, Abraham and Banks of the British Red Cross in Skoplje to discuss the situation and devise a remedial plan. As a result, Dr Barrie of the British Red Cross was despatched to Nish, the seat of the Serbian Government, to obtain powers to combat the situation. There the Serbian Prime Minister, appointed a Committee of Serbian and British representatives to oversee the sanitary control of Skoplje. Acting as their executive, Dr Knobel of Lady Paget's Hospital and Dr Suskalovitch, were appointed Medical Officers of Health for the town with powers to enforce compulsory notification and isolation of cases, disinfection of houses and clothing, *'scrutinization of all passengers leaving trains'* and closing of all public places including churches, mosques and theatres. Most importantly, two buildings outside the town were immediately offered for use as an isolation hospital.[65]

Situated on a hill about a mile outside Skoplje on the road to Kumanovo, the buildings consisted of a newly built cadet school and a group of three pavilions, also originally built as a cadet school, but now in use as a hospital. The situation was high and wind-swept and well away from

Nursing in Serbia with Lady Paget in 1915

the town. Dr Johnston Abraham walked out to view the proposed site:

'It was a beautiful spring morning with the sun high overhead in a sky of fleecy blue, and the walk across the Vardar up past the Citadel on to the high level plateau above the town was most exhilarating ... Beyond the Tekkah [Saint's tomb], on the brow of the hill, a half finished carriage drive led to a large white, many windowed building, which was the former palace of the Turkish Governor; and behind it some six or eight long barrack-like buildings were arranged... The Palace I found was already a hospital. The other buildings behind were still occupied by troops...'[66]

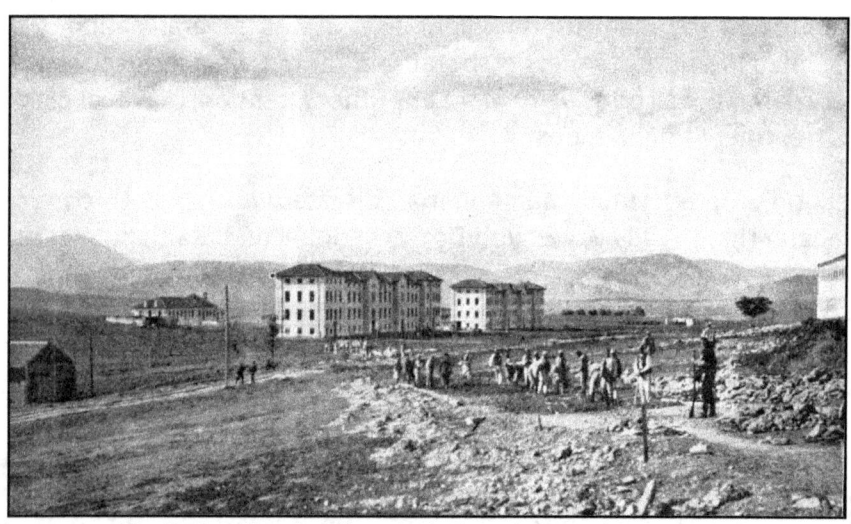

The Typhus Hospital (from Lady Paget's Second Report, 1916

Although the site was ideal for an isolation hospital, there were many bureaucratic obstacles to overcome before the buildings were finally handed over *'after much pressure and repeated promises'* about 28th February. Lady Paget later recalled the frustration in her report:

'The difficulty of getting things to move has been the greatest obstacle we have had to contend with all the winter; and so it was that, while we were promised the two isolation blocks immediately, there was much difficulty and delay in getting them handed over...'[67]

The Typhus Epidemic

Not least was the problem that the barracks were still occupied by troops and there was a cadet course in progress at the school. The commandant of the school flatly refused to hand over the building. It was only when the British Red Cross contacted the Serbian Prime Minister, M Pasitch, that opposition collapsed. Dr Johnston Abraham who was part of one of the delegations to the Government at Nish, interviewed the Prime Minister and was deeply impressed:

'The only person who seemed to have any grasp of the situation was the Premier, M Pasitch. We heard that he had cabled to France and England asking for a Sanitary Mission of one hundred doctors from each country, and that these were being sent. In the meanwhile, Sir Ralph Paget and our Chief were given almost autocratic powers in Uscub...'[68]

When Lady Paget and Dr Maitland first visited the Cadet School and barracks, before the buildings were officially handed over, they were shocked to find typhus cases mixed up with other patients. In the stables below the pavilions, they were appalled to discover many Austrian soldiers, huddled on dirty straw, in a terrible state of neglect. Since the crisis of the typhus outbreak, no one had taken responsibility for feeding these unfortunate men.

'There were long lines of buildings, long and airless, the smoke from the open furnace on one corner hanging always in the roof because there was no vent for it. At the entrance, we had to step through pools of filthy water which collected in the holes of the mud floor, and all along the sides and down the middle wretched figures in foul old uniforms were huddled together on dirty straw. Many were lying hidden under greatcoats, some shuddering, some quite still. As we lifted the coats to look under we found six dead bodies in a single building, and no one to carry them away...'[69]

Whilst Flora cannot have been with them on this first occasion, she described the scene vividly in her memoirs and was probably later involved with taking typhus victims from the basements once there was space for them in the wards above:

Nursing in Serbia with Lady Paget in 1915

'...in the basements below our wards, were several hundreds of these Austrian prisoners. To get at the entrance to these stables and basements you had to step through piles ankle deep of filthy snow & water. Then you opened a door into a long room, dark & airless & all along sides & down the middle were wretched creatures, in full old Austrian uniform. In one room almost 400 were found & only 40 out of this number were able to stand. They had been without food, water or light for 5 days. The living were making pillows of the dead, those too ill & dazed to know what they were doing. Oh these dreadful places, all too dreadful to picture to you & here it does not seem possible such places could exist...'

From then on Dr Maitland spent his time at the site, superintending food supplies and directing Austrian prisoners in the construction of stone causeways through the deep mud which lay between the pavilion buildings.

Once the buildings were relinquished by the Serbs, Dr Barrie of the Red Cross took charge of the new cadet school and Dr Maitland of Lady Paget's unit moved in to the large hospital. A further building, like the new cadet school, with amazing innovations- for Serbia- of hot and cold water, laundry and latrines was promised within four or five weeks.

Meanwhile, Dr Maitland took up residence in what Flora identified as the *'old Turkish Barracks'* and set about cleaning and disinfecting the wards. Lady Paget travelled out each day in order to oversee equipping the kitchen and staffrooms. She was aided by Dr Knobel who was unable to start upon any of his other plans until suitable accommodation could be provided for typhus cases from the town. With a fever nurse and a ward maid as assistants, the party laboured late into the night, preparing the first ward. By 1 March, one pavilion had been cleaned and prepared and a staff of Austrian prisoners who had already survived typhus had been selected. The hospital was now ready for its first patients and the ward was filled the same day. By 5 March, when disinfection of another pavilion had been completed, a further ward was opened. Sister Henry and Nurse Isherwood who had been travelling up to the site each day, now took up residence. Since there were no suitable rooms available at the hospital, the British Red Cross kindly allowed Lady Paget, the Doctors

The Typhus Epidemic

and nurses to live in the cadet school.

Dr Johnston Abraham, who curiously seems to have thought himself in charge, recorded:

'Meanwhile, our old friends, the Paget unit (No 1 Serbian Relief Mission) had taken over the building next to us, and some barracks across the campus which they proposed to run as a typhus hospital. In order to do this, they had turned half their unit into a typhus staff, leaving the rest to carry on their surgical hospital in the town. This made us feel less isolated...'[70]

All at the Paget unit was not quite as organised as he believed. In their haste to open the hospital and remove infectious cases from Skoplje, little time was left for other aspects of nursing. With a staff of only two doctors, two nurses and Lady Paget herself, the most that could be achieved was to see that every patient was thoroughly cleaned and disinfected before being admitted to the ward. All clothes were destroyed regardless of the fact that replacement clothing was in great shortage and not always available. All that the nurses could really hope to do was *'provide fresh air, ice on the head and supporting treatment...'*[71] Despite the evident limitations of the Hospital, the Vice President of the Serbian Red Cross Colonel Soubotitch, when he visited on 8 March was greatly impressed declaring that this was the only adequate scheme of isolation in Serbia and a model for all.

'Oh now I often shudder when I think of these days but there was no time to think of one's own feelings...'

Back in Skoplje, Flora was not initially involved: *'No one was asked or invited to do this fever work, as it was considered as dangerous & contagious. The D[octo]rs decided all going to it must be voluntary. As far as one heard then, everyone coming into direct contact with it, caught it.'*

All the British were well aware that there had already been many fatalities not only amongst the Serbs but also amongst the British and American

Nursing in Serbia with Lady Paget in 1915

nurses. Two orderlies at the British Red Cross hospital in Skoplje had already died and Flora was well aware of the tribulations there:

'The British Red [Cross] had a unit in Skoplje. They had the tobacco & cigarettes factory as a hospital. They were fearfully unfortunate. Most of their patients fell ill & all the staff except the matron. At one time all the D[octo]rs were down together. A Russian lady Dr went to their help & had charge of 300 patients alone. She poor thing also fell & until a Sister from our hospital went to her, there was not a soul to nurse her...'

The nurse who went to help is not named although Dr Johnston Abraham also recorded the incident:

'We had moved the little woman [Dr Kadisch] over from her quarters to my old room just before a furious downpour of rain; and she was so ill after it, we decided much against our will, that we must really beg a nurse for night duty from the other unit. Of course they sent us a nurse at once, and we felt most absurdly grateful.'[72]

This was not the first occasion that a member of staff from the Paget unit had come to their aid. Sister F A Fry who was serving as matron with the Paget unit, in the company of her brother, James Duncan Fry, an orderly, had been a former hospital sister of Dr Johnston Abraham. When she visited his hospital in Skoplje, she was appalled at the conditions and lack of nurses and obtained permission to help out in the afternoons. Later, Sister Fry, always jokingly referred to as 'Sister Rowntree' by Dr Johnston Abraham (deliberately confusing the names of chocolate manufacturers), eventually worked full time at his hospital: *'Our one and only nurse Sister Rowntree remained smiling through it all . She looked after all our people...'*[73]

On her return to England in May, Sister Fry told a representative of the *British Journal of Nursing* how she had organised the nursing in the British Red Cross' tobacco factory *'consisting of three blocks, one surgical, one medical and one convalescent, with three floors in each'* and superintended the theatre under the English Doctors.[74] She had relied for assistance on Serbian ladies and Austrian prisoners:

The Typhus Epidemic

'All sorts of diseases were rife, and, in the hospital cases broke out of smallpox, typhus, diphtheria, enteric and scarlet fever...'

Mr Morrison described the problems amongst other missions with obvious horror:

'I had opportunities of observing the zeal and self-sacrifice displayed by the various foreign missions, and can only regret that too often the impossible was attempted, and with tragic results, for the death toll was heavy...'[75]

He was not impressed with the large factory in Skoplje in which the British Red Cross had established themselves. Besides the *'inherent unsuitability of the premises'*, he noted that the hospital was *'detestably insanitary'* and overcrowded with over a thousand medical and surgical patients:

'On the ground floor, I saw 250 men lying on sacks of straw packed closely together, covered only by their ragged uniform under a blanket. Gangrenous limbs and septic compound fractures were common, the stench being overpowering; yet every window was closely shut. The hospital was credited with being the starting point of the epidemic of typhus which ravaged Skoplje; be that as it may, the disease secured a firm foothold on each of the four floors before it was recognised. Of the 16 members of the British staff two doctors and five orderlies went down with typhus, and two of the latter died; other victims were a Russian Doctor (Miss Kadisch) and a medical Austrian prisoner, and of these two the Austrian died...'

When the remnant of the unit was withdrawn due to ill health, it was the Russian Doctor, Dr Esther Kadisch, who remained behind and worked single handed. This intriguing woman had impressed even the redoubtable Mr Morrison who singled her out as *'a courageous member of our profession'*.[76] She had been educated around Europe in places as far from her home in Riga, as Dublin, Germany and England, and had met Morrison previously in 1913 when she had been a student at Queen's Hospital in Birmingham. The pair had met once again in November 1914,

Nursing in Serbia with Lady Paget in 1915

when Lady Paget's unit took over the Serbian hospital in which she was working.

Dr Johnston Abraham also recalled this remarkable woman and confessed:

'Looking back on it now I do not know what we should have done without the Little Woman. She was so wonderful, so enthusiastic, so energetic, so fiery, so emotional, so very brave, so wrongheaded at times, so intensely feminine. We were all on the strain to keep up with her...' [77]

The British Red Cross had found Dr Kadisch already labouring in the Serbian hospital in Skoplje when they took it over. She had been running the hospital for two months single handed. Her fluency in English, French, German, Russian and Serbian proved of enormous value. She clashed with the English doctors principally over her fatalistic refusal to take measures to avoid catching infection. For a woman of only twenty two, she exhibited remarkable courage and determination, showing herself afraid of only two things... the dark and Serbian oxen,

Dr Johnston Abraham, like Mr Morrison, was open in his admiration:

'She acted as an intermediary between us and the patients, explaining, re-explaining, calming their suspicions, making them feel what we could not express to them in words, our overwhelming desire to do every possible thing we could for them. She apologised for our foibles to the Serbian authorities, especially to our courteous old Commandant, Major Suskalovitch, explaining that our attempts to get open windows and cross ventilation were not absolutely criminal, but only an English fad, to be more or less humoured...' [78]

To return to events in Skoplje in 1915, Mr Morrison had himself left Lady Paget's hospital by the end of January declaring himself unfit due to a fever which was variously described as 'Uskubitis' or typhus. (The British Red Cross referred to the same recurrent illness amongst their staff as 'Relapsing Fever'.) As part of his convalescence, Morrison toured hospitals on behalf of the newly appointed Typhus Commission.

The Typhus Epidemic

Meanwhile, his colleagues were left behind to cope with the immediate crisis...

Sister Fry also left the unit soon afterwards:

'When the need arose for the care of 200 typhus cases in a big barracks taken over by the British Red Cross up in the mountains, Miss Fry obtained permission to transfer from service under the Serbian Relief Fund to that of the Red Cross. She was the only Englishwoman there, and with the two English doctors and four orderlies, who were admirable men, ran the hospital. They appealed to the military authorities for the services of 40 to 60 Austrian prisoners as orderlies, and could not have done without them. Miss Fry states they were for the most part willing and excellent men, who expressed themselves as having no quarrel with the English. The head Austrian orderly, who spoke eight languages, was quite invaluable...'[79]

'Hundreds are dying of typhus & the poor fellows are without a soul to look after them'.

Understandably, Flora felt that she should avoid visiting the Fever Hospital although she was deeply troubled by the suffering she witnessed around the town:

' I heard such pitiful tales & when out saw many many poor creatures (especially among the Austrian prisoners) trying to drag themselves about, no one daring to go near or offer help, I felt I could not visit. Then one afternoon, I was taking a walk & met 2 poor fellows trying to struggle across asking for the nearest hospital. One died before we could get him there. The other a few hours afterwards, their ghastly faces & dejected hopeless condition haunted me day & night. I could not rest, so I volunteered to go up to the Fever Hospital much against everyones advice...'

In a letter to her sisters, dated 10th March, Flora intimated only that she had left the first hospital:

Nursing in Serbia with Lady Paget in 1915

'The Nurses are still there but there is such terrible distress among the Austrian prisoners. Hundreds are dying of typhus & the poor fellows are without a soul to look after them. Ill ones, no food or water for days & days. Lady Paget heard of this. Went to see if it was true & found things too dreadful to describe so she & the D[octo]rs have got permission to have some old Turkish barracks among the mountains... so 2 other nurses & I are here...'

Flora was keen to stress the beauty of the surrounding mountains with only passing reference to the ankle deep mud. Although the new bedrooms had been *'dreadful'*, they were now much improved by white wash and a good scrubbing. Each of the nurses was allowed a fire but there was the additional concern that the roof was infested with rats and birds: *'I am just terrified at night'*. After a *'big rat'* had fallen from the roof onto one of the nurse's bed, all burnt a light in their rooms at night. Notwithstanding such problems, Flora had now obviously adapted well to the primitive conditions. She boasted proudly to her sisters that she had never yet missed a bath at night, having schooled herself to wash one limb at a time in a *'thimble full of water'* inside a large tin, placed before the fire. The tins, she later recalled, were exactly like the lard tins used at home and measured only *'24 or 5 inches across & 8 or 9 ins deep'*.

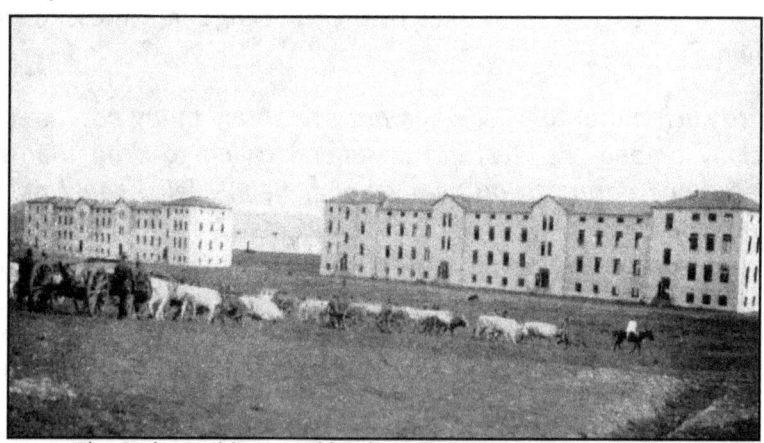

The Cadet Building used by the British Red Cross, 1915 (from My Balkan Log by J Johnston Abraham)

The Typhus Epidemic

The situation of the new Typhus Hospital was ideal and the scenery *'almost beyond description, so wild & lonely.'* Flora found the *'old barracks'* to be *'very picturesque'* consisting of four large buildings in a square with a large court yard of mud in the centre:

'One building we used as offices, dispensary, linen room, kitchens etc the other 3 pavilions as wards. These had been beautiful places built of white stone with basements, almost 14 steps in centre leading to wards which went right & left, each taking 48 beds.'

On her first morning at work in the Typhus Hospital, it was the mud that caused the initial problem. Since it was known that typhus was caused by body lice, it was decided that all working in the fever wards should wear protective suits to cover all their clothes. The Doctors had white calico suits with feet made in one piece, buttoning across the shoulders. As there was no time to obtain a nurse's suit, the Doctor asked her to wear one of his own suits and Flora wisely complied:

'I can never forget the first morning I went into the ward, white trousers with feet covering gum boots, a mask to cover face & head, with exception of eyes & rubber gloves. My feelings were strange & oh, how D[octo]rs & other sister laughed...'

Flora had become stuck in the mud as she struggled across the courtyard and her mud bespattered suit testified to her difficulties. She noted, with not very well disguised satisfaction, that the nursing colleague who found her plight so amusing had refused to don any protective clothing and was to succumb to typhus within the week.

At the British Red Cross hospital, close by, staff smeared themselves with crude paraffin oil from head to toes twice a day and found that the smell repelled lice quite successfully. Sister Fry later described the countermeasures to a journalist: *'In regard to personal precautions, Miss Fry, who certainly looks the picture of health, states that she took daily an antiseptic bath, and rubbed herself all over with petroleum. It was found that the lice which are generally supposed to be responsible for the disease would not come near petroleum...'*[80] The alternative course

Nursing in Serbia with Lady Paget in 1915

pursued by the Paget nurses was viewed with more suspicion:

'Most of the nurses of the Paget Unit were now dressed in pyjamas, wore rubber boots into which the lower ends of their trouser legs were tucked, had rubber gloves which went over the ends of the sleeves, and wore face masks. They were therefore practically lice-proof...'[81]

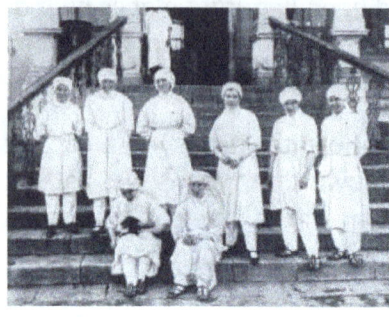

Illustrated London News, *July 1915*

Flora soon had more important problems to tackle:

'It would be impossible to describe my feelings when I first entered the wards. They were so long & bare looking. The beds so uninviting & oh, the patients, poor souls lying huggled up, lots of them quite unconscious , some talking, some singing, some walking about, all with a strange look (which one soon got to recognise as the typhus expression). It was really gruesome...'

Faced with a pavilion containing ninety eight such cases, Flora wondered where on earth she should begin. She had no experience of typhus fever and looked to the Doctors for direction. She commenced by giving drinks and taking temperatures. Lady Paget was about the hospital looking ill and exhausted. She retired to bed early and the following day was too ill to get up. Before the day was out, all knew that she had contracted typhus.

Lady Paget's own account of this time is understandably vague. In her report, she recorded that she had been taken ill with typhus on 8 March and that Sister Scott joined the Typhus Colony on the following day. This seems unlikely since Flora clearly remembered her working in the hospital wards on her first day. What is certain is that Flora found herself suddenly faced with a crisis even worse than she had feared. Whilst Sister Henry and Nurse Round undertook to nurse Lady Paget by day and by night, Nurse Isherwood and Sister Scott were the only nurses left in the wards. Then the Doctors started to go down with typhus, Dr

The Typhus Epidemic

Knobel on 13 March and Dr Moon down in Skoplje on 20th.

When on 17 March, Nurse Isherwood too succumbed to typhus, the third pavilion had just been opened and Flora found herself, alone, in charge of three hundred cases.

Although Lady Paget later described the situation in her report under the heading *'One Nurse – 300 Patients'* she makes no special commendation of Sister Scott, noting simply that *'...after Nurse Isherwood began the typhus on the 17th, Sister Scott remained alone in charge of 300 men until the 24th...'*[82]

Only Nurse Isherwood, who had initially helped nurse Lady Paget, was singled out for special attention:

'So great was the strain on our nursing resources that for two days and nights Nurse Isherwood, with a temperature of 104°, was putting ice on her own head, as Dr Knobel and I were both unconscious and needing constant attention.'[83]

Miss K. Isherwood had come out with Lady Paget's unit in November 1914 as a ward maid but had by now obtained the status of Nurse. It was natural that there should be a strong camaraderie between those who had served together from the start but one cannot help wondering whether Nurse Round and Nurse Scott who had both joined the unit barely a month before, were still viewed a little as outsiders.

Flora wrote in her memoirs about the horror of the disease but was modestly reticent about her own role, only referring briefly to the fact that she was alone: *'I have often said to the Dr when he came in, I have 14 or 16 new patients for you to see. One day when I was on alone, 42 were admitted...'*

In her memoirs, Flora confessed that the suffering caused by this *'horrible disease'* was *'well past description'*. The course of the fever involved three or four days of delirium: *'It was dreadful to be in the wards, naked men wandering about. Some sing, some shouting make absurd face laughing loudly etc...It was a mad rush from the time you went on duty*

Nursing in Serbia with Lady Paget in 1915

until you went off too tired & done up to think of own feelings.'

Sister Fry later described the symptoms of the disease to a representative of the *British Journal of Nursing*:

'Typhus, Miss Fry emphasises, is a disease which needs good nursing and careful feeding, and unquestionably many Serbians died for the lack of them. The symptoms are headache, backache, and rising temperature. After the spots come out it rises very highly, often up to 106°. There is great prostration and often delirium. Complications, due to the fact that typhus is a very septic disease, are embolism, and sloughing off of extremities, such as noses and toes. Treatment includes the application of ice-bags to the head (plenty of ice obtainable in the mountains) and cold packs; also flushing out the kidneys with fluid to help to eliminate the poison. Fresh air is essential, and it was difficult to induce Serbians to believe it ...'[84]

An odd souvenir of these times survives amongst Flora's papers at the Imperial War Museum. Amongst the photographs, letters and miscellaneous papers is the table of temperature for 'Marco' a twenty three year old Austrian who was admitted on 5th April 1915 *'from the basement where he had been ill five days'.* His illness from 5th April to the 20th is traced through brief annotations concerning temperature and bowel movements, recording that he reached his highest temperature of 105° on 8th April when he was delirious, the purple rash appearing six days later. A similar record relating to the twenty-nine year old' 'Lipel Hermann', chronicles the progress of his illness from 28th March to 19th April, his highest temperature reaching 104.5° on 28th March. Such records convey a rare sense of reality to the cold facts and statistics of the appalling epidemic. A letter home written around this time, perhaps explains why Flora kept such a reminder of suffering:

'Typhus is a very distressing disease, and generally patients are delirious for a day or two. Their cries and groans are fearful. Yet it repays one to see them getting better, and you feel all your worry and work have been worth something. I cannot possible describe to you the gratitude and looks of these men. Their eyes seem to follow you everywhere you move

The Typhus Epidemic

in the wards, and wherever I go every man I pass stands and salutes...'[85]

'Oh, it was terrible to see & know this was done, but we were helpless and could do no other...'

Flora was appalled too by the apparently callous way in which even those close to death were shaved and bathed in hydrogen peroxide. As they gradually cleared the basements, the Doctors and any Austrians who were fit enough to help, sorted the living from the dead and carried them to a courtyard where they were put into a strong disinfectant bath, shaved and scrubbed in the open air. All patients whether from the town or the basements, received the same treatment:

' However ill, they were obliged to go through this process, for you must remember, all were covered with lice & our only hope of getting this fever under hand was to keep the wards free of vermin. It often seemed a cruel & terrible thing to put dying men in to a bath, shave & scrub them & what was even worse, all this had to be done in the open air. When first we started, we were without towels & sheets, so these poor souls were left on stretchers in the courtyard to be thoroughly shaved, then their clothes cut off & taken naked up the steps to entrance of wards, where a bath of hydroperoxide was ready. Here they were scrubbed quickly down, if there was such a thing as a towel, dried & run to bed (without sheets often)...'

Once in the wards, an effort was made to give drinks and some degree of warmth, although shortages made even this difficult:

'Many and many a time after these just few things I felt it seemed useless to attempt nursing. Food & drinks were so short. Then we were often without fires & water & not even an extra blanket for a bed, just the one army blanket for each patient. One could see them shivering & not be able to help in any way. Beds were never empty. As one poor soul died, another was laid on the bed at once. Always the steps were covered with poor fellows waiting for admission. We just took in as fast as possible...'

The unreliability of the water supply was a constant worry. Lady Paget in

Nursing in Serbia with Lady Paget in 1915

her report recalled that this was one of her chief causes of anxiety. The water supply would be cut off without warning sometimes for several hours, *'often for the day and once for two days'*:

'To me personally, the days when there was no water were days of mental torture – a nightmare of remembrance. Never shall I forget going round the wards from bed to bed, seeing the flushed, fevered faces and the dry, parched mouths and hearing the incessant cry of ' Water, Sister! Water!' from every corner of the room. Those too ill to speak raised trembling hands in supplication. It was heartrending, and enough to drive one mad, when we knew we had not a drop of water to give them. We used to send the ambulance in to the town loaded with small vessels to bring us back water, and also bought oranges and lemons, cutting them up into quarters and giving them to the men to suck.'[86]

Flora too recalled rather more concisely that water was *'very very scarce. A tap was placed in the court yards but very often no water could be got from it.'* In a letter of Flora's which was published in the *Leicester Daily Post* of 23rd April 1915, she described the horror more fully:

'Another day when I was on duty, all were craving for a drink. There was not even a glass full of water in any ward, and for eight hours we could get nothing but snow water. No one until they had lived up here, could in any way realise the difficulties one has, and continually I have asked myself: Is it doing a scrap of good to stay here? Then when I go into a ward and see their faces light up, and hear them say in their Austrian language 'Sister, a drink', I feel I must stay.'[87]

Another constant headache was the problem of sanitation. Behind the pavilions were two overflowing cess pits. Since their level was above that of the basements where Serbian orderlies were now accommodated, sewage leaked frequently into the entrance. From the start, Dr Maitland struggled with Serbian officialdom as he made strenuous efforts to have the cess pits pumped out but in every case his attempts were thwarted. A suitable pump was never supplied for a sufficiently long time to accomplish the task and in the end, in something of despair, he cabled the Serbian Relief Fund urging that a sanitary engineer should be

The Typhus Epidemic

sent out to plan and organise a scheme of sanitation for the hospital. With the loss of Lady Paget and Dr Knobel, he now found himself solely responsible not only for supervising the buildings but also the staff and patients.

Flora acknowledged sadly that there was *'no pretence of sanitation'* in the hospital but what exercised her more was the shortage of food. In the same letter published in the *Leicester Daily Post*, she described the problem:

'Also we are terribly short of food. Honestly, for three days every one complained of being hungry. We could not get food up. Even now our stores are short. The cocoa, chocolates, Bovril, prepared foods and biscuits which we brought out, have been a real godsend to me. Often I have made the patients these on my little spirit stove, and it has been grand to see their look of gratitude.'

It was a theme which she returned to in her memoirs:

'Foods also we got from the Serbian allies at the rate of 6 ½ sue a day for food., so you may guess, these poor souls never got a real good meal. I used to be fearfully worried by the small quantities that came up & was always worried and going for the cook & secretary. Patients on milk only were allowed less than 1 pt for 24 hours, nothing else. Meal times were full of anxiety. One could not make food go round & every morning as the Dr went round, the continued cry was for more labrus (bread)...'

The Secretary mentioned by Flora was Lady Paget's cousin Richard Chichester who had stepped in to help Dr Maitland when Lady Paget fell ill. Flora had been impressed by him when he met them at Salonika and in her letter to her sisters of 10 March she described him in glowing terms:

'He is the Hon R Chichester. He 2 Drs & we nurses have meals together & great fun we have had. Often we have to use same plate for 2 or 3 courses. Today we all sat & drank soup out of enameled [sic] mugs..'

This presumably was before food supplies became so stretched but it is

Nursing in Serbia with Lady Paget in 1915

clear that Flora was not at this stage revealing the true state of affairs in her letters. In a letter of 12th April [in Serbia 31st March], she mentioned the shortage of food for the first time:

'Yesterday I could not get enough for them to eat. Many of them said they were so hungry. I felt so miserable & wondered if it was worth staying here trying to get them well. Then I was going round & one poor man beckoned me to him. (He had been terribly ill & I have looked after his food & fed him myself.)He lifted my hand to his heart, kissed it, then raised it to his head & kissed it again. Poor fellow, he is so grateful but too ill to speak. I think he noticed how worried I was over the food.'

As in the first hospital, Flora found the beds to be *'funny low iron things'* which were liable to collapse with the patients lying on them. Mattresses consisted of large sacks of straw, with straw pillows and sheets - when they could be obtained - all covered by a single army blanket. Beds were arranged around each side and down the centre of the ward.

Heating was also erratic with *'quaint stoves'* situated in the centre with *'piping'* pushed through the windows. Much to everyone's discomfort, these makeshift chimneys would only permit the stoves to burn when the wind was in the right direction. More often than not, it was in the wrong direction. There was often a shortage of wood too, since the heavy snow occasionally prevented oxen from pulling loads up from the town. The cold was *'intense'* often with very deep snow. Her letter to a friend, reprinted in the *Leicester Daily Post* emphasised the point:

'For instance, the weather a fortnight ago was intensely cold, with deep snow three days. Unfortunately we were without wood, and could not get it up here. The roads were too bad for the oxen to pull heavy loads up here through the thick snow. These poor men lay without fires, and only one army blanket each. It was too shocking. Yet we were helpless, and could not in any way give them warmth. There was no fire to heat water. Oh! Never have I felt so cold and wretched.'[88]

Back down in the town, Miss Gertrude Smith, one of the original team of nurses, also reported the cold weather in a postcard which was

The Typhus Epidemic

published in *The British Journal of Nursing*:

'We are working very hard under trying conditions. We are up to our knees in snow! The country is very lovely. I have charge of the theatre. Getting very good work. I have no idea how the outer world is getting on.'[89]

'I often said these first weeks at the Typhus Colony, we were in one of the most beautiful spots in the earth, but I honestly could not conceive any place more sad & sorrowful.'

Flora recorded that the death rate at first was enormous and estimated the figure at around thirty to forty a day. Lady Paget was a little more conservative suggesting a mortality rate of between twenty and thirty a day.[90] It was difficult amid such appalling conditions to keep any sort of record:

'... Oh the sadness of those deaths. At first we had no way of finding out names, address etc of these poor Austrian prisoners & as they died one after another without the comfort of a friend & in such pitiful conditions, my heart would ache, when I thought of wives, mothers etc [who] would never know how & when they had died & for years or their lifetime, be looking & praying for their return. Many of these prisoners had been men in good positions, a few gentlemen & it was terrible to see their last days & manner of living...'

When Nurse Isherwood succumbed to typhus, Flora was left alone nursing some three hundred patients for almost ten days, with no help on the ward apart from Austrian prisoners. In addition to the typhus cases, there were two cases of small pox, a few dysentery , and one or two cases of diphtheria and scarlet fever: *'I don't quite know how I managed these days. I seemed only able to go around giving drinks, medication etc...'*

Flora described the situation in a letter home to a friend in Leicester which was reprinted in *The British Journal of Nursing* in May under the title *'In a Serbian Hospital'*:

Nursing in Serbia with Lady Paget in 1915

'...for about ten days I was left alone, with only the convalescent Austrian to nurse these poor souls. Never can I forget it. I felt so helpless. I could get little else done than just give medicines drinks and other necessaries. But those men are so grateful. Although I seemed the only woman about the place, neither day nor night die I feel in any way nervous...'[91]

It was the indefatigable Dr Maitland who now stepped in and brought to Flora a present in the shape of a tall, lanky twenty two year old Austrian known by the rather unlikely name of 'Mick'. The boy, who could speak a little English, was instructed to take care of Flora and undertake any errands. He turned out to be an *'invaluable friend'* who would scarcely allow her out of his sight:

'Poor Mick, I am real fond of him. He just follows me about like Tiny does. Lights fires for me at night in my room, sweeps & dusts it, carries my water, sees to my lau[ndry], cleans boots (a terrible job these dirty days), puts them on & off for me, lights fire for me to dress by & gets my bath water. Honestly, I believe he would feed me, if I would let him...'

Flora was greatly moved to hear the boy's story and that he too had links with Canada, where he had been farming for four years. At the outbreak of war, he had, unluckily, been spending four months in his former home in Austria and had been promptly conscripted. More misfortune ensued when he was taken prisoner on the battlefield and brought to Skoplje. With his fellow prisoners he had suffered greatly, without any food or clothes during the harsh winter. It was when he contracted typhus that he *'crawled up to see the English'*. The boy was terribly home sick and continually talked of his parents and sisters, wondering if they were alive. He had sent them twelve letters but received no reply. Flora resolved to use her family in Canada to try and make contact and later wrote to her sisters enclosing a letter from the Austrian for Sydney to post in Montreal. It is frustrating not to know the end of this particular story but the conclusion is likely to have been tragic.

Flora was delighted to have someone to talk with and regarded the boy as a *'godsend'*, although his efforts at interpreting were hampered by his poor English: *'We all used to get in great muddles'*.

The Typhus Epidemic

As Mick carried the medicines and stimulants around for Flora, he tried to discourage her from trying to feed unconscious or delirious patients especially if they were moribund:

'Often he would say as I put the spoon to their mouth, no good, why feed him, he going green die soon. Poor fellows they all seemed to think it strange, we tried to give brandy or water to very very ill patients...'

Flora seems to have found this an amusing feature of her companion. She did, however, have rather greater concerns. Her biggest fear, she confessed, was that a patient should be taken out of the ward before they were actually dead: *' I knew one man who had been in a Serbian hospital in the town, he told me, he was so ill they said he was dying so about 8 o'clock at night he was put in a coffin & taken into a shed. He recovered consciousness & found himself there in the early morning, managed to crawl back to the ward & to a bed. This was not at all an uncommon occurrence in Serbia, I was told.'*

This story obviously circulated quite rapidly amongst the three hundred or so British workers present in Serbia at the end of March. Monica Stanley recalled that later it was even reported in English newspapers by Dr Percy Dearmer, Chaplain to the British Units in Serbia.[92]

The fear of something like this happening whilst she was in sole charge, haunted Flora. She was only too well aware that her patients were left alone at night with only Austrian prisoners to look after them. Her solution in the end, was to insist that *'our head man'* should go early to the mortuary each morning and examine the dead carefully.

Although she declared that there was no place *'more sad & sorrowful'* Flora was sustained amidst all the suffering by the gratitude of those she tried to help:

'Our only comfort & happiness was the gratitude of those poor sufferers. Often as I passed, they would catch hold of my coat & kiss it. Their thankfulness was pathetic. Until the very day I came away, whenever I passed them, they stood aside & saluted.'

Nursing in Serbia with Lady Paget in 1915

Although in the first three weeks of Flora's stay at the hospital, the only patients were Austrian, they would later be joined by Serbs, Germans, Greeks, Turks and Italians. By then, help was at last in sight with the advent of Dr Bellingham Smith and the nurses of the 2nd Serbian Relief Fund, known as 'Lady Wimborne's unit'. The name arose from the fact that it was Lady Cornelia Wimborne, the well known philanthropist who had raised the funds for the unit. Her efforts could not have been more welcome...

According to Lady Paget's account, which contains several contradictory dates, four nurses, one lady bacteriologist and two orderlies from the Wimborne Unit, went up to the Typhus Colony on 24th March. Dr Bellingham Smith was said to have joined Dr Maitland a few days earlier. Flora recorded however, that two new sisters had joined her first after she had been on her own for around ten days and she had been mightily relieved since this now meant that each nurse was responsible for only ninety eight beds: *'It was wonderful what a little nursing and attention did.'* This was possibly two of the nurses who had been sent out with Dr Moon on 18th February to assist the Lady Paget unit and advise on a site for a future unit. The party had travelled overland via Brindisi and had arrived well before the Wimborne Unit.[93] A note in the *British Journal of Nursing* in February had recorded the departure of Nurses A D Beaton, Lilian Gerard and Jane E Peter to join Lady Paget and this is perhaps the group that accompanied Dr Moon.[94]

In fact, the Wimborne unit, under a Mr W P G Graham, the former Director General to the Public Health Department of Egypt, as administrator, had left London on 9th February but had spent some five weeks travelling via Malta, Athens and Salonika. When they had set out they had not known their destination. Mr Graham, as a sanitary expert was expecting to tackle the sanitation problems in Nish and the Serbian Relief Committee had objected strongly to the Serbians when it became clear that they were to be sent to Skoplje.

The party consisted of three surgeons, Messrs Barrington Ward, GH Sinclair and Edmund B Jones, Dr Bellingham Smith as physician and Dr J Dalyell *'the lady doctor'* as bacteriologist and anaesthetist. Mr Graham

The Typhus Epidemic

had as his assistant a Miss Monsie Scott, the sister of the famous explorer Robert Falcon Scott, as well as a matron, nine nurses, nine female orderlies, twelve male orderlies, a cook with assistant, a laundry maid with assistant, a dispenser and quartermaster.[95] This unit of forty four people clearly did not perceive its role as a support for Lady Paget's Hospital but rather as a separate unit with its own objectives.

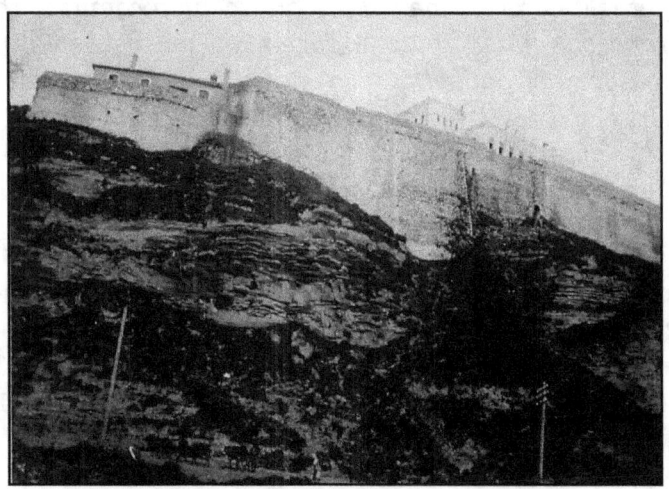

Postcard of the 'Grad' at Skoplje, c. 1915

Lady Muriel Herbert who served as a rather unlikely orderly with the Lady Wimborne unit wrote home with enthusiasm after the unit had arrived in Skoplje on 24th March, that they had established a new hospital in 'The Grad' the old Turkish fort situated on *'the old citadel rock overhanging the river, and high above the town.'*[96] At Salonika, where they had arrived on 2nd March, she had met *'a convalescing Paget orderly'* on leave who had reported *'that things are not too bad at Uscub'*. He had been *'seedy, and one of their nurses had had a slight go of Uskub fever, which is really typhus, but otherwise all are well.'*[97]

Apparently unaware of the crisis at the Typhus colony in Skoplje, the party remained in Salonika until 24 March whilst Mr Graham and Barrington Ward looked for a suitable hospital in Skoplje, Nish and finally, Belgrade. Eventually, having rejected several offers, Mr Graham *'found a nice building [in Belgrade] which he has been promised if any fighting takes*

Nursing in Serbia with Lady Paget in 1915

place'. In the mean time, he agreed to take *'some quite good buildings in Uscub'* which would make a good hospital for surgical cases. Like others, Lady Herbert was disappointed to learn that they were not bound for Nish where the typhus was *'pretty bad'* but for Skoplje *'the same place as Lady Paget.'* She was inclined to refer rather disparagingly to *'the town hospital (ex Paget)'* but she did at least note in a letter of 19 March: *'Leila Paget is a heroine, she started an isolation camp for the typhus patients, and one nurse and one doctor are up there with hundreds, nearly thousands of patients...'*[98] In her letter of 29 March, from the Hotel Liberty in Skoplje –no schoolrooms for this orderly – she wrote: *'Bellingham Smith, De Dalzell [sic] and four sisters are out at the fever place now, where the conditions are pretty bad- 100 patients in a ward with one nurse; no chance of proper nursing...'* [99]

Flora wrote enthusiastically that with the advent of the *'Lady Doctor'*, they began to do *'a little real nursing'*. The *'lady doctor'* whom Flora never mentioned by name, was Dr Elsie Jean Dalyell (1881-1948), an Australian bacteriologist who had qualified in Sydney in 1910.[100] She arrived with the Wimborne unit and served under Dr Maitland from March to April 1915.

On 17th March, far away in London, the Serbian Relief Fund committee were struggling to find a destination for their third Relief Unit which was to be led by the redoubtable Mrs St Clair Stobart. They resolved unanimously *'that a cable should be sent to Lady Paget instructing her unit to return on 31st March with the exception of individuals who elected to remain under the control and with the sanction of Mr Graham'.*[101] In Skoplje, on 29th March Lady Herbert wrote *'next week we take over the Paget Town Hospital, which will mean more work again.'* Although Lady Paget was too ill to return, it does seem as if this timetable was adhered to by most of her staff. On 6th April, Lady Herbert wrote further: *'Taking over the Paget Hospital has made lots more work, as it all has be cleaned and washed, and generally refitted, as they want their stuff for the fever place as soon as we can replace it...'*[102]

In her memoirs, Flora recorded that the surgical hospital was handed over to Lady Wimborne's unit on 1 April and that most of Lady Paget's

The Typhus Epidemic

unit, apart from six who remained, sailed for England on 31 March.

Flora recalled that most of those leaving were *'very very tired & ill. Winter & the poor conditions had tired them greatly.'* On the night before they were due to depart, all were invited to a *'banquet of honour'*, hosted by the Serbian General of the District. Lady Paget was still too ill to attend but Flora and one or two from her hospital went down to enjoy the entertainment. Mr Morrison was also there :

'The proceedings were enlivened by the music of a military band, and speeches were made beyond our deserving in French and Serbian'[103]

Flora described the scene rather more vividly:

'It really was a fine & interesting ceremony given in the Picture House with a full band. The tables (& linen) were beautifully laid & decorated. A very delicious repast & specially served dinner of many courses, real good champagne & wine flowed like water, lots of speeches, toasts (both in Serbian & English) winding up with pictures & dancing until between 3 & 4 the next morning...As the train for Salonique left Uscub between 5 & 6 there was no sleep for that night for those starting to England.'

Flora sent a menu to her sisters, noting that there was *'heaps of champagne'* and the dinner *'very nice'* although she had probably not comprehended much of the speeches: *'Several toasts & speeches, in Servian language sounded strange to us...'*

To her sisters, Flora also wrote of the carriage ride down to Skoplje that evening: *'I think I have never seen the moon so beautiful, big & bright as was that night.'* The rough roads provided the usual entertainment, with all holding on for dear life. Whilst she wrote in glowing terms of the dinner and beautiful band, enclosing the menu card, it was really the journey there and back which made the deepest impression upon Flora. Leaving 'early' – at 1.20 am – she and a fellow nurse returned home, delighting in the moonlight and snowy landscape: *'The snow mountains in the far distance were lovely. The sky so blue but we were followed a long way by a pack of wolf dogs (lovely creatures) & they made such a*

Nursing in Serbia with Lady Paget in 1915

noise...'

Calamity struck some ten minutes' walk from home, when one of the two horses stumbled whilst crossing a big trench full of water. All were thrown from the carriage with apparently little injury although the poor horse had to be left in the ditch until men could be summoned to rescue it the next day. Characteristically, it was the fate of the animal which concerned Flora most.

Flora was one of the few to remain in Skoplje. In her letter to her sisters, confusingly dated 12th April [in Serbia 31st March] but probably written much earlier in March she explained: *'We hope to have a big unit of Sisters out from England shortly but they have not yet started and I really could not leave here until someone could take my place'*. The arrival of twenty five nurses and five doctors, with stores, clothes and food transformed the situation. At last equipped with good supplies of linen, pyjamas, bed socks and slippers, Flora and her colleagues could really help their patients: *'How we wished there were 24 working hours each day. One always left unsatisfied'*.

The Serbian Relief Committee had resolved to send out thirty additional nurses as soon as news of the crisis in Skoplje reached them on 17 March. So urgent was the matter, that they agreed to send fifteen by the quicker overland route if no transport were available.[104] A note in the *British Journal of Nursing* issued on 10th April 1915 recorded the names of several nurses who had left London on Sunday 4th April to work in Serbia at Mrs Hardy's Hospital in Nish and *'the Typhus Colony'*:

'The Misses L Kelley, R M Ridge, T Crombleholme, L Sturt, C Gowans, B L Robinshaw, R Mansell, C L Norman (Norwegian), M T O'Neil, M Coleman.

Also mentioned were *'Miss K N Fitch, Miss E Lyn Jones and Miss V Lüders (Danish) who left London on 1st April.'*

The remaining party of nurses, all widely experienced in fever nursing, left London on 11th April: Miss Louisa Ball; Miss Sara Bonser; Miss Maud E Bullock; Miss Roberta Parsons; Miss Eva E Egerton; Miss Helen Smith

The Typhus Epidemic

and Miss M E Skertchley.[106]

The nurses are not mentioned again in the minutes but many of the above names reappear on the back of Flora's personal photographs and it is clear that the majority ended up working with her at the Typhus Hospital. Their names are recorded alongside Flora's in the list of supplementary personnel for Lady Paget's first unit and most remained for the second phase of the hospital [see appendix 2 and page 290].

Further help for the Paget Hospital also eventually arrived in the shape of a unit organised by a certain Dr J Hartnell Beavis, fresh from running a similar medical unit in Belgium, which arrived in Salonika on 15 April. The unit had travelled out from Liverpool on 1 April on board the *Saidieh*, on the same vessel as Mrs Stobart's Unit. With him sailed his assistant, Gerald Sim, Mr Fergus Armstrong as surgeon and Dr G Landsborough Findlay as physician with his wife Lady Sybil acting as one of the nurses.[107]

The well-staffed unit included, in addition to *'a staff of most capable nurses'*, dressers, orderlies, chauffeurs, a cook, washerwoman and interpreter. Also in tow, were the writers Alice and Claude Askew as special correspondents for the English newspaper *'Daily Express'*. Together they composed 'the First British Field Hospital for Serbia' attached to the Second Serbian Army.

Since there was no serious fighting in progress, Dr Beavis' unit was sent first to Skoplje to *'mark time'*. The unit had arrived by 26 April when Lady Herbert reported that *'a new unit- Dr Bevis in charge- is taking over the town Hospital (ex Paget) from us'*.[108] Claude Askew wrote with his usual hyperbole:

'Conditions were better when we reached Skoplje, and this was owing to the brave men and women who toiled devotedly through those dark winter days to combat the grim spectre – they who went out fearlessly, their lives in their hands, and all too many of whom fell victims to their devotion.

A few of those who had fought this stern fight were still at Skoplje when

Nursing in Serbia with Lady Paget in 1915

we arrived. Lady Paget, convalescent from a severe attack of typhus, left for England a few days later, carrying with her the love and gratitude of the whole nation...'[109]

Lady Paget's death had been prematurely reported by a news agency in Berlin but by the end of March, her mother, Lady Mary Paget had cabled the Associated Press with a denial and even the *New York Times* was correcting the rumour:

'Lady Paget is most touched by the kind sympathy of her friends in America, and cables saying that the rumor is false. Her daughter is out of danger in Serbia.'[110]

Not all were so fortunate. Although, Dr Maitland could be proud that no member of the British staff died from typhus, this was not the case with the Serbian staff. Between 6 and 24 March, sixteen workers went down with typhus and the deaths occurred of a Greek and an Austrian doctor; a Serbian inspector and a Serbian officer acting as a voluntary assistant.

'As far as Skoplje is concerned, the result of our two month's hard labour was that at the time of our departure on May 6th, the town had been entirely cleared of typhus, not a single case being recorded'[111]

In her report to the Serbian Relief Fund, Lady Paget recorded that once the hospital was fully staffed, the death rate fell dramatically. When no death occurred on three consecutive days, the Serbian authorities rang up in some concern to ask why they had not received the usual daily return of deaths. Although Lady Paget acknowledged that under such trying circumstances, it was difficult to work out accurately the rate of mortality, she estimated that a death rate of thirty per cent when no nursing was available had fallen to around fourteen per cent with a staff of twenty five nurses.

It is unclear whether she is quoting the English or the Serbian date but Lady Paget's report, although subject to erratic proof reading errors, records that she left Skoplje for England on 6th May. Dates of English letters from Serbia are often confusingly contradictory but her late

The Typhus Epidemic

departure is certainly confirmed by other sources.

Mrs St Clair Stobart, leading the third Serbian Relief hospital unit on its way to Kragujevatz, left Salonika on 20th April and recorded that she called at Skoplje in the evening. The party was greeted by Sir Ralph Paget who offered light refreshments - *'soup floating with grease and omelette as tough as leather'* if Monica Stanley is to be believed - and reported that Lady Paget was now recovering from typhus. Lady Paget was evidently back in England by 2 June when she was welcomed back by the Serbian Relief Fund Committee.[114]

Flora herself explained the difficulties of having two calendars to her sisters, pointing out that dates in Serbia were thirteen days behind those in England. This problem of differing calendars had existed since 1582 when an edict of Pope Gregory XII had very sensibly acknowledged the increasing divergence of the calendar year from the solar year by reforming the calendar with the loss of ten days. Future difficulties were to be avoided by introducing the concept of the Leap year. Whilst this reform was widely accepted in Catholic countries, political rivals in Protestant states were understandably more reluctant to adopt the change. Britain did not adopt the Gregorian calendar until 1752 when Parliament decreed that that 2 September should be followed by 14 September.

The Orthodox churches of the East were even slower to adopt the new style of calendar with the result that in 1915, Russia, Greece and the Balkan states were all still operating under the old 'Julian calendar'. By this stage the discrepancy in dates had increased to thirteen days. This confusion does not explain all the contradictions in dates but may in part explain the source of the problem. The difficulty of remembering dates correctly, particularly amidst such chaos and horror when diary keeping was the last concern, is probably also an important factor.

When Flora wrote on 2 April, pointing out to her sisters that it was 15 April in England, she was still very short staffed. The hospital was expecting another three hundred patients, bringing the total number to seven hundred and fifty and there were still only three nurses. In

Nursing in Serbia with Lady Paget in 1915

addition, she was concerned that the other two sisters might have to leave any day *'so I look as though I am going to have my hands very full again...'* It would appear that the Wimborne unit still anticipated moving on to Belgrade. The doubt was only finally settled with the arrival of the additional fever nurses and Dr Beavis' unit on 26 April.

In any case, by the time of Lady Paget's departure for England, life was a lot more relaxed at the Typhus hospital.

> **'I only hope I shall get back safely to England without typhus, but so [far no one] nursing it seems to escape...'**

Even at the Typhus Hospital, Flora wrote home with enthusiasm about the beautiful surroundings and the opportunities afforded by living out of the town. Although the mail from home was erratic, she endeavoured to send a letter home each week, resorting to postcards when she was too busy for anything of length. Amidst much love sent to her nephews and nieces from their 'Auntie Tod', there was still a deal of anxiety about the pets at home: *'I had a nice letter from Miss Corah the other day, telling me of Vanity. She is in clover no doubt & of course Nurse Pickering hears about Tiny. She seems to have settled but I know they would make a fuss of her...'*

Flora was still concerned about the *'poor old puss'* and whilst she was pleased to hear that the bulbs were doing well in Victoria Road, she was very alarmed about the presence of a mysterious *'Mrs Viles'*, imparting the earnest instruction: *'Be sure if ever Mrs Viles go to V[ictoria] R[oad] you lock my lavatory. There is a lot of soap & crockery in the cupboards. Also lock my bedroom & store room. She does not mind what she takes.'*

Financing the nursing home in Victoria Road was a constant concern for Flora. In a rare display of her Christian faith, which obviously mattered deeply to her, she wrote to her sisters:

'I often wonder what the future will be for V[ictoria] R[oad]. It often worries me when I think, well so far, God has given me work, food & home & He will no doubt guide my future & work things as He thinks

The Typhus Epidemic

best. Evidently this was all planned for me. I have so enjoyed it & been so happy. I only hope I shall get back safely to England without typhus, but so [far no one] nursing it seems to escape...'

Although, Flora was a regular church-goer there is little else in her writing to suggest a deep Christian faith. Amongst her papers at the Imperial War Museum, a reference from William Williamson, minister of St Stephen's Presbyterian Church in Leicester *'warmly'* recommending her as a member in full communion and a further letter from him dated 15th April 1915 sent to *'all our members in service at the front'*, are the only evidence for her spiritual life.

Incongruously, Flora was also full of advice for her sister Aggie who was about to set out for Canada, suggesting that she should make several large pockets to hang on the wall of her cabin with drawing pins to accommodate brushes and combs, as was the practice of officers' wives struggling to cope with a lack of drawers in a poky cabin. She had advice about what to wear on the voyage too: Dressing gowns were unnecessary as most went to the bath in coats or mackintoshes. Evening dress was not required. An afternoon dress and a change of collar was quite adequate, perhaps with a *'pretty evening cloak'*. As soon as dinner was over, you would require a big coat once more so as to sit on deck. In fact, by this time the increasing fear of submarines meant that most passengers slept in their clothes and there was certainly little time for social niceties like changing for dinner.

Flora was also very concerned to hear news of *'Dear old Leicester'*. She was grateful to receive newspapers from home even though by the time they reached her, they were at least three weeks out of date. She read with interest of plans, not actually ever realised, to use De Montfort Hall as a hospital along with several school buildings in Leicester, realising that this meant the expectation of *'a tremendous amount of wounded'*.

As well as letters from her immediate family circle, Flora received letters from nursing colleagues and several former patients who had seen her address in the newspapers. Mr Cavan wrote weekly enclosing newspapers and Flora was somewhat astonished to see her letters

Nursing in Serbia with Lady Paget in 1915

appearing often in a somewhat distorted form:

'Con, did you see one of my first letters to you girls in the papers. How did they get it? It was rather a funny letter, so many things put wrong. The letters seem to have been copied from paper to lots of different papers, for the Nurses have shown me them in their papers from home....'

It is easy to imagine Flora's surprise, reading in her letter published in the *Leicester Daily Post* of 9 March, that Skoplje was *'really in Albania and belonged to Serbia until the last war.'* She was probably less amused to find in the *Derbyshire Advertiser* of 15 May 1915 that her constant admiration for the work of the Austrian prisoners at the Typhus Colony had been transformed into: *' It was impossible to do much else with such few helpers, for the Austrians who were assisting seemed very callous and ignorant...'*

Mistakes - or deliberate distortions - it seems, were not confined to the provincial papers:

'Do keep a good watch on the picture papers. I am sure our hospital & work will be in some of them. Did you see the picture of Lady Paget? It is not our Lady Paget but her mother. Mr Cavan cut it out of Daily Mirror & sent me. We did laugh, so did she...'

'What a treat it would be to get a glass of good milk or a cup of tea with cream...'

As the weather improved, the food supply became more reliable and the menu began to return to its former not altogether welcome style:

'Don't ever know quite what we are eating, only that we have lots of vegetables, loads of rice, chickens, turkey (did I tell you chickens are 8d each turkeys 1/2 here) goats , sucking pigs, occasionally sheep. We never drink water (except bottled german mineral waters) just wine or lemonade. I very much doubt if my biscuits will hold out until I return. They are dreadfully expensive here 1/8 per lb. Tea I shall [have] enough to last me. I do so long for some bread & butter. We get such dreadfully strong butter. I cannot bear it near. The bread is coarse brown & I never

The Typhus Epidemic

cared much for brown bread. Fish we never see. There are no fish shops anywhere, so when I return I shall first want to live on water & bread & butter for a few days... Milk (oxens buffalo or goats) is not nice so we use condensed milk & I hate it...'

At the height of the typhus epidemic, the two staff cooks at the Typhus Colony had fallen ill and staff were left to cook their own meals or have food sent up from the main hospital. Flora's hopes had been raised when a new chef had been sent over from the officers' mess and announced himself in German, with a great smile, as the new cook. However, on his first evening he evidently *'forgot dinner'*. Flora and her hapless companions appeared at seven in great expectation but discovered after a long wait that the chef was nowhere to be found.

The heroic Mr Chichester took the carriage down to the other hospital to find some dinner for his colleagues: *'He arrived back with some about 9. We then found that he had lost the pudding. The carriage nearly fell into a ditch so no doubt the pudding got out then.'* Fortunately, the chef on subsequent days proved to be very good.

The improvement in conditions within the Typhus Hospital also meant that Easter, which fell later in the Orthodox calendar, could be celebrated in style and Flora enjoyed herself immensely, as she reported to her sisters:

'We were awakened between one & two Sunday morning by guns & found it meant Resurrection morning. Here Easter is made a great deal of, more than any other time. All the patients got a lovely red egg each, [loaf] of bread & cigarettes. I was allowed to take them all around & give to each. It was lovely. You should have seen their expectant faces...'

Flora was very concerned that there were so few cigarettes available *'for my dear men'*- the Austrian prisoners. She noted how delighted the men were with just one cigarette:

'Still they are delighted with even that...I must own I love them & they do not hate us but they are made to fight us. Oh I do so hope our English

Nursing in Serbia with Lady Paget in 1915

men prisoners in Germany are not in half the pitiful condition those poor fellows are. Anyway, our men could not possibly stand hardships like these people stand . Both the Serbs & Austrians must be terribly tough & hardy. They seem to live on so little yet have such wonderful constitutions...'

It was not possible to buy any cigarettes locally and the problem moved Flora to send a telegram to her sister, Aggie, eagerly requesting her to send cigarettes out. Aggie had written to say that she would be glad to give to the Austrians and Flora had acted quickly, evidently greatly relieved that her sister perceived no moral problem in giving to the *'enemy'*. She urged her sister to send the cigarettes out as soon as possible in a wooden box, bearing a large red cross, with definitely no mention of the word 'cigarettes' on the outside.

Flora had *'another very great friend'* amongst the Austrians called 'John' who seemed to be the leader of the prisoners. He was twenty seven and well educated and spoke several languages including English. He knew England well and had travelled extensively in Europe and the United States. Like, Mick, he looked after Flora and was very protective: *'He greatly objected to me working & was terribly upset those 10 days I was alone here. He thinks I had not ought to run the risk of catching typhus (he has had it twice) & has worried & worried until today'*. It was to John that Flora urged her sister to send the cigarettes in case Flora herself had by then returned home.

'I love living in these barracks. It is just grand to hear the bugles, bands etc among the hills & see the sham fights etc'

As staffing improved and the regime at the hospital became more relaxed, Flora took full advantage of the surroundings. To her sisters, she reported that she was learning to ride and had access to a horse or a mountain pony from the nearby barracks whenever she liked: *'Oh these ponies are lovely, but such brisk shy creatures.'* She also had access to the carriage and horses for drives, but organising this seemed to entail a

The Typhus Epidemic

good deal of patience:

'No one is in a hurry and men just do things when they think. I asked it [the carriage] to be ready about 9 and of course they said 'Dobra Sister' meaning 'Good' and that he would. I have sent several times & he keeps saying 'he is coming'. At 11 I went myself and he said 'Checker utura Sistia' (Wait I am coming). There is no use getting cross, for they just come when they think & do not understand us if we scold, so one just shrugs their shoulders & waits. I put my coat & hat on about 11. It is now 5 to 12 & he has not yet turned up...'

Needless to say, Flora did not get her drive that day but her sisters did receive an inordinately long letter as a consequence.

Flora, as ever, was deeply interested in the animals around her. To her nephews and nieces she sent the news that she had, rather unwisely, adopted *'a wolf dog'*: *'Oh, he is lovely, about Vanity's size, sort of white & yellow, rather long tail & such beautiful eyes.'* His disappearance for three days had caused great concern but he had now returned, allowing only Flora to approach. Not content with this canine friend, she had also adopted a *'dear little puppy'* who was half-wolf : *'The children all love him. He is like a ball of soft wool & so playful. He will make such a big dog & ofcourse will be tame...'*. Others, apparently did not share her enthusiasm. In her letter written around 6th May, she imparted the sad news: *'Tell the children I am very sick today, for I have lost my pet dog. He was such a beauty & it has taken me all this while to tame him. A wolf dog, beautiful white, yellow, great brown eyes. They are very savage & yesterday & the day before he followed me about & even played with me & let me stroke him but today, I cannot find him anywhere, so I am afraid he has been shot...'*

'How I wished you were with me'

With the new staff from Dr Beavis' unit in post, Flora was able to enjoy sightseeing once more:

'Last Friday, 3 other Sisters, 2 orderlies & I went to see a most funny

Nursing in Serbia with Lady Paget in 1915

religion, called the Diervishers [sic], It was so weird . The men all stand in a circle, shout & throw themselves about, dance, wail, sigh & are so peculiar & just keep on until they drop. Some of them, we are told, dance etc until they drop dead. There was a screen for the women to look through & everyone took off their boots or shoes, but of course we English did not. Also we were allowed to go right into the chapel not as the other poor women behind the screen...'

There was time for shopping too, evidently an enthusiasm which Flora shared with her sister, Constance. On a recent Saturday, Flora and another sister had driven down into the Turkish quarters for what she termed a *'real good shop fuddle'*: *'Oh how I should just love you & I to go there. Con, I scarcely think though, I should ever get you away...'*. She reported purchasing a large brass tray and the great fun she had enjoyed *'beating down the old Arab'*. She eyed the beautiful silver ware with regret knowing that it was beyond her pocket.

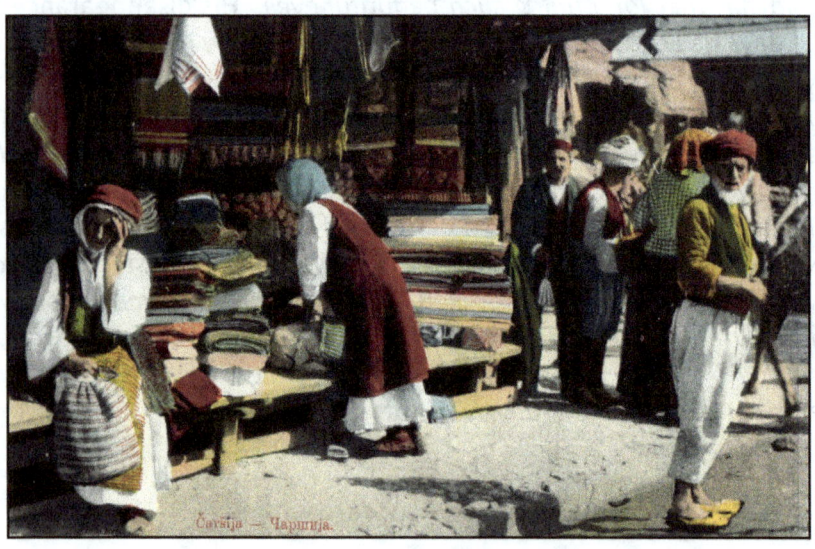

Postcard of carpet-sellers in the Old Bazaar, at Skoplje, c. 1915

Other members of the British community talked of encountering the Paget nurses on their shopping sprees. Dr Johnston Abraham of the

The Typhus Epidemic

British Red Cross recalled:

'Half of the nurses from the Paget Unit seemed to be in the market. They went into ecstasies over certain native costumes, and constantly called upon us to approve their choice, or mitigate the demands of would-be sellers. It was obvious the market was rising owing to the presence of the English community...'[115]

Other visitors to Skoplje viewed the market with more cynicism. When Jan and Cora Gordon visited a few months later, fresh from a tour of western Serbia and Montenegro, they observed:

'The stamp of the English was on Uscub. Prices were high. One Turk offered us a rubbishy silver thing for fifteen dinars; and Jan laughed, saying that one could see the English had been there. Without blushing, the man pointed to a twin article, saying he would let us have it for five dinars...'[116]

Money was beginning to be a problem for Flora. She eagerly awaited not only gifts of cigarettes for distribution amongst the patients but also money from her brother in law, Neil, for her own needs:

'Oh dear, here I am without a thing now. I have today paid away my very last para (penny). Had to have my shoes mended. They charged 6'20 . That is about 5/3 & they are mended with wooden nails not stitched. My rubber boots are worn out long ago. I bought a pair off a nurse leaving for England...I gave about 9/- so I hope to manage until I return...'

Flora was rather proud that she was now wearing men's clothes and sleeping in pyjamas. The recent heavy rain had left the fields and roads in a terrible state which made long rubber boots a necessity and rendered it almost impossible to get about in skirts but Flora was unabashed: *'Honestly I love wearing trousers'.*

There was also time to socialise with the nurses at the main hospital. Flora went down to see Nurses Pickering and Cluley and found them very happy, both having resolved to stay on after their three month term was completed. Rather ungenerously, Flora attributed their dedication

Nursing in Serbia with Lady Paget in 1915

to the fact that they would be paid £1 a week, an apparent improvement on their previous arrangement with Lady Paget. She had not seen them for over a month since *'They dare not come up here & I have had no time to go down to see them'.*

She noted that Nurse Pickering looked *'dreadfully ill'* but did not voice her doubts about the wisdom of her staying on: *'I wont say a word'.* An element of strain had obviously crept in to the relationship between Flora and her former employees, with Flora sadly concluding: *'They have not been nice to me in many ways.'*

Presumably, neither party had adjusted well to their new roles under Lady Paget and the nurses perhaps resented Flora's continued assumption of leadership.

'At first I felt rather cross but really I am getting tired...'

In her letter of 10 March, before Lady Paget fell ill with typhus, Flora had speculated about the date of her return home. She stated that the greater part of the original staff at the hospital were due to leave on 31 March but there was still doubt as to whether Lady Paget would continue. Presumably the typhus epidemic and Lady Paget's own illness meant that the date for her departure was subsequently postponed. Flora was well aware that there were other British units in Serbia who would welcome her as a trained nurse but she felt strongly that she should not stay after 1st May:

'I do not think it wise for English nurses to stay here longer than three months at a time. Summer will be dreadfully hot & trying. Even now when the sun shines, it is real hot...'

However, after this, she was rather overtaken by events. When the Typhus Hospital was dangerously understaffed, it was obviously unthinkable for Flora to leave her post and even when the new nurses began to arrive, she felt obliged to stay: *'When I asked the other day about returning home, they asked me to stay & I said I felt I must return, but they made me promise I would stay until other Sisters came from England. I simply*

The Typhus Epidemic

could not come until there was some one else here...'

Later, Flora wrote to say that she was very well and very happy, but that Lady Paget, two doctors and one Sister were still terribly ill with typhus. More staff had arrived and now Flora found to her annoyance that the doctors had decided that she was not to work on the wards anymore. Instead, she was to superintend work and oversee feeding: *'At first I felt rather cross but really I am getting tired & as he [the doctor] points out, I can still go in & out to see the men but shall not run the risks as I have been doing...'*

There was a clearly a certain amount of tension with the new nurses too, as Flora confided to her sisters:

'These new sisters are rather jealous of me, because all the Austrians seem to speak & salute me. They forget that I nursed them alone for some time & just when most of them were down with it...'

Although Flora longed for England, English food and above all for cleanliness, she also hated the thought of leaving. Understandably, she enjoyed the attention she received from her adoring Austrians:

'What I shall do when I get back home & get none of these attentions I do not know. Honestly, although we live very rough & ready, I am waited on hand & foot & when ever I say I would like, as far as possible to get it, I have it. If I am ill and have this terrible typhus, these boys will nurse me & you need not worry in the least over me...'

Only one comment in her letters, suggests the physical effect upon her of the recent ordeal. When discussing her current predilection for trousers, she added *'Also my hair, did I tell you, went quite grey on the boat..'.*

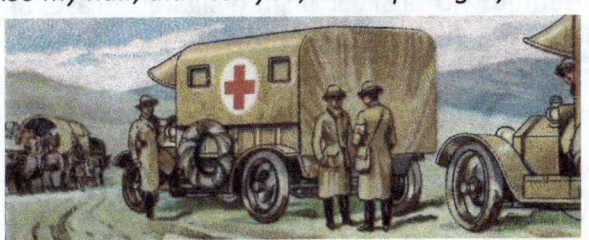

Nursing in Serbia with Lady Paget in 1915

Chapter 6

Home to Leicester

'I was very sorry to leave and I believe they were all very sorry to lose me...'

On Thursday 20th May, Flora wrote her final letter from Serbia to her sister Constance. She wrote from the train carrying her to Salonika on the first leg of her journey home, having left Skoplje that morning. She confessed herself to be very sad at leaving and related with enthusiasm, the farewell parties of the last few days. On the previous Monday, a party of nurses in the caps and aprons of their indoors uniform had piled into two boxes at the local Picture House but Flora had been less than impressed: *'It was a rotten show though'*.

'Everyone' had, apparently, urged Flora to stay and now took trouble to ensure a memorable send-off. On the Wednesday, she had been taken on *'a lovely drive'* delighting in the sight of storks which she longed to share with her nephews and nieces. When she returned at four, she was somewhat flummoxed to be asked by a doctor whether she could *'manage a few extra to dinner'* to share her last meal. Flora was a little reluctant since she had not yet packed and had planned a simple milk pudding, but wisely she threw herself upon the mercy of the cook who agreed to prepare pancakes for the unexpected guests. In the event, there were thirty nine at the impromptu pancake party and Flora enjoyed herself immensely: *'Well, it was a very jolly dinner & I have never been so important or made so much of & what is more one of the D[octo]rs got up [to] make a long speech.'* All drank Flora's health before she was presented with a silver filigree cigarette case, an occasion for much hilarity since she could still only bring herself to smoke a very little, despite everybody urging her to do more. Flora had admired the cigarette cases on a shopping trip and she was now delighted: *'I do feel proud of it.'*

Overcome with emotion, Flora resisted calls for a speech and could

Home to Leicester

manage only to thank everyone thoroughly. There were further gifts too. After dinner, one of the American doctors thanked her for all she had done and bestowed a gift of *'loads of chocolates'* whilst another doctor plied her with further *'delicious'* comestibles: *'It was a great night & 1.15 when I got to bed.'*

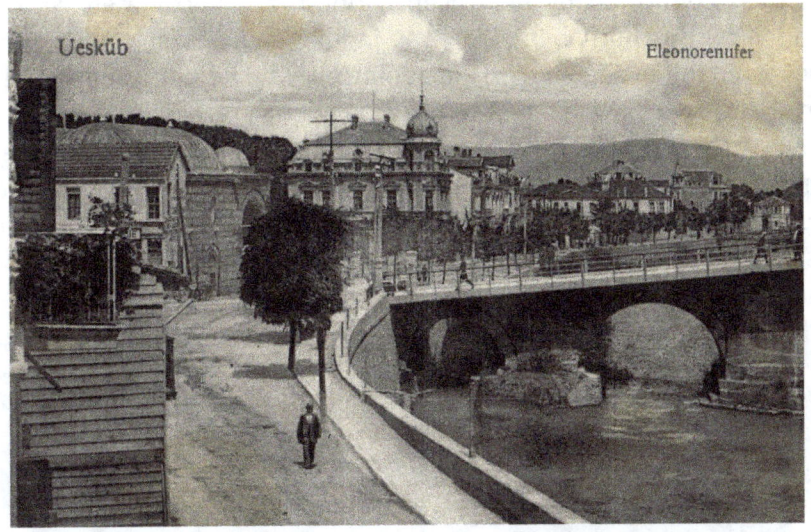

Postcard of the bridge over the River Vardar, at Skoplje [Uskub], c. 1910

Since the only train left Skoplje at 6.15am , Flora faced an early start next morning. At 4.30, her beloved Austrian orderlies called her to a good breakfast which they had lovingly prepared. Whilst her luggage was taken to the station in one of the ambulance motor cars, Flora made the two mile journey to the station in a carriage, which the Austrians had decorated for the occasion with poppies, cornflowers and other wild flowers: *'It was a perfect picture. Even my feet were on a carpet of flowers. Was it not sweet & good of them? I did hate saying goodbye.'*

Flora had ample time to reflect on her final goodbyes for she would not reach Salonika until nine that night. There a carriage waited to take her to her hotel.

Nursing in Serbia with Lady Paget in 1915

'It was a great trouble & bother'

It was in Salonika, that Flora encountered the first of many problems regarding her passport. With dismay she heard from the English Consul that she would require a new passport to travel through Italy and this was then confirmed by his Italian counterpart. Fortunately, she was aided in all this bureaucracy, by the indefatigable Honourable Richard Chichester and even Sir Ralph Paget himself, who helped her correctly to sign all the appropriate documents. Finally, she was required to visit the French, Italian and English Consuls once more to receive the seal of each dignitary on her troublesome passport. When at last, Flora was able to return to her hotel, she was deeply disappointed to find that she had missed an invitation to lunch on the steam yacht *'Erin'* from none other than Sir Thomas Lipton (1848-1931). Instead, she was able to have tea with the distinguished gentleman:

'He was so nice & made such a fuss. Made me sit beside him & said he would like to take me home & I could wait in the yatch [sic] if I would stay, but he may be 2 or 3 weeks in Serbia & I could not possibly wait all that time. Made me promise I would see him in England when he returned? Is he not a duck?'

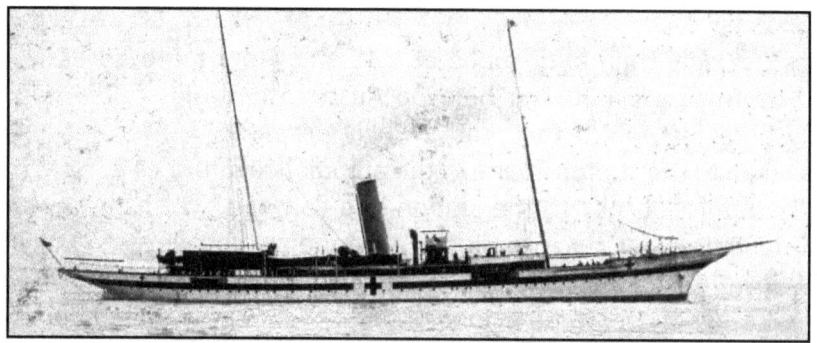

The luxury steam yacht Erin, *in her later role as a hospital ship, c. 1916.*

It was natural that Flora and Sir Thomas should have got on well. He had been born into poor circumstances in Glasgow to parents who had been driven from Ulster by the potato famine. All asserted that he remained a very modest man, having built his fortune from a humble grocery shop

Home to Leicester

in Glasgow. Lipton, by the time he met Flora, was a self-made millionaire with tea and coffee plantations in Ceylon and had received a baronetcy in 1902.

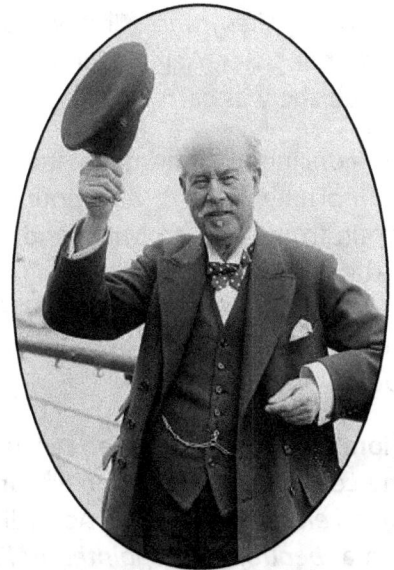

Sir Thomas Lipton
(1848-1931)

Throughout the early part of the war, Sir Thomas used his steam yacht to transport supplies and personnel between Marseilles and Salonika for medical units in Serbia.[117] Many members of the British Red Cross units were privileged to travel out to Serbia in this fashion. However, his support for the hospital work went further than supplying free transport.

Mabel Dearmer, after the fateful church service in which she learnt with some surprise that her husband had agreed to accompany the Stobart Serbian Unit as Chaplain, attended a meeting at Lady Cowdray's house where Sir Thomas Lipton spoke. His address in which he described a hospital at Skoplje where three hundred deaths occurred in a day and *'only two suffragettes'* were there to tend them, thrilled the audience: *'He left us convinced of misery and need beyond words, and with a thrilling sense of the joy of service'*.[118] He was certainly a busy man, for after leaving Flora in Salonika he travelled up to Serbia in the company of a crowd of reporters and three Serbian officers, arriving at Mrs Stobart's unit in time for breakfast on 1st June.[119]

Nursing in Serbia with Lady Paget in 1915

Flora was clearly in demand and finished her exciting day with dinner in the company of the Honourable Richard Chichester, Sir Ralph Paget, General Lauvenuvitch [sic] and *'another big pot'*. *'So'* she proudly proclaimed *'I have been doing the grand'*. She was also rather pleased to be enclosing a letter to her sister, Aggie, stamped *'For Active Service Only'* in the mail bag which she was carrying.

Flora's final letter was concluded aboard an Italian ship which left Salonika at ten on the morning of 22nd May, bound for Messina. She intended to travel by train from there to Milan and home. At least this boat was preferable to the French boat by which she had arrived, for she reported *'This boat is lovely. The food is magnificent'*. She promised to provide all news when she reached home but also warned: *'Be sure & let me have my own room'*.

The sole evidence for Flora's return journey is an account which appeared on the front page of the *Leicester Daily Post* on 8th June 1915 under the subtitle *'Adventures of a Leicester Nurse'*.[120] According to this source, she had left Salonika on a *'beautifully appointed Italian steamer which carried 30 first class passengers'*. The ship was bound for Brindisi on the Adriatic coast of Italy but having called at Piraeus, was diverted to Messina in Sicily after receiving what the newspaper termed *'an exciting Marconigram'*. The telegram announced to the general joy of the Italian passengers, that Italy had declared war on the Austro-Hungarian Empire and apparently warned that the Adriatic had been mined as a result.

Flora had been delighted once aboard, to discover a fellow Leicester resident, a certain Mrs Elliott, formerly Miss Bailey, whose husband was working in Belgrade. She told the newspaper both of this encounter and a somewhat more alarming one with a French warship. The great *'man-of-war'* drew alongside and Flora and the other passengers were summoned on deck, many still in their night attire, to have their passports examined. A thorough search of the ship lasted over two hours, delayed by a moment of alarm when one passenger, named as Mr Basil Clarke, unwisely decided to take the opportunity for a swim, still clad in his pyjamas. He was unceremoniously hauled back up the steps *'by the scruff of his neck'* and Flora thought him very lucky to have

Home to Leicester

escaped arrest. The French were obviously very active in the area, for Flora also recalled the memorable sight of a fleet of nineteen cruisers and battleships, apparently practising their gun drill.

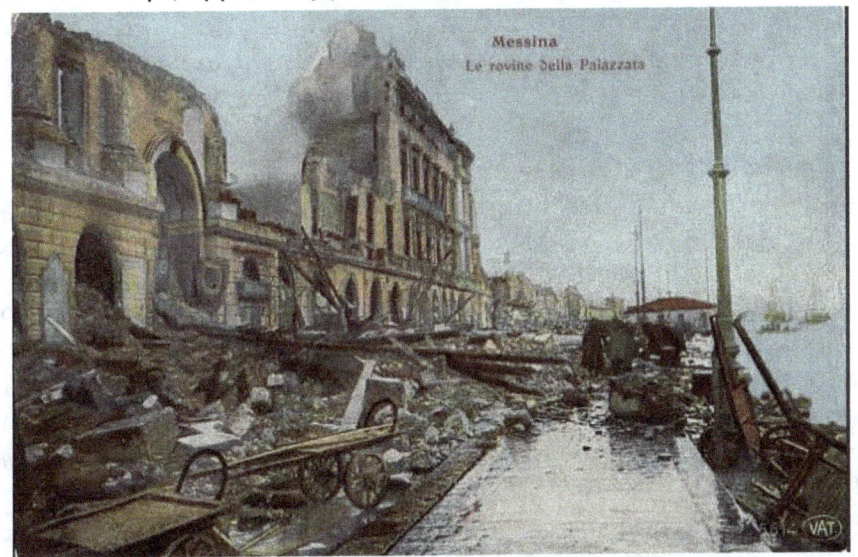

Postcard of Messina after the earthquake, c. 1908

At Messina, Flora inspected the *'heap of ruins'* which had once been a proud city. The earthquake of 28th December 1908, which had almost completely destroyed the cities of Messina and Reggio Calabria had resulted in the loss of between 75,000 to 82,000 lives and the disaster was still fresh in the mind of Flora and her fellow passengers as they disembarked and found their way to a newly rebuilt hotel, on a hill above the harbour. The town had been partially rebuilt about a mile or so from the quay, mostly in wood in a style reminiscent of Canadian log huts or Swiss chalets.

From here Flora travelled to Naples where she stayed two days, battling once more with the authorities over her passport. On this occasion, the bureaucrats were not satisfied with her photograph and she had to have a new photograph taken. Despite these problems, she was seeing Naples under the best of circumstances since the weather was beautiful. It was clear that the city was anticipating large numbers of casualties,

Nursing in Serbia with Lady Paget in 1915

and Flora, attracting much attention in her khaki uniform adorned with a Red Cross, was even invited by the British Consul to stay to help since it was feared that there would be a shortage of skilled nurses. Flora, however, whilst content to assist the Italian Red Cross when a minor accident occurred at the station, was definitely not to be persuaded to stay any longer. She observed, with interest, the excitement of the local population at the declaration of war amidst an atmosphere akin to that of a gala day, with flag bedecked streets. She noted with surprise that the women seemed as enthusiastic as the men and must have wondered at their naivety.

Over three days, Flora travelled to Switzerland by train and thence on to Paris, spending two nights there, still required to report daily to the police and military authorities, before finally reaching home by way of Boulogne and Folkestone. The *Leicester Daily Post* reported that the remainder of the journey was *'enjoyable but comparatively uneventful'*. Flora herself was in *'perfect health'* and although glad to be home and among friends again she conveyed *'the impression that the experience had been one which she would not readily have missed...'*. Of the two nurses who went out with her, one -Nurse Pickering- was already home and now only Nurse Cluley remained in Skoplje. She apparently followed not much later.

'I do thank everyone in Leicester who has given so fully to the Serbs.'

Once safely back in Leicester, it appears Flora reopened her Nursing Home in Victoria Road. Stray references to her in the local newspapers, suggest she embraced civic life once more. She was much in evidence at the Serbian Flag Day in September 1915 and a newscutting amidst her papers at the Imperial War Museum which shows Flora out with her dogs collecting in Leicester for the *'Wycliffe Society for Helping the Blind'*, makes it clear that she did not confine her charitable efforts to the Serbian cause.

Flora also spent some considerable time writing letters of thanks to all those who had supported her in Serbia. This may well have been the original motivation for writing the notes which now survive with her

Home to Leicester

letters from Serbia. Typical is an article which was published in a Burton-on-Trent paper, submitted by her cousin *'Miss Cotton of Belvedere Road'*. It opens : *'Many times since my return to England from Serbia, I have tried to write and thank all the kind people in Burton-on-Trent who helped my cousin to send out such a splendid gift of money...'*[121] She went on to describe her work in Skoplje and her trials in the Typhus hospital, concluding: *'When I left the last week of May, typhus was practically over, and the Hospital looked almost English. I was very very sorry to leave, and would love to go back. Again, I thank you for your help and sympathy.'*

Serbia was never far from Flora's thoughts. Despite her duties as matron of a busy nursing home, she clearly kept in close touch with nurses who were still out there.

In October 1915, Flora was the author of an article published in the *Leicester Pioneer* under the heading: *'Serbia and its Difficulties. Urgent Assistance Required. More Ambulances Needed'*. It opened: *'Lately I have had several interesting letters from Serbia, and it will no doubt interest Leicester people to hear a little of them...'* [122]

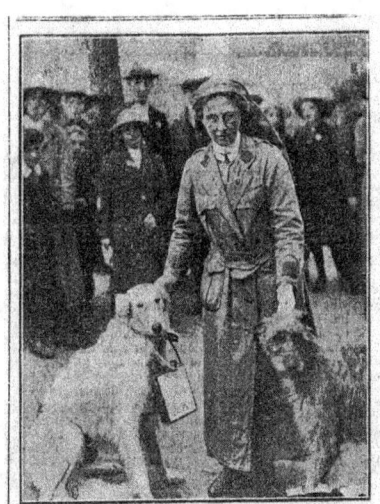

Collecting for Blind Soldiers.—Many of our soldiers have been blinded while fighting their country's battles, and various efforts are being made to provide for their future. Our picture shows Miss Scott, who has just returned from Serbia, after nursing there for six months, with her dogs, making a collection at Leicester, as an agent for the Wycliffe Society for helping the blind. (Photo: Illustrations Bureau.)

She recounted her own experiences, struggling against typhus, adding that the situation was saved when the American Red Cross came to their aid with Doctors and appliances including two large refrigerator carts for disinfecting patients, which were transported from town to town by motor vehicles. No mention of such an intervention occurs in Flora's memoirs although she does mention American doctors at her leaving party. Perhaps, she is referring to developments after her departure.

Nursing in Serbia with Lady Paget in 1915

Most attributed the successful eradication of typhus to the measures set in place by a British mission led by Colonel Hunter. It certainly seems a little unfair that all the measures carried out by Colonel Hunter and his team of thirty Royal Army Medical Corps doctors are largely ignored in her account. Perhaps this reflects the number of Americans in Lady Paget's second unit.

In fact, Sir Ralph Paget had chaired a conference of the British Units in Nish at the beginning of April in order to discuss the typhus epidemic. Colonel Hunter and his doctors had been sent out by the British Government specifically to tackle the problem.

Dr Johnston Abraham of the British Red Cross, recalled encountering Colonel William Hunter and his RAMC officers on a street corner in Nish, in March 1915:

'*Standing at a street corner, looking rather cold and lost were six British RAMC, all young lieutenants, very smart and trim in their neat well-cut khaki, making me feel how shabby I must appear in my battered old Red Cross uniform...I remembered that we had advised that 200 doctors should be asked for from France and England, and came to the conclusion this must be the British response. I looked at these clean-cut, fresh looking boys, and wondered what earthly use they could be...*'[123]

Abraham took the new arrivals under his wing, and later dined with Colonel Hunter and his second in command, Major Stammers, at the Colunna restaurant where most of the British seemed to congregate. Later, in his memoirs, he recalled his bitter disappointment at the small size of the mission:

'*Now, six years later, I can freely admit I was wrong, for the twice-told tale of the wonderful change they wrought on the whole situation is known to every student of the great epidemic...*'

Others were more immediately impressed with Colonel Hunter's measures. Edward Alabaster, a dresser with Lady Paget told the *Birmingham Post* on his return:

Home to Leicester

'*One of the most fruitful sources of infection for the fever are the railway carriages, and but for these Mr Alabaster believed that the typhus would have been very much more localised instead of being rampant all over the country. He mentioned the good work of Colonel Hunter, of the RAMC under whose superintendence a large number of trains had been fumigated, and who was also providing sterilisers for use in the hospitals...*'[124]

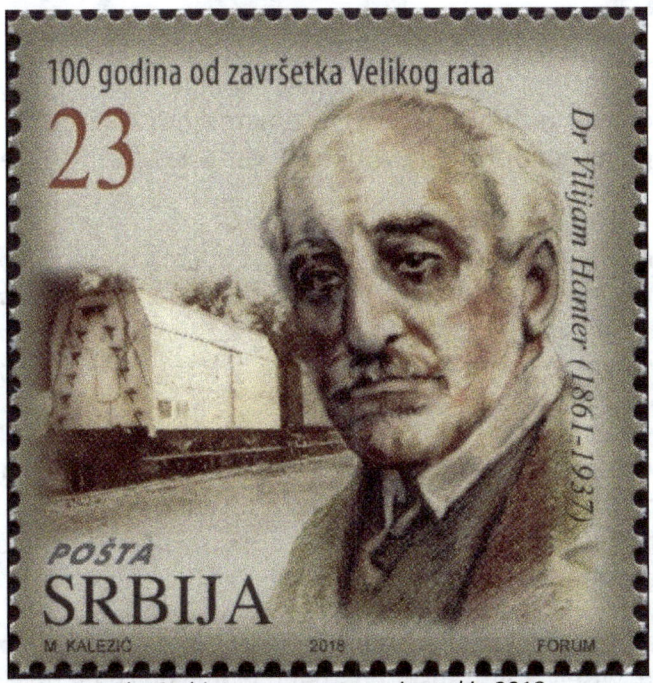

The Serbian postage stamp issued in 2018 to honour Colonel William Hunter

At Colonel Hunter's recommendation, the Serbian Government agreed to break the line of infection by cancelling all army leave and suspending railway communications for a two week period whilst quarantine stations were established behind the lines.

Here suspect cases would be retained for fifteen days. Under Colonel Hunter's guidance, a programme of disinfection, aimed at eradicating

Nursing in Serbia with Lady Paget in 1915

the typhus carrying lice from all public places was embarked upon. In line with this, all fabric was ripped out of railway carriages and the bare wood was disinfected daily for fifteen days. In towns around the whole country, restaurants, hotels and places of entertainment were all compelled to close for several hours each day so that floors, furniture and walls could be scrubbed. It was undoubtedly the success of these stringent measures which led to dramatic improvements in Skoplje and the final disappearance of typhus by the end of June.[125]

Flora had also been warned that cholera would take over from typhus in the summer but this threat was fortunately not realised. She recalled the disappointment of the new nurses who joined Lady Paget's unit in May:

'The last batch of English Sisters who came out in May while I was there, said how disappointed they were to find things so English... Each letter I receive tells me there are no hardships to go through now, the country keeps healthy, and they grumble the work is not sufficient for the number of English out there...'

Flora saw a further improvement too in that there were now many English ambulance motor cars and even a well fitted ambulance train- all a great improvement on the haphazard transport of wounded at the beginning of the conflict.

She praised the recent collection in Leicester for Serbia as *'magnificent'* and hoped, wisely as it transpired, that it would be spent on clothing for the soldiers in the coming winter. She appealed particularly for knitted goods, remembering how highly prized had been the three dozen balaclava helmets provided by one lady, and concluded with heartfelt thanks:

'I do thank everyone in Leicester who has given so fully to the Serbs. You have never given anywhere before where it is more needed, or appreciated. If the Serbs were here, they would kneel to you, kiss your hand, put it on their heart, then their forehead, then kiss again, very gracefully.'

Chapter 7

Lady Paget's Return to Serbia

It is a measure of the success of the Serbian Relief Fund, that the small disparate group of individuals of September 1914, had by May of the following year grown into a formidable organisation, with receipts amounting to some £85,965.6.5.[126] Oversight of various projects that month resulted in the expenditure of £48,724.91. There was however, a problem. The executive committee just couldn't quite make up its mind as to what they should be doing in Serbia, now that the fighting had apparently ceased.

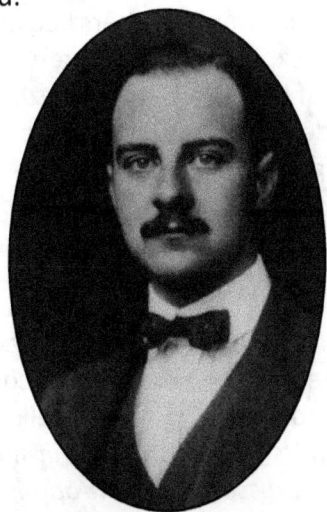

Hon Richard Chichester
(1889-1915)

At the end of April, on 28th, Richard Chichester had attended a committee meeting and read a report on Lady Paget's unit, suggesting that the hospital should be converted in to a surgical hospital once the typhus crisis was over. He also suggested the formation of local committees to alleviate distress amongst the local population. At the same meeting, Mr Graham, also apparently back from Serbia on a brief visit, delivered a report on *'the condition of Lady Wimborne's unit and the general sanitary conditions of Serbia'*.[127]

Nursing with Lady Paget in Serbia in 1915

Although, Chichester's plans were approved, there seems to have been some indecision over plans for the hospital in Skoplje, about which the minutes of the meeting are frustratingly silent. There is only a rather puzzling note that the Chairman announced that he would resign from 30th April and Edward Boyle, the Treasurer, would take over as acting Chairman.

On 5th May, Mr Graham's report was considered and it was resolved to send a cable to Sir Ralph Paget to enquire as to the desirability of extending the sphere of Lady Wimborne's Unit and making it the main military hospital in Serbia. A few days later, on 12th May, Mr Bertram Christian resumed the Chairmanship and no more was said about his reasons for resigning. Lady Wimborne's feathers had also evidently been ruffled and she demanded an explanation of the return of Mr Graham to Serbia without consultation of the committee. Was Mr Graham proving himself rather too high handed? The apparent power struggle between Mr Graham and the Sir Ralph Paget ended with the resolution on 2nd June *'that the committee could not sanction Mr Graham's scheme for the establishment of a base hospital at Skoplje'*.[128] Was the attendance at that meeting by the newly returned Lady Paget a deciding factor?

The future of Lady Wimborne's unit was now to be decided by Sir Ralph Paget and Lady Wimborne herself. By 23rd June, the committee resolved in accordance with Lady Wimborne's expressed feelings, *'that having in view the present state of affairs in Serbia, the Unit no 2 (Cornelia Lady Wimborne's Hospital) shall be dissolved as an administrative unit and the members of it who wish to remain in Serbia should , if approved, be encouraged to join other units; that the stores, equipment and buildings so far as possible, of Lady Wimborne's unit should be left at the disposition of Sir Ralph Paget'*.[129]

Meanwhile in Skoplje, Lady Herbert of Lady Wimborne's unit was blissfully unaware of any power struggles in London. On 25th May, just after Flora's departure she wrote:

'Time is getting on, and here is the end of May, and when I started I thought I should probably be home about now; but I expect if all goes

Lady Paget's Return to Serbia

well, I shall stick on here now till about the end of the Unit, which is August 6th, I believe...'

Things moved faster than she expected. Chichester -or *'Sir Chichester as the people here call him'*[131] - had wasted no time in returning to Serbia and implementing his ideas for relief committees. On 9th June, Lady Herbert returned from nine days trekking to Novi Bazar, during which she had been involved in forming relief committees in areas where poverty was particularly pressing . She returned to find that their surgeon, Barrington Ward, was on his way home on the following day and the whole unit was breaking up at the end of the month.

Lady Herbert hoped to stay on *'doing either relief work entirely, or if we can possibly, forming a small Unit out of the debris of this one...'*[132] She expressed the thoughts of many members of British units when she wrote *'...we are feeling very unsettled and cross, but there is no work to do at the present, and lots of them think they would be more useful in England...'*[133]

By 17th June, Lady Herbert was further lamenting that the hospital was nearly empty and that there was no likelihood of more work. As a result, the Unit was shutting down a month early and the first group was departing next week:

'The Paget fever hospital is also shutting up, no more work there either and the only thing left to do is relief and this is urgently wanted. No one [ie no Serbian] is paid here, let alone any family allowance given, and the poor things are starving in every part.'[134]

With this in mind, Lady Herbert, her friend Elia Lindon and the Honourable Richard Chichester set off on a three week tour of Albania and Montenegro. Lady Herbert's letters recorded an adventurous but clearly very happy journey for the threesome:

'Very loth we were to get back to Skoplje and people and fusses and worry...Three weeks in which we had gone far, seen much, learnt a great deal, and done something for the people we had met, some of them,

Nursing with Lady Paget in Serbia in 1915

anyway, and hoped to do more when our reports reached headquarters...'[135]

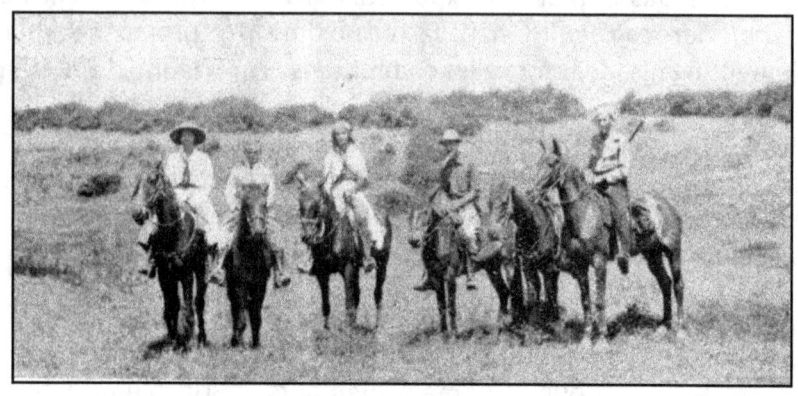

Lady Herbert and her trekking companions (from Serbia and the Serbians by Lady Herbert, 1915)

However, there was to be a tragic sequel. Somewhere on his travels that summer, Chichester who seemed beloved by all who met him – including Flora - contracted a virulent form of typhoid fever. He died nine days later on 31st July 1915 . This might well have signified the sad end of Lady Paget's Unit were it not for one individual – Lady Paget herself.

'As this Report was already going to press, the Committee to its deep regret, received a telegram announcing the death of Mr Richard Chichester, from typhoid fever at Nish, as he was on the point of leaving Serbia. As acting Secretary to his cousin, Lady Paget, at Skoplje since last November, Mr Chichester rendered quite invaluable services to the Serbian Relief Fund and to Serbia and his name will always be associated with the desperate and successful struggle against typhus. The Committee's deepest sympathy goes out to his father and mother, Lord and Lady Templemore, in their bereavement.'[136]

Although Lady Paget, still convalescing after her attack of typhus, had been present in London, to present her report to the committee in June, she did not tarry long and by July she was back in Skoplje. She

Lady Paget's Return to Serbia

had returned to see for herself whether it was justified to continue to maintain a hospital with Serbian Relief funding and whether in fact there was any point in remaining in Serbia at all.

Fighting in Serbia had ended in December 1914, and many individual members of hospital units were now leaving the country believing that hostilities had ceased for good. As she travelled up from Salonika, Lady Paget witnessed many British travelling in the opposite direction, but she for one, was not convinced by the present calm.

In the hospital, she found about 350 cases in the wards, roughly equal numbers of soldiers and civilians. At the typhus hospital, she found the hospital was now assuming the role of a general hospital. Staff there were restless, unwilling to stay longer if there was not enough work. Many felt that the Serbians were now well placed to look after their own.

Lady Paget, however, was well aware of the strengths of her own hospital:

'When I reviewed the splendid advantages and resources of our colony-hospital, its ideal situation on a sunny hill outside the town, its laundries and workshops, its great storehouses filled with every kind of supply and equipment, when I thought of all the labour and expense which had been bestowed upon it, it seemed a great pity it should be allowed to disintegrate prematurely.'[137]

She was conscious too of the great ally she enjoyed in the form of General Popovitch, the civil and military Governor of Macedonia, who had bestowed full powers upon the British to carry out any reform in sanitation and medical organisation which they advised.

The question of whether her unit should remain, depended ultimately, on the likelihood of fighting breaking out once more in Serbia. In an effort, to secure the answer, Lady Paget went on a tour of hospital units in the North of the country where she found the same degree of unrest as amongst her own staff. On 24th July she and her husband visited the British Fever Hospital in Belgrade where she met Monica Stanley, a

Nursing with Lady Paget in Serbia in 1915

Stobart nurse who was recovering from typhoid:

'Sir Ralph and Lady Paget called to see one of their nurses who is at this hospital with typhus (so they came in to see us). Lady Paget still looks very ill after her illness of typhus. I had a long talk with her; she is a charming woman, and Sir Ralph is very nice...'[138]

Lady Paget was thorough in her investigations and even made a point of interviewing the Crown Prince himself. She heard from him that this would be the worst possible moment to leave Serbia. Soon, it was feared, the troops would require more help than ever before.

With this in mind, Lady Paget arranged for the transfer or loan of various members of other British units who were not now *'actively employed'* agreeing with each individual as to whether they would be paid by their own unit or the Serbian Relief Fund: *'We thus saved the expense of having a fresh staff sent out from England'.*[139]

It was when she returned to Skoplje from this mission, that she suffered the terrible shock of the loss of her cousin and secretary, Richard Chichester. He was buried on the following evening with full military honours *'amid touching demonstrations of affection and respect on the part of all ranks of the civil and military population.'*[140]

In her subsequent report of the unit's final months, she sadly concluded:

'There was no member of the unit whose absence could have left a greater gap, or whose presence during the indescribable difficulties of the following winter would have been a more effective aid to us all...'[141]

It was the end of an appalling month for the Serbian Relief Fund which had seen the death of two members from Mrs Stobart's Unit: Nurse Lorna Ferris and the popular playwright and children's author Mabel Dearmer, who had volunteered as an orderly in order to accompany her husband Percy, the chaplain to the English units.

Help at the Hospital had also arrived from more unusual quarters. In June, a relief party, under the auspices of the Committee of Mercy of

Lady Paget's Return to Serbia

New York had sailed from America.[142] The principal organiser appears to have been Professor Pupin, a Professor at Columbia University and a native Serb. When he lectured at Princeton, urging students to join the party, he succeeded in persuading three members of the wrestling team: William Prickett, Angus M Frantz and Montague A Tancock to join the mission. With them also went George B Logan, a recent Princeton graduate and former editor of the Nassau Literary Magazine and Elmer Elsworth Childs. The team engaged in relief work at the Lady Paget Hospital throughout the summer but when the party returned for the new semester, Logan and Tancock elected to remain with Lady Paget. Logan's letters home to his family, provide an interesting commentary on subsequent events.

In September, work at Lady Paget's hospital steadily increased as the unit benefited from a new surgical theatre and the advent of Dr Fergus Armstrong, a former surgeon with the First British Field Hospital. Whilst the hospital prospered, Lady Paget once more found herself at odds with the medical staff who were now intent upon establishing a well organised general hospital, before handing it over to the Serbians. Lady Paget admired their work but could not but feel that their efforts amounted to *'the building of a palace on a volcano'*.[143]

As a result of this evident conflict in policy, she withdrew from administration for a while, and instead toured Northern Serbia. Despite her detachment, she took a keen interest in everything which affected her hospital. When the Serbians issued an order that all Austro-Hungarian prisoners of war were to be removed to a safer distance from the front, Lady Paget was swift to make strong and ultimately successful representations to the Governor and Commanding Officer in Skoplje protesting against the idea. The hospital was still utterly dependent on the prisoners as orderlies.

It was whilst in Valjevo, attending a banquet given by the Serbian Army, that Lady Paget witnessed the first bombs dropped from an Austrian aeroplane. The air raid was part of a series across the country that formed a prearranged signal for the advance of German and Austrian troops against Serbia. She returned at once to Skoplje, arriving on 24th

Nursing with Lady Paget in Serbia in 1915

September, to find the Serbians eagerly awaiting the arrival of Allied troops to assist them to repel this new invasion. Delegations of Serbian and British gathered at the station each evening to welcome the train from Salonika. At the beginning of October, when news reached Skoplje that Allied troops had arrived in Salonika, the town was festooned with Allied flags to celebrate:

'Little bunches of box, the traditional sign of rejoicing, were tied on the station lamp-posts, and a row of lanterns ready for illumination decked either side of the bridge over the Vardar...'[144]

Such was the confidence that the Allies would stand by Serbia that arrangements were even made for the quartering of the troops in the town. All was in vain. No such aid was ever forthcoming...

There were obvious reasons for the apparent perfidy of the Allies. The landings at Gallipoli had not been the success that had been anticipated. The ill fated campaign had persuaded Italy to enter the war on the side of the Allies but had achieved little more. Bulgaria was still bitterly eyeing the territory in Macedonia which she had won and lost in a short space of time after the Second Balkan war in 1913. Now she recognised a huge opportunity to join the Central Powers against their old foe of Serbia. The Allies certainly perceived the danger and even went so far as to offer Bulgaria a share of Macedonia- an offer which would have appalled the Serbians had they known about it. The offer, however, came too late and on 6th September, Bulgaria signed treaties with the Germans and Austria, agreeing to go to war within thirty days in return for a financial subsidy and the future transfer of territory from Serbia.[145]

The stalemate in Gallipoli had also done nothing to encourage Greece to join the Allied cause. For a brief moment there was hope, when the Greek Prime Minister Eleutherios Venezelos suggested to the Allies that he could bring his country in to the war if the British and French would send 150,000 troops to Salonika to aid Serbia in her new plight. The Allies agreed at once, sending at first a token force and later an expeditionary force, withdrawn in part from Gallipoli. These were the troops expected so confidently in Skoplje in September. However, on 5th

Lady Paget's Return to Serbia

October, the King of Greece dismissed Venezelos from office, insisting that his country would remain neutral. The Allies, intent now only on turning Salonika in to a huge military camp, sent only a small advance guard into southern Macedonia, too little, too late. By early December, both the French and British Division which had crossed in to Macedonia had been driven back by the Bulgarians into Greek territory.

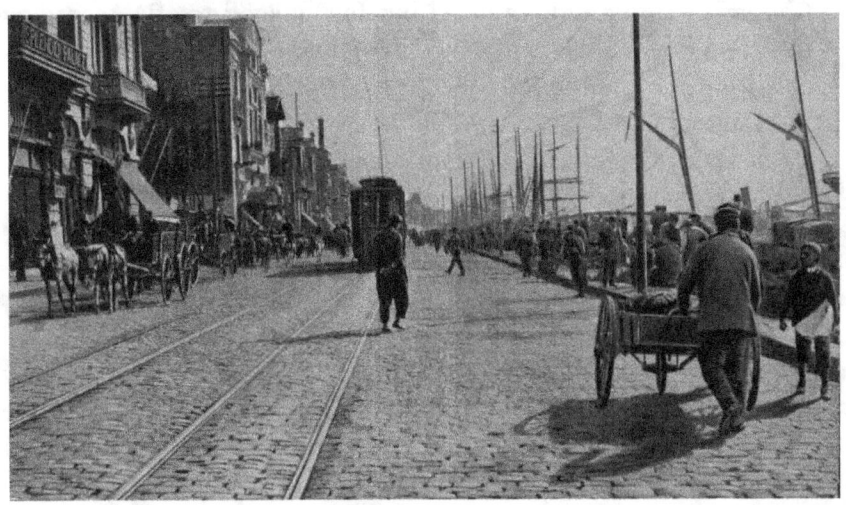

Postcard of the quayside at Salonika, c. 1916

It was also on October 5th that the Germans and Austrians commenced their bombardment of Belgrade and the first trickle of wounded began arriving at the hospital. By the 15th, the hospital had received over two hundred wounded and a second surgical theatre was quickly brought in to action. It was at this moment that the Germans and Austrians launched their long feared invasion from the north, whilst the Bulgarians swept in to Macedonia from the east. All available Serbian regiments had been sent north since the Serbians had remained confident that Allied troops would defend the south. Their trust, it transpired, was badly misplaced.

On 16th October, the staff of the British Naval Mission of Belgrade arrived at Skoplje on the last train to get through before the Bulgarians blew up

Nursing with Lady Paget in Serbia in 1915

the railway bridge at Vranja. The telephone and telegraph lines between Nish and Skoplje were cut and the Governor informed Lady Paget that the situation was now desperate. He had been sending regular reports to the Allies at Salonika requesting immediate reinforcements but had received no satisfactory reply. Now he urged Lady Paget to travel to Salonika and persuade the French and British Generals to come to their rescue. Lady Paget had her doubts about her ability to persuade the Generals to do anything at all but felt obliged to try. Accordingly, she travelled down to Salonika, accompanied by the staff of the Naval Mission and two wounded marines, on a special train laid on that night for the National Bank.

The party arrived at midday on 17th October but, predictably, Lady Paget received no offer of help from the British or French Generals whom she interviewed. She left again at seven the following morning. All she had secured was two large motor lorries which the British had offered to help with the evacuation of the hospital. These reached Ghevgeli on the Greek frontier but no further. The train was too heavy for the Serbian engine to pull and officials insisted that the vehicles should be unloaded. There they were left in the tender care of the Army Service Corps with instructions to follow if possible on a later train or return to Salonika.

On the journey back to Skoplje, Lady Paget witnessed scenes of appalling panic as refugees and wounded jostled to find a place on the already crowded train . At Veles, two hours south of her destination, she was alarmed to hear nearby gunfire. The station was in great disorder as refugees competed with wounded soldiers who had struggled in from the nearby battlefield:

'... before the train finally drew up, wounded and unwounded alike tried to rush it, hanging on to the footboards and struggling to get up on to the roofs, the one idea of the crowd being to escape no matter how. Little children were trampled underfoot, and others were hurled by their parents over the heads of the affrighted crowds into the horseboxes, where the sick and wounded soldiers were huddled together. Willing hands were outstretched to catch these little ones, but many of them were injured. The scene was horrible...'[146]

Lady Paget's Return to Serbia

In a gesture typical of her compassion and authority, she intervened in the scenes of confrontation at the station, making fellow passengers stand so that the wounded could also be accommodated and taking sick women and children into her own carriage so that she could tend them. What the Serbians thought of this regal English woman's interference, is not however recorded. She reached Skoplje at ten thirty in the evening, to be met by Dr Maitland and her secretary Mr Davies amidst a scene of chaos on *'a far greater scale'*:

'The station was besieged with throngs of terrified people fighting round the open trucks of the train, leaving for Prishtina next morning, counting themselves fortunate if they could only sit there through the night in the pelting rain. There was weariness and desolation everywhere, to which the incessant rain and mud contributed in no inconsiderable degree.'[147]

Lady Paget had been away only for forty eight hours but in that time the order for the immediate evacuation of the hospital had been received and the staff had resolved to retire to Salonika with patients, stores and equipment, hoping to set up a temporary hospital at Monastir. When, the military authorities had been informed of this decision, and transport requested, it was found that their plan was somewhat different. The military were preparing for a last stand and offered transport to Prishtina or Mitrovitza in the west. Accordingly, it was agreed to send an advance party to Prishtina to look for a suitable building for a hospital. When on the following day, all was packed and arrangements were in hand for transport of staff, it became clear that there was no rolling stock available for transport.

Worse still, the order came once again for all Austrian prisoners to be taken away and sent further from the frontier for safe custody. Yet again, hospital staff remonstrated that it would be impossible to maintain the hospital without their labour and eventually, a compromise was reached whereby only those Austrians *'known to be trustworthy'* were permitted to stay.[148] Two hundred prisoners had been marched away to an uncertain fate.

Lady Paget examined matters carefully. She had been deeply shocked by

Nursing with Lady Paget in Serbia in 1915

the scenes which she had witnessed on her journey north. She had no desire to abandon patients and stores to the Bulgarians. She knew too that Prishtina was little safer than Skoplje. She had the wisdom to see that congestion and distress there would be extreme and once there, the only route of escape would be across the frozen mountains of Albania. She would not allow her nurses to face that ordeal and although she herself had already resolved to stay *'whatever happened'*, she determined that they should retreat to Salonika rather than the west:

'I knew the chances were that I, and any who stayed with me, would be safe in the hands of the Bulgarians; that if I stayed it might mean protection for all the Serbians, both wounded in the hospitals and civilians in the town; that we should possibly save our stores, which would be of inestimable value to our troops if they came, and in any case, later on, to the Serbians.'[149]

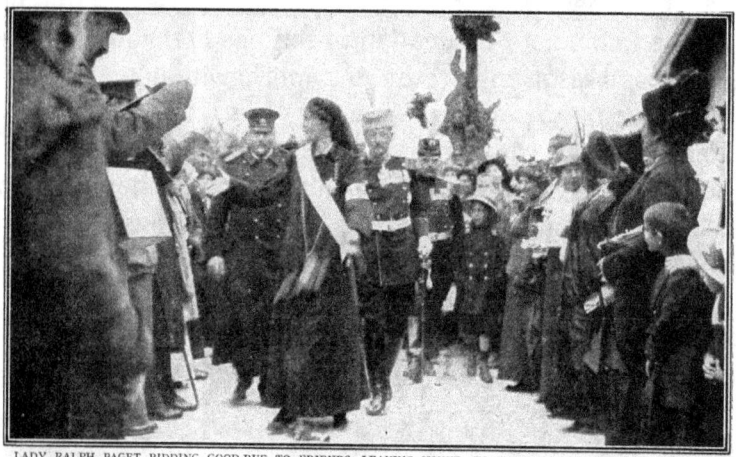

LADY RALPH PAGET BIDDING GOOD-BYE TO FRIENDS LEAVING USKUB, IN ANTICIPATION OF THE CITY'S FALL. When the Bulgarians captured Uskub, Lady Paget decided to remain behind with her wounded Serbian patients and staff of nurses. She is here seen, wearing the Serbian decorations conferred on her by King Peter, in front of General Popovitch and another Serbian officer.

Lady Paget in Skoplje, 1915 (from The Great War V, p. 185*)*

Lady Paget was apparently not one to brook opposition. She overcame the objections of the Serbians to her hospital remaining fairly easily but interestingly, it was her own nurses who alone resisted her plans. In her subsequent Report, she wrote vividly of the scene at a midnight when she addressed the staff assembled in the dining room: *'a motley crowd, some travel stained and splashed to the eyes with mud, some of the*

Lady Paget's Return to Serbia

sisters in dressing gowns and plaits, just waked out of uneasy slumber.'[150]

To the men, she gave the choice of going to Salonika or remaining in Skoplje and all elected to remain. To the nurses, however, she offered no choice. She feared most of all the 'Comitadji' or irregular troops- *'lawless and brutal plunderers'*- who would be swift to take advantage of the present anarchy. In view of the risk of violence from this quarter, she refused to take responsibility for her nurses staying. The nurses, however, were evidently not persuaded and made it clear that they thought their responsibility was to remain with their patients *'rather than run away from danger'*.

When Lady Paget attempted to bludgeon them in to obeying orders, the nurses resisted further, one nurse even saying that she would take up residence in Skoplje and nurse Serbians independently. Lady Paget appealed to the men but to her astonishment found them in favour of the women remaining once the dangers had been fully explained. She looked to the other hospitals in the town which had already been evacuated, leaving patients without medical attention or protection:

'It was this consideration, and the hope that our refusal to leave would do something locally to dispel the feeling of bitterness and disappointment at the non-appearance of the Allies, that finally determined us. I think we all felt that the sisters were making a noble choice and that we none of us had the right to forbid them this sacrifice...'[151]

At two in the morning of 20th October, *'amid great enthusiasm'* the decision was made. Cables were sent to recall the staff who had been sent ahead to Prishtina, together with the Austrians and stores. The last member of staff returned on 21st October, the day before the Bulgarians entered Skoplje. The provisions had to remain in Prishtina, where they were in any case very much needed and only three of the Austrians made it back. Most died from cold and hunger as they were force-marched across Serbia.

To their credit, the Serbian General and the Senior Medical Officer in Skoplje, strongly opposed the decision of the British to remain but once

Nursing with Lady Paget in Serbia in 1915

they realised that Lady Paget was not to be persuaded, made every effort to assist. All Austrian orderlies who were still in the hospital were allowed to stay and some who had just started on the road returned. Now the nurses, still adamant that they would not leave, laboured hard to restore the hospital to its former state and gather the wounded from the other hospitals.

On 21st October, Sir Ralph Paget, unable to reach his wife by telegraph, made a hazardous journey to Skoplje by motor car and train. He found the town *'almost entirely deserted'*. Met by his wife at the station , he learnt , presumably with some misgivings, that she had been entrusted by the Serbians *'to take charge of the situation generally and with her unit to give assistance to any Serbians who might remain, and to preserve order as far as in her power lay.'*[152]

After consultation with Lady Paget and Dr Maitland it was agreed that there was no purpose in Sir Ralph remaining with the unit and *'that the interests of the other units still in the north of Serbia demanded my return to Nish'*. Whilst her husband returned to aid the other British hospital units after a visit of only four hours, Lady Paget turned to matters in the town.

In the hospital located in the Citadel, known as 'The Grad', occupied formerly by Lady Wimborne's unit, there were still over a hundred severely wounded cases, tended by a Mrs Ada Barlow, an English woman, who had refused to leave when the Serbian staff fled. In the confusion, no food had reached the hospital and hunger had been added to the trials of the patients. Now the wounded were transferred to Lady Paget's hospital in motor ambulances and Mrs Barlow joined the staff there.

Ada Barlow is an interesting example of the remarkable and still largely uncelebrated, set of British women who were to be encountered battling singly and in groups all over Serbia at this time. She had left for Serbia on 12th August 1914 as part of an Anglo-American Unit which had been hastily assembled by Mabel Grujic the American wife of the Serbian Under Secretary for Foreign Affairs.[153] The group had included Flora Sandes who would later establish fame not for her nursing activities as a VAD —which

Lady Paget's Return to Serbia

were short lived – but for her role as a combatant in the Serbian army. Ada, following a less romantic but probably more useful course, served first in the First Reserve Hospital in Kragujevatz but somehow found her way to a hospital in Nish. There she was encountered, at the start of the typhus epidemic, by Dr Johnston Abraham of the 1st British Red Cross unit, when she was working in a hospital with two Greek doctors and two other English nurses who were leaving for England the next day.

Together this exhausted team was struggling to look after around one thousand and sixteen patients in appalling conditions. When asked why she too was not departing with the other nurses, Ada apparently replied in dejection: *'I have nothing to go back for'*.

Dr Johnston Abraham, with the unconscious sexism of his age, described Ada in unnecessarily unflattering terms:

'It was the drab grey tragedy of the unwanted woman. She was fat and plain, elderly and rather pasty. Personally I did not take to her. She was a piece of flotsam on the tide of life; but she was an Englishwoman, and the thought of her made me wretched all day...'[154]

Later, Dr Barrie the chief of the 1st British Red Cross unit, also met Ada in Nish and brought her back to help in his hospital in Skoplje where she laboured untiringly even after Dr Abrahams and the rest of the unit had withdrawn. It was here that Lady Paget found her and apparently recognised her worth.

Ada Barlow remained with Lady Paget for the rest of her time in Serbia and was listed in Lady Paget's subsequent report as one of the two masseuses in her unit.

Whilst any able bodied wounded were ordered to walk to the nearest station thirty miles away, Lady Paget and her staff watched helplessly as the long line of refugees and exhausted soldiers marched North through the hospital grounds. The regular soldiers were ill clad and unprepared for a march over the mountains in freezing conditions, and staff at the hospital had to content themselves with handing out clothing and

Nursing with Lady Paget in Serbia in 1915

blankets from their stores.

Sir Ralph on his brief, rather unromantic visit to his wife had expressed concern that large amounts of stores at her hospital were falling into enemy hands. She reassured him that she had *'distributed a large amount of these stores to the Serbian soldiers during the last days*

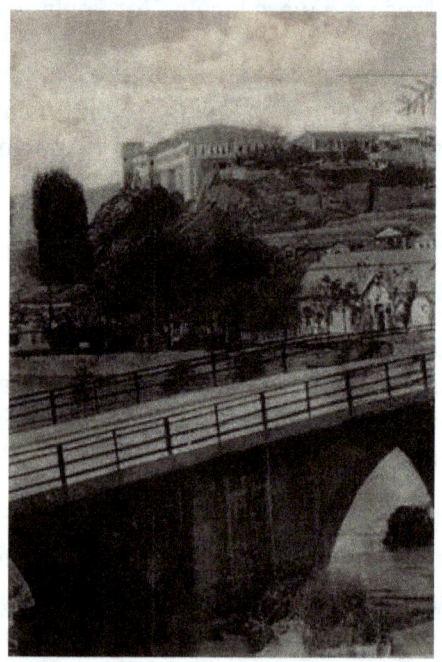

View of the Grad, or citadel, at Skoplje, c. 1916

who had passed in front of her hospital in their retreat'.[155] Now, as they awaited the arrival of the enemy, motor ambulances from the Hospital rushed back and forth *'bringing in the last of the wounded as well as food, stores, drugs, surgical instruments, and hospital appliances from other hospitals in the town'.*[156] At the Grad, they found big barrels of wine in the vaults and with considerable regret, poured the contents over the rocks, fearful of the effect it might have when found by victorious troops. It was a wise precaution. That night Skoplje was like a *'city of*

Lady Paget's Return to Serbia

the dead' with no light in any window, and the only noise the occasional *'howling of a dog far away in the Turkish quarter'.*[157]

George B Logan, who was also involved in the ransacking of the other hospital stores, recalled *'days of uncertainty and suspense, while the town lay silent and deserted but for galloping gendarmes in the streets and the flare of burning magazines...Meanwhile, I had been looting the magazines of all the Serbian Hospitals in town which were being abandoned, and carrying their stores here for safety...'*[158]

On a last trip to The Grad, he ran the gauntlet of a battle raging between retreating gendarmes and Turks:

'I drove to the hospital with 1000 pounds of sugar in my car, six people handing on the mudguards, three wheels and the drum of the axle on the ground and two dead Turks lying on the steps of the building we had left... Halfway the car gave its last gasp so we abandoned it and ran the rest of the way...'

At nine the following morning, the Government train left for Prishtina and Lady Paget rushed down to the station with cases of food for the departing military staff. Chests of tea were unceremoniously thrown aboard the train as the train pulled out of the station. The grateful officers warned Lady Paget that she should return to the Hospital at once since 'comitadji' were already present in the town. Instead, her thoughts turned to some of her nurses who had gone to help at the old fever hospital – the Polimesis- *'a little way down the river bank in the direction from which the Bulgarians were advancing'.*[159] Two cars set out to rescue them, taking different routes in order to ensure that at least one reached the hospital. They drove through excited crowds and *'maddened Albanians who had armed themselves and were shooting at random'.*

At the Fever Hospital, they were appalled to find a group of around a dozen Serbian patients who had just been admitted and were awaiting transfer to Lady Paget's hospital. There was room only for the children and the more seriously injured patients.The remainder had to be left with

Nursing with Lady Paget in Serbia in 1915

the Greek and Swiss Doctors who were left in charge. It was heartrending to turn a deaf ear to the entreaties of the patients left behind, but shells were falling ever closer and there was clearly little time left.

By midday, the Bulgarians were shelling the town itself. A committee of Bulgarians resident in the town had been hastily formed to take over the town provisionally and Lady Paget arranged with them that her ambulances would go out to meet the advancing Bulgarians, announce that the British Hospital had remained and seek permission to collect the wounded. Logan recalled that Lady Paget was greatly concerned that the Bulgarians might mistake her hospital buildings for a barracks. In the cars were one Danish doctor, Logan and three other Americans and several Bulgarian residents. Shells were now falling close to the Hospital and one shattered the windows of the pavilions:

'It was a truly dreadful experience to watch the shells bursting overhead and then to see the wounded struggling to reach the hospital. .. Now came the crowning horror of the day. The Albanian civil population of the town ran amok; they armed themselves with rifles which they took from the dead soldiers, and as the wounded Serbians dragged themselves over the brow of the hill in a vain attempt to reach the hospital they were shot at by these maddened and merciless fanatics...'[160]

Concerned that orderlies fetching the wounded and nurses passing from one building to another would fall victim to these snipers, Dr Maitland and some of his Austrian orderlies took control of the situation, rounding the Albanians up and locking them in the stables. This heroic action was hardly noticed, as the staff of the hospital struggled to cope with the wounded pouring in from the surrounding battlefield: *'The corridors and staircases were soon full to excess; we therefore placed forms at the back under cover of the buildings, on which they* [the wounded Serbian soldiers] *sat with their ghastly wounds, waiting till they could be attended to...'*

Lady Paget was deeply impressed with *'the cool practical way in which the whole staff went about their work'* but singled out for particular praise the role played by the Austrian orderlies:

Lady Paget's Return to Serbia

'Our Austrian orderlies had always won my admiration by their loyalty and devotion to duty, but never did their behaviour better merit our respect than now. Though it was their Allies who were coming, though after long captivity the moment of their deliverance was at hand, and though they knew we were absolutely at their mercy, they stuck to their work and took all risks with us, bringing in wounded Serbians from the battlefield and helping to wash and dress their wounds...'[161]

Before dusk, to the great relief of all, the motor ambulances returned with the assurance of the Bulgarian commander that the hospital would have his protection. The vehicles were garlanded with flowers but also bore the mark of many bullet holes suffered when the party had been caught in the crossfire and forced to take cover in a ditch: 'Three of the four ambulances were more or less out of action'.[162]

Logan later described the adventures of the ambulance party to his parents:

'Next day, three of us, Tancock, Osborn and I went out in our cars to meet the advancing Bulgarian Army as shrapnel had begun to burst over the hospital ... we did not start quite soon enough and drove between the two lines [Serb and Bulgarian] just as the infantry battle was beginning. Again we had to abandon the cars and lie in a ditch until the Bulgarian attack had passed over us. All of our cars were hit, as the men used them as temporary shelters, and the engine of one was wrecked, but during a lull we drove the other two behind the lines, where we found the artillery and the commanding officer who promised to respect the hospital. Our return was in the nature of a triumphal procession. We filled the cars with wounded and drove into town at the head of the first body of troops who were marching through the streets. The Turks pelted us with flowers and pushed our car along; and as soon as the Serbs had retreated past the hospital we drove back with an officer who took control of it, freeing our Austrian Bolinchars ...'[163]

In the evening, Lady Paget retraced her steps to the fever hospital to check on the condition of the Serbian soldiers whom they had been forced to leave behind. She found the hospital miraculously untouched

Nursing with Lady Paget in Serbia in 1915

but overwhelmed with Bulgarian wounded. The doctors had run out of dressings, food and even basic necessities and there were no nurses or orderlies to assist them. The Greek doctor in charge, however, was less than grateful when Lady Paget suggested that the seriously wounded should be transferred to her hospital for surgery. He had been entrusted with their care by a Bulgarian officer and was understandably reluctant to relinquish the responsibility to the interfering English. The unseemly argument which ensued, conducted in raised voices, might have continued some time had not a wounded Bulgarian officer intervened in broken French and gratefully accepted Lady Paget's offer.

It was an uneasy night for the hospital staff as they worked in the red glow of a nearby powder magazine, set alight by the departing Serbs, to the sound of exploding cartridges.

On the morning of 23rd October, Lady Paget sought out the Bulgarian commandant to seek permission to gather the wounded and put her hospital and its stores at his disposal. Ever mindful of the impression which the British presence made on the native inhabitants, she drove about the town advertising her hospital's continued presence. When people stopped her to give details of those wounded in the recent shelling, she arranged for ambulances to collect the victims. She noted that most were young children injured by shrapnel.

To the new Commandant and his Chief Medical Officer, Lady Paget made it clear that she and her staff had chosen to stay and become prisoners rather than abandon their work. Whilst she offered immediate humanitarian aid to the Bulgarians who had as yet no medical facilities, she pointed out that her unit was supported by a public fund raised in England and could not help the Bulgarians once their own medical arrangements were in place. She put in a formal request to be sent home with her staff *'as soon as it was practicable'*.[164] The Bulgarians agreed to this readily enough, promising to send the party home once the railway was reconstructed.

There were still some three hundred Austrian orderlies at the Hospital and now a Hungarian Oberleutnant, finding himself the highest ranking

Lady Paget's Return to Serbia

officer of the Austrian army in Skoplje took charge and demanded their release. The tables had been neatly turned and it was Lady Paget and her staff who were now the captives. However, the orderlies had only remained at the Hospital because of Lady Paget's determination to keep them, and now she found herself arguing with their Officer that they were mostly unfit for further military service and would render the most help to their Bulgarian allies by remaining in service at the Hospital. The Oberleutnant, heedful of the aid that his fellow prisoners had received in the recent typhus epidemic, undertook to consult the powers in Vienna and leave the Austrians in place whilst he awaited a reply. Once again, this disparate group of Austrians, Hungarians, Czechs, Croats, Slovenes and Moravians who had suffered so much as prisoners of war, felt the iron hand of Austrian military discipline. It was an evident shock for them, as well as the British staff who witnessed soldiers who had forgotten how to salute their officers *'soundly cuffed'*.

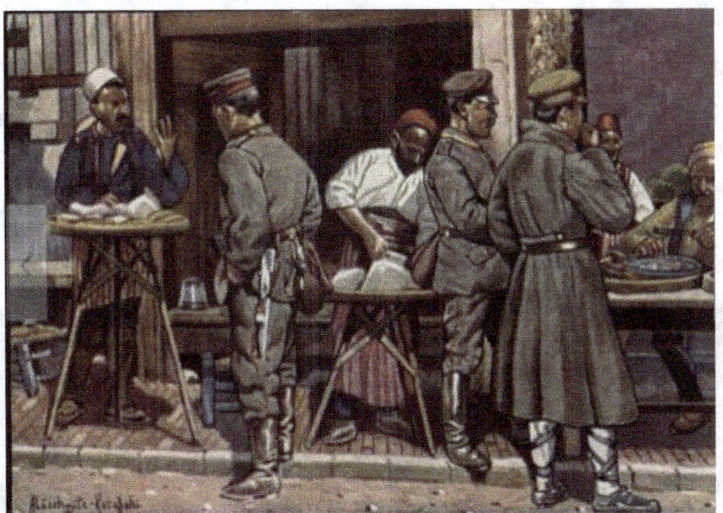

Postcard of street life in Skoplje under enemy occupation, c. 1916

Now began a tense period of chaos within the newly occupied town, with the British constantly under suspicion of spying. Lady Paget deftly walked a tightrope, always asking the permission of the Bulgarians for

Nursing with Lady Paget in Serbia in 1915

any activity and soon realising the vital importance of securing written consent, sealed by an appropriate authority. Famine was the new threat since the Serbians troops had taken all food away with them, burning their crops as they left. The Bulgarians found little food and fuel and were unable to bring in supplies because the railways had been destroyed. What little remained, was commandeered for the Bulgarian troops and the civilian population, their numbers swollen by crowds of refugees, was without bread or any form of subsistence.

On Wednesday 27th October, the hospital opened its first centre for distribution to those in need in the town. Now the stores of flour and that rice which had been so resented earlier, proved of immense value as did the *'endless'* supplies of clothing which they had amassed. The Bulgarians watched jealously, constantly afraid that the Serbians were being favoured, whilst Lady Paget made conspicuous efforts to distribute her largesse fairly amongst all those in need, regardless of their nationality. There followed constant harassment from the authorities who regularly attempted to halt the distribution.

In particular, the new Governor proved himself objectionable even to the mild Lady Paget. She had already angered him by refusing to allow herself to be photographed when she was invited to view evidence of Serbian atrocities. She and Dr Maitland with several other doctors, had attended the small cemetery just below the hospital on 25th October, as bidden, and had there been shown recently exhumed bodies purported to be Bulgarian victims of Serbian atrocities. Reluctant to be used for Bulgarian or German propaganda, she had taken care to keep behind the camera despite the increasingly angry entreaties of the Governor. She bravely defied the Governor pointing out that even her own government would not force her to be photographed against her will.

Lady Paget wisely took the line that only an expert's evidence would be of use in confirming a war crime. Privately, however, she noted her suspicions, commenting that the corpses, all wounded by bullets to the front, had probably been damaged in the process of exhumation and looked as if they had been bound after death. Since they were all in Macedonian dress, they could as easily have been Serbs as Bulgarians,

Lady Paget's Return to Serbia

except in five cases where they were *'partly'* clothed in Bulgarian uniform.[165]

By good fortune, Lady Paget was saved from this particular conflict when she was able to appeal to some high ranking Bulgarian officers who were travelling to the front through Skoplje. She not only succeeded in convincing them of the urgent need of the refugees but also of the advisability of moving the Governor to *'another sphere of action'*.[166] Her friendship with the Queen of Bulgaria, whom she had met whilst nursing Bulgarian troops during the first Balkan War, was evidently paying dividends.

At the beginning of November, as the number of refugees rapidly increased, the decision was made to set up a separate distribution centre for refugees at the hospital whilst maintaining the first centre in the town purely for local inhabitants. Rations for two days were distributed simultaneously at both centres every other day. The numbers of those receiving aid in this way was then around eight hundred but to their number were soon added a group of three hundred Macedonians and members of the Roman Catholic Croatian population. By mid month, there were over a thousand receiving support in this way and numbers continued to escalate. At the end of January when stores were almost completely depleted, accounts recorded the overall provision of relief to 55,255 individuals.[167] In addition a dispensary was opened in the town for the civilian population and two of the American doctors on the staff undertook house to house visits, thus providing the only medical care available in Skoplje.

Money was soon a pressing problem. Although the Bulgarians had at first announced that Serbian money would remain current until a settlement, the dinar was quickly devalued. Since there was no Bulgarian money available, Lady Paget planned first to raise a loan from the Bulgarian Red Cross but in the end found help from an unexpected source. When she explained that, without money to buy flour, she could not prevent starvation in the town, the military authorities arranged credit for her with the National Bank of Bulgaria for a loan of one thousand levas (the equivalent of one thousand francs) until such time as the Serbian Relief

Nursing with Lady Paget in Serbia in 1915

Fund should remit money to her credit in Sofia. Lady Paget cabled the committee of the Serbian Relief Fund accordingly, but received no reply. Later, she noted ruefully in her report, she learnt that the cable had been received but since it was thought inadvisable to send money to an enemy country, *'no steps were taken'*.[168]

A brighter moment occurred in November when a telegram arrived from the Queen of Bulgaria, expressing her admiration for *'your charitable and unceasing work amongst the needy and suffering in Scopié'* and enclosing a gift of five thousand levas.[169] Lady Paget recorded her gratitude in her report:

'This was only the first of many times that Her Majesty showed her practical sympathy with us and our work; from beginning to end, both while we remained in Macedonia and later in Bulgaria, she was untiring in the exercise of her influence for our comfort and also for the expediting of our departure for England...'[170]

Meanwhile, the hospital still functioned with wards crowded and the theatre often working from ten to fifteen hours a day. Logan, who had evidently come out as an ambulance driver, more often found himself dressing wounds:

'The bathroom is not a pleasant place these days with its bloody stretchers and steaming shrapnel wounds and huge heaps of dirty dressings...Most of the time I spend there dressing the wounded as they come in and I have almost forgotten how to run a Ford...'[171]

As a harsh winter set in, it became a constant struggle to find sufficient fuel and other essentials:

'Those were strange times, and in the common struggle for mere existence it did not occur very much to anyone to consider who were friends and who were enemies. At the military and municipal Headquarters, we forced our way into the stores along with a jostling throng of Bulgarians and Macedonians, all clamouring for supplies, and on the whole we were quite as successful as they.'[172]

Lady Paget's Return to Serbia

Despite the hardships of everyday life, there was also some discontent amongst the staff that they were treating so many Bulgarian patients. Some felt that it would be better to return home and tend their own wounded. Lady Paget's report of this time is understandably defensive, seeking to justify a position which some questioned. She would later receive considerable criticism for the closeness of her cooperation with the Bulgarians. Logan summed up her dilemma well:

'The British are prisoners of war: until the Kaiser wills and until the trains run again from Skoplje they remain here binding the wounds of their enemies, and we four are going to stay with Lady Paget as long as she wants us... Czar Ferdinand rode to the door today in a great gray automobile and kissed her hand on the steps, but none the less she cannot move without permission...'[173]

However, at the beginning of December, the situation changed once more with the arrival of the Germans who now effectively took possession of

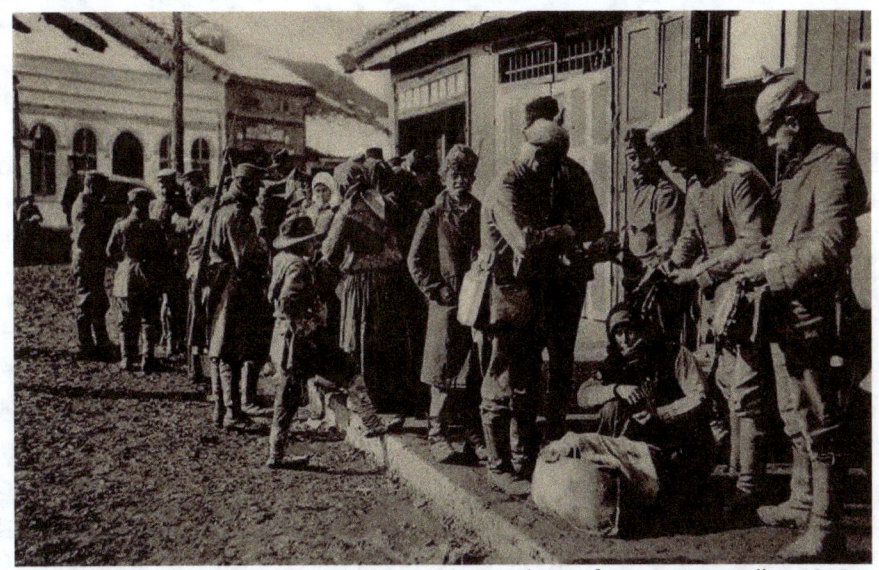

German soldiers purchase tobacco from a street seller, 1916

the town.

Logan recalled the arrival of *'the spike helmets'* as he termed them, in an uncensored letter dated 18th December, which he smuggled out with

Nursing with Lady Paget in Serbia in 1915

three Americans who were leaving the unit. The happy trio, Charles E Fox, Dr Stanley H Osborne and Richard Schellens were members of the American Red Cross Sanitary Commission who had been sheltering at the hospital but now judged it wise to make a tactical withdrawal. Logan reported that two weeks ago, after the battle of Krivolak, the Germans had arrived *'ploughing through the mud with bicycles slung over their shoulders, to sweep the French into the sea at Salonique.'* Now, he reported gloomily: *'Today there is half famine in the town, the hospital is overflowing with wounded from the battle of Krivolak and the spike helmets are everywhere. The end is not yet...'*[174]

Lady Paget, fearing that the Germans would take over the hospital and worse still, intern the British in Germany, felt that a closer association with the Bulgarians would be the best way of resisting German ambitions. She accordingly took the controversial step of agreeing that the Bulgarian flag should fly over the hospital and a Bulgarian medical officer should be nominally appointed as director. Management of the hospital remained firmly in the hands of the British and subsequent events seemed to justify her pragmatism.

Around the middle of January, an epidemic of typhoid broke out in the Orphan's Home in Skoplje and Lady Paget persuaded the Bulgarians to allow her to admit the children to her hospital. Despite the efforts of the nurses, several of the orphans died, proving too weak to withstand the illness. The incident must have brought back terrible memories of the previous winter.

By now the supply of flour and rice was exhausted, and hospital staff found that all they could supply to the refugees was a little money to purchase potatoes and onions. In individual cases, they even paid rent so as to prevent landlords throwing them into the street. They had always investigated each case to check that it was genuine, before giving money, flour or clothes and were confident that they were helping those most in need. This thorough attention to detail had an additional value, as Lady Paget later recalled:

'As each person came for relief we wrote the name and history down in

Lady Paget's Return to Serbia

a book, a copy of which has been sent to Serbian Headquarters, Corfu, for reference, so that Serbian families who escaped from the country can get news of those who remained behind. We have named this book 'The Tragedy of the Women of Serbia' and its contents would, I think, wring tears from the stoniest of hearts.'[175]

It was also at the beginning of January 1916, that the Bulgarians issued a proclamation ordering all Serbians to return to their homes. Although, some regarded this as inhumane and callous, Lady Paget for one, thought it wise. Many refugees had remained in Skoplje rather than returning home, and their presence together with several thousand Serbian prisoners and over one hundred thousand enemy troops, meant that the spectre of famine was ever present:

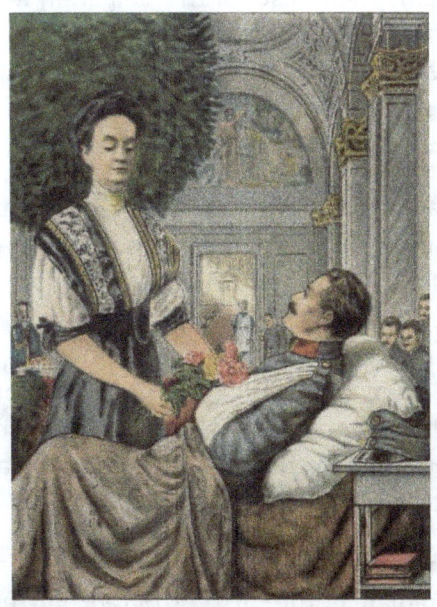

Queen Elionora of Bulgaria at the besdside of a wounded Hungarian officer

'Had the Bulgarians not taken this step, many hundreds more people would have died of starvation than was actually the case.'[176]

As early as 5th December, Lady Paget had written to Elionora the Queen

Nursing with Lady Paget in Serbia in 1915

of Bulgaria telling her that the strain of work was now telling upon the staff of her hospital and requesting that she should use her influence to arrange for her unit's departure as soon as the railways were open. After much delay and amidst strong opposition from the Germans, the party finally left Skoplje on 17th February 1916. By now the stores were almost entirely exhausted and many of the refugees had been moved on to other cities so that at last the numbers of applicants for relief were falling.

The railways had been operating for a full five weeks before the departure of the Paget unit but in the end, the Bulgarians provided ten large motor ambulances to take the party first to Sofia. Such was the distrust of German intentions, that it was judged safer to return via Bulgaria. After four weeks in Sofia as the guests of the Bulgarian Red Cross, the party, still avoiding German territory, departed via Bucharest and Petrograd, Sweden and Norway, arriving in Newcastle on 2nd April and in London the following day, seventeen months after first starting out to Serbia in the Autumn of 1914.

Logan wrote a final letter home aboard SS Irma as it steamed towards Newcastle, describing their triumphal progress, as the fifty three members of the unit made their tortuous way home *'feted and dined and deluged with flowers'*.[177] With evident glee, he recorded that the Queens of Romania and Norway gave them all signed photographs and the Crown Princess of Sweden showed them round her palace. In Moscow, he and one of the sisters had taken a sleigh ride in order to see the Kremlin . Despite such highlights, they felt grimy and ill prepared for such a reception, clad only in *'Skoplje made mufti'*.

They had spent around eleven nights aboard trains and travelled by car from the Rumanian border to Petrograd and from Hagarauch to Bergen. Now as they neared the English coast, most of the party were laid low with seasickness, confined to their bunks whilst Lady Paget *'like a ministering angel'* went round delivering seasickness pills – possibly a little too late. All the talk at this stage was of plans to go out once more to help the Serbians, to tend to the surviving army in Corfu, Salonika, or perhaps even further afield. Logan was in no doubt about his loyalty to

Lady Paget's Return to Serbia

his leader: *'If Lady Paget asks me to go out, I certainly will do so.'*

On 13th April, Lady Paget made her final appearance before the committee of the Serbian Relief Fund:

'Lady Paget made a statement on the work of her hospital at Skoplje and elsewhere, giving a vivid account of the conditions under which her unit worked, first under the Serbian Government, then during the Bulgarian and German occupation, and of its return home through Sofia, Bucharest and Petrograd.'[178]

The committee responded with a *'hearty vote of thanks'*, expressing gratification at her safe return and pride in being associated with the work of her unit, which was duly *'carried by acclamation.'*

Despite muttering in the popular press about her apparent collaboration with the Bulgarians, Lady Paget was appointed a Dame Grand Cross of the British Empire [GBE] in August 1917. Many others were in no doubt about her achievements. Barbara McLaren, author of 'Women of the War' published in 1917 was typical when she enthused:

'As a monument to human endurance and courage there can be no more wonderful record than that of Lady Paget's Hospital Unit in Serbia...'

She had no doubts either about Lady Paget's role during the Bulgarian occupation:

'It is a remarkable tribute to her personality that the enemy, though not too plentifully equipped themselves, should yet have allowed her to retain possession of this large quantity of stores, trusting as they did to her scrupulous sense of fairness and straight-dealing...'

Perhaps more eloquent still is a tribute written by a Hungarian soldier and former prisoner of war in Skoplje, which was subsequently circulated by the Press Association under the title *'Lady Paget's work in Serbia. A Hungarian tribute'* :

*'Being ill, he writes, I was left behind in Uscub, instead of being transported

Nursing with Lady Paget in Serbia in 1915

to Albania and saw all the fighting there. I cannot sufficiently express my gratitude to Lady Paget. She saved many of my comrades from death, going out herself and collecting such prisoners and bringing them in to her hospital. She helped the convalescence with food and clothing, visited the prisoners' camps, and being held in high esteem by the Serbians she was able to do a great deal for the prisoners. She took care the gifts sent to them reached them safely.'

'You cannot imagine what we all felt when Lady Paget caught spotted typhus from us and what joy it gave us to see her restored to health again. She taught many of us nursing and it was the height of our desires to become a nurse in the hospital of this noble lady.'[179]

Lady Paget would have been honoured by a testimony such as this and so would Flora and those that served with her. For them, Barbara McLaren's tribute to the nurses of the First World War seems more appropriate than any other:

'To the nurses of the war, it will be admitted by all, belongs the crown of women's war service. Their ranks contain many heroines whose names and deeds will never be chronicled; but their selfless devotion, their courage, their unquestioning acceptance of any risk, and their willing sacrifice of personal comfort, health, even life itself, will stand for all time in the proudest memorials of these tragic years.'

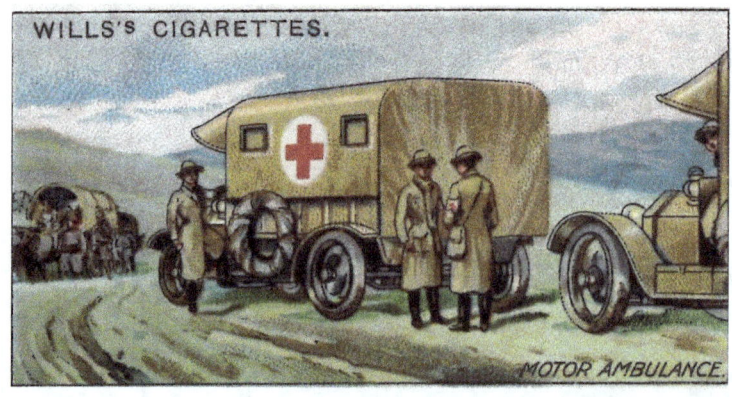

Lady Paget's Return to Serbia

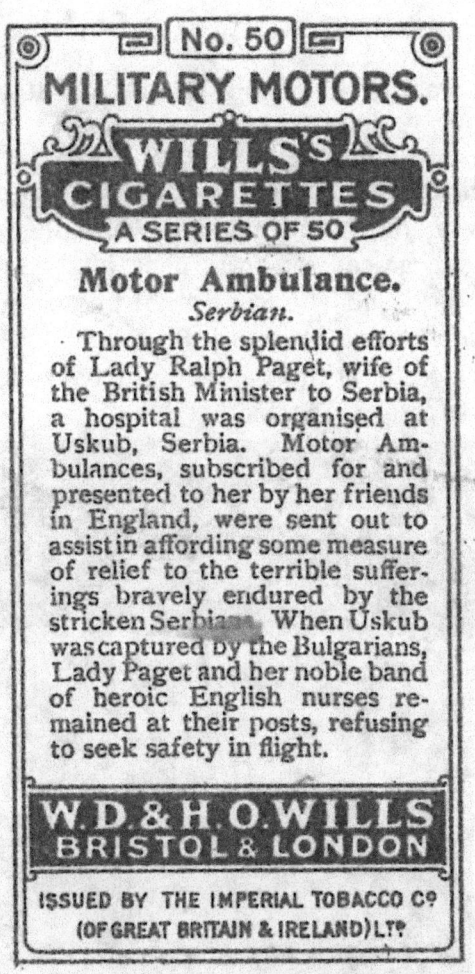

Left and above: cigarette card from the series on 'Military Motors', c. 1916

Chapter 8

Nurse Scott after Serbia

Back at the nursing home, April 1916

Tracing Flora's movements during the rest of the war, becomes increasingly difficult. A large photograph of her with members of the Leicester Pioneers and the pet monkey which she was bestowing on them as a mascot, graced the front page of the *Illustrated Leicester Chronicle* on 1st April 1916. The scene of the photograph is the garden of Nurse Scott's nursing home in Victoria Road and it is clear that Flora was still working in Leicester at this date, despite her repeated declarations that she longed to return to Serbia.

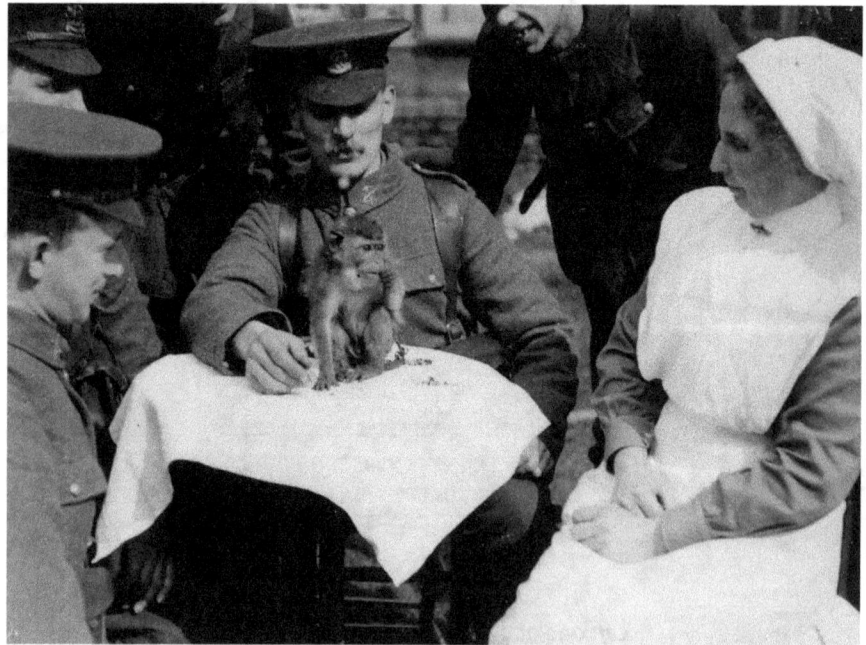

Flora introduces her monkey to men of the 11th Battalion, The Leicestershire Regiment (The 'Leicester Pioneers')

Flora apparently remained at her nursing home throughout 1916 and most of the following year. One tantalising glimpse of her may possibly

Nurse Scott after Serbia

be seen in *'The Dandy Hun'* a book written at the end of the war, by an Austrian Officer named Konstantin Maglic who was imprisoned during the war at Donington Hall, not far from Castle Donington in the northern reaches of Leicestershire.

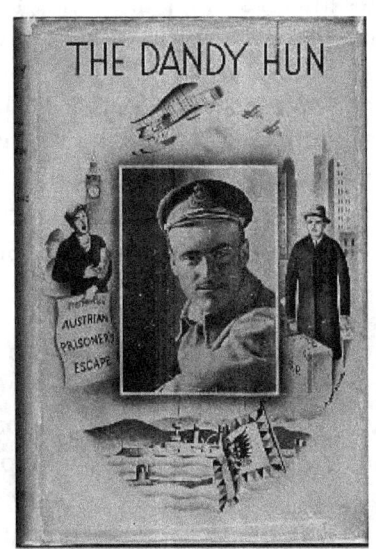

Dustjacket for the English translation of Maglic's memoirs, published in 1932

Early in 1917, Maglic became ill and was transferred to the military Base Hospital in Leicester which then existed at the former mental asylum, in Victoria Road, just a short distance from Flora's nursing home.[180] The Officer recalled that whilst he was a patient there, he was visited by *'an English lady, a Scotchwoman by birth, who had worked in Serbia during the first year of the war, when there was the great typhus epidemic. In 1915, she had been taken prisoner by the Austro-Hungarians and in February 1916 released. As she had (of course), been treated very well during her imprisonment, she lavished upon me the wealth of gratitude she felt; she brought me fruit and at Easter sent gifts to all the prisoners-of- war in the hospital. When she could not come herself, she would always send me flowers with the wish: 'May their scent help you to sleep, to gather strength and to recover!' Kindly soul, dear sister, I thank you.'*[181]

Could this be Flora? The details of her imprisonment are not correct

Nursing in Serbia with Lady Paget in 1915

at all but it sounds very like Flora's love for the Austrians and it is quite possible that linguistic problems contributed to the confusion. It would also be easy to understand if Maglic was a little vague in his recollections of a time when he was, after all, seriously ill and often delirious. It is certainly tempting to see in this story, Flora trying to repay her debt to her beloved Austrian orderlies...

In fact, by 1917, Flora's beloved Serbia, apparently deserted by the Allies, had already suffered the catastrophe of invasion and occupation by Bulgarian, German and Austrian forces. The surviving remnants of the Serbian army, having endured a disastrous retreat over the mountains to Albania, were in exile, recovering in Corsica and Greece or fighting in support of the Russians on the Rumanian front.

With return to Serbia now no longer an option, Flora did not apparently relinquish her ambition to return to the war zone. One clue as to her plans at this time, survives amongst her personal papers. Amidst the newscuttings and letters is a typescript list of equipment required for women relief workers and nurses in Russia, issued by the Friends' War Victims Relief Committee. This Quaker organisation had been founded in 1870 during the Franco Prussian War in order to bring relief to civilians in distress. At the beginning of the First World War the organisation had undertaken some work amongst Serbian refugees but by this stage in the war, they were planning to concentrate on aiding the 34,000 Polish and Belarusians who were trapped and facing famine in the Volga region. Events were overtaken by revolution in Russia and in the end, the plans came to little. However, for a time at least, Flora seems to have seriously contemplated joining their efforts. A newspaper account written about Flora at the end of the war, stated:

'After the terrible retreat of the [Serbian] army, she came back to England, and after an interval tried hard to get back to South Russia and Rumania to be with the Serbian troops again. Many difficulties cropped up, and she was obliged to give up her desire ...'

It is to be assumed that at least one of these difficulties was the violent upheavals of the Russian revolution but probably another was the not

Nurse Scott after Serbia

inconsiderable problem of what to do with her nursing home. Whilst unable to do anything about the former, Flora certainly found a way of extricating herself from her role at the Nursing Home for by the end of 1917, she was to be found applying for the position of matron at the Disabled Soldiers & Sailors Hospital in Nottingham. The final letter to her family preserved amongst her papers is dated Friday 29th December 1917 and was written at Welbeck Auxiliary Hospital , Welbeck Abbey near Worksop in Nottinghamshire. In this, she explained to her family that from a field of ninety two applicants, she had been shortlisted for interview by the Duchess of Portland who was funding the hospital. When the Duchess could not finally decide upon Flora or the other successful applicant , the scientific method of choosing names out of a hat was adopted: 'The other ladies [sic] came out first & I lost. Rather hard luck but I am used to it by this [time].'

Christmas at Welbeck Abbey, 1917

The Duchess was apparently most apologetic to Flora and offered the slight compensation of a temporary post over Christmas at her own home of Welbeck Abbey where the Duchess was opening a hospital for thirty wounded soldiers. Since the matron appointed to this hospital was still in France and unable to leave before the New Year, Flora was asked to help open the wards in time for Christmas. Flora, never one to resist the aristocracy's charm, *'jumped'* at the opportunity. So it was, that a week before Christmas, Flora, having once more packed in a hurry, found herself in the Duchess of Portland's car under *'heaps of furs'*, travelling from her sister's home in Nottingham on the twenty five mile trip to Worksop in thick fog and bitter cold. With her this time came her beloved hound 'Tiny'.

Flora wrote with gushing enthusiasm of the luxury of her new bedroom which was pretty and comfy: 'well heated, electric candles etc, down quilt, all cover, quilt etc Indian work; white & blue curtains & hanging rose pink, white walls etc, rose pink down quilt.' Did she spare a thought for her former home in a Serbian classroom?

The hospital, located in a wing of the house, was *'most beautifully fitted*

Nursing in Serbia with Lady Paget in 1915

up':

'Most luxurious couches, all covered in blue & white Indian embroidery. Books every kind & loads in every room; all sporting pictures; a lovely toned grand piano (in Fox Hall an immense room) gramophone, writing tables, bagatelle table, cards – all kinds of games; immense arm chairs, large palms & glorious flowers; then there is [a] large billiard room, another large recreation room, several smaller, an immence [sic] dining hall, very high ,decorated in ordinary way, with shields & large flags (now of course especially decorated for Xmas) kitchens, boot rooms etc. Staff rooms are also very pretty & most comfortable; high easy chairs, chesterfields all covered in embroidery; lots of plants, flowers etc'

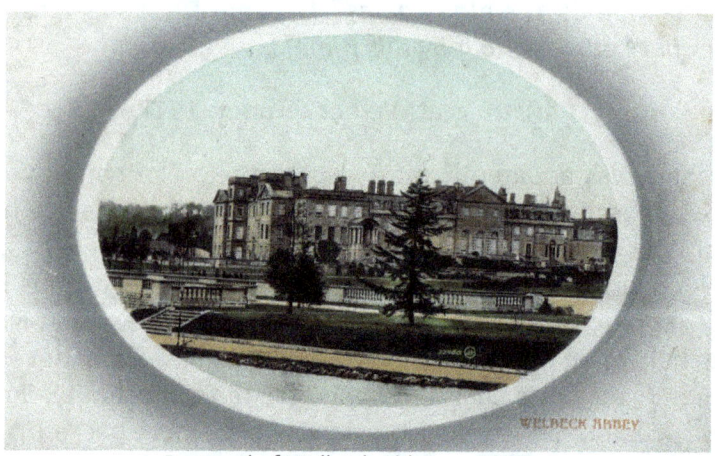

Postcard of Welbeck Abbey, c. 1920

Food, always a source of great interest to Flora, was also *'splendid'* with *'venison, game and rabbits etc'* and no sign as yet of rationing. The twenty- seven patients who arrived on the Saturday before Christmas day were indeed, as Flora, observed *'lucky men'*. Flora had worked hard to prepare everything for them, finding that she had to instruct the VAD nurses in everything. In charge as Commandant, of course, was *'Her Grace'* who was always planning something *'fresh & nice'* for the men. The regime seemed fairly relaxed with the provision of two donkeys and carts, four bicycles, several wheelchairs for exploring the park and a large gas motor car with seating capacity for fourteen. The latter was useful

Nurse Scott after Serbia

for trips to matinee performances in Nottingham and picture houses as well as conveyance to and from the station: *'Oh, they have everything one could wish for'.*

Flora was very impressed with the Duke and Duchess of Portland who were *'kindness itself'*. Not only were they prepared to shake hands and talk freely with the proletariat but they never addressed their servants by surname and were *'very , very Liberal'*. Better still, the noble family were *'dog people'* and the Duke in particular took great care of Tiny: *'She has a most luxurious feather bed, in padded basket with a canopy, most picturesque'*. With Flora, she attended every concert and entertainment, of which, apparently there was a great number.

Festivities opened on Christmas eve with a whist drive in the *'underground*

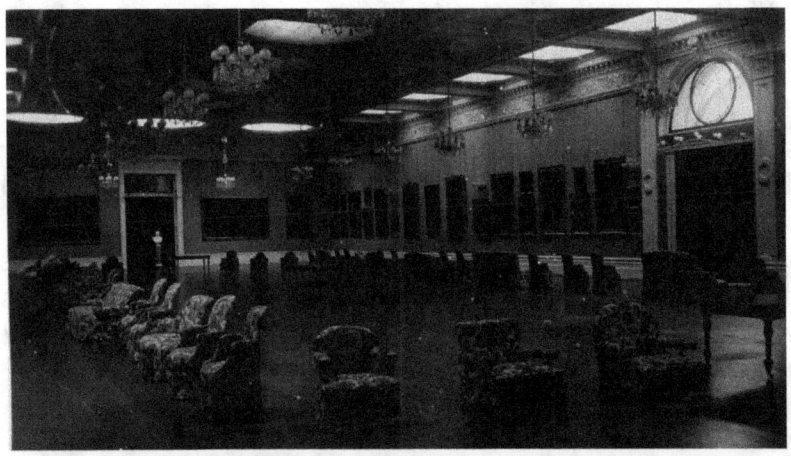

Postcard of the underground ballroom at Welbeck, c. 1905

ball room'. Here Flora, realised that she must explain that the 5th Duke of Portland (1800-1879), whom those who are kindly disposed might have called 'eccentric', had designed and constructed miles of underground apartments and tunnels beneath his home: *'You know, there are whole suites of exquisite rooms etc underground here ... so we are safe from air raids...'* Flora thought the ball room a lovely room and was particularly pleased because she came away with first prize: *'a lovely little jewel case'*.

Nursing in Serbia with Lady Paget in 1915

After this social success, there followed a dance with three musicians providing the music and light refreshments. The Duke and Duchess were joined on this occasion by Lord and Lady Lichfield, Lady Victoria etc and all the Abbey's Christmas guests. Patients retired to bed at eleven but Flora and her staff remained another hour or so. At this point, an unlikely Father Christmas team of *'Her Grace and Lady Victoria'* laid stockings at the foot of each patient's bed amidst much laughter and enjoyment. Flora was duly impressed by their generosity: *'Every man had in [the stocking] a plated cigarette case with His Grace's monogram on, leather treasure & photo case, leather purse, gilt pencil, apple, orange, nuts etc. Was it not splendid?'*

Flora was touched to find that the largesse had also been extended to herself and the other nurse. Outside her bed room door she found *'a beautiful purple leather bag with gilt fittings'*.

Christmas day commenced with breakfast at 9.15 followed by a service in the Abbey Church attended by the Duke and Duchess, patients, nurses, maids and people off the estate. The choir of boys and men, all paid, obliged with carols and Flora found the whole affair *'grand'*. There followed dinner with three *'immense'* turkeys, eight plum puddings and fruit. The Duke, Duchess and guests helped serve whilst the butlers, no doubt a little confused by the whole affair, did the carving. This was all very far from the meagre meals being served in Leicester in 1917, let alone Serbia...

At 4.30, tea was served in the large banquet hall, with scones, cakes, crackers, fruit and sweets. There were two large tables for the patients and one for the Duke and Duchess and nurses. Flora happily poured out tea for her benefactors. In the centre of the room, on a table , was the *'immense'* Christmas cake, beautifully decorated. This he Duke proceeded to cut and the Duchess handed out to everyone: *'Oh, it was rich, like real good bride cake. Then all tables crossed hands with crackers & pulled together. After tea a bran tub, with a present for every one in the room. Then a concert in big Hall [which] the Duke greatly enjoyed & clapped. Auld Lang Syne & patients off to bed, like tired happy children'*

Nurse Scott after Serbia

The fun had not finished. On the Wednesday, all went by motor to Nottingham for a pantomime and the day concluded with whist and music. On the following day there was *'a very grand concert'* in the big ball room with *'paid artistes comic & otherwise'*. On the Friday the patients enjoyed a big tea, games and music, followed on the Saturday by a motor trip to Worksop Picture House: *'Sunday , thank God, a quiet day...'*. New Year's eve on the Monday involved yet another whist drive and a dance in the Ball Room to see in the New Year of 1918. Flora had enjoyed it all and was especially pleased that the Duchess was satisfied with all proceedings. The new matron was due to arrive on 1st January and Flora was due to return to her sister Aggie's residence in Nottingham. Her final comment in her letter suggests that at this point she had still not relinquished the hope of working abroad again:

'My passport really came this morning & I definitely said by middle of January...'

'Why Sister, you have given us chicken meal.'

Whatever, her intentions, Flora did not go abroad again. Although, the Royal College of Nursing's registers list Flora's residence as the Nursing Home, Victoria Road, Leicester for 1919, 1921 and 1923, it is would appear that Flora had left someone else in charge whilst pursuing her own career. The final register notes that mail sent to the Victoria Road address had been returned unopened but Flora had obviously begun her travels long before that date.

A newscutting amongst her papers, as often, it must be confessed, a source of confusion as of accurate information, records that having been forced to give up her desire to rejoin the Serbian forces in South Russia and Rumania, Flora had *'obtained immediately'* the post of matron in charge of the Duchess of Portland's Hospital in Welbeck Abbey and later of a VAD Hospital outside Nottingham. The latter post cannot have lasted long for by the 2nd March 1918, she had been appointed to another post in Leicester but it is possibly to this period that some out of place notes amongst her memoirs refer.

Nursing in Serbia with Lady Paget in 1915

On two sheets of notes, filed incongruously with her account of life in Serbia, is Flora's description of her struggles as matron to control a hospital of thirty beds, filled with boisterous and mischievous soldiers. The notes probably formed part of a letter of which the remainder has not survived but they afford a brief glimpse into a hospital very different from Welbeck. The most likely candidate for this hospital listed in the history of the 5th Northern General Hospital, would seem to be Eastwood V.A.D. Hospital, which is the only hospital in Nottinghamshire of the right size which was open at this date. The situation of this coal mining town just eight miles north west of Nottingham and only a little further from Derby would fit well with Flora's description of frequent visits to picture houses and other entertainments.

The rooms at this unidentified hospital were *'large, lofty & bright'* and strict discipline was imposed by *'the Colonel'* who seemed to hold the Matron responsible for any lapses in discipline. If the patients left the grounds, it was Flora's responsibility to write them a pass: *'each man that can walk is allowed one from 1 until 6.30 every day.'* Many of the patients tried to stay out later and were accustomed to return through mysteriously unlocked doors and windows. The previous Matron had been dismissed over the matter and Flora had a great deal of trouble establishing her authority in the first week:

'...they played every trick imaginable on me, I suppose to see how I took things. Well, I met them every way, caught them stepping through windows, coming in through the lav[atory] window, pushing back locks etc & each one I talked to straight & pointed out how silly it was...'

In the end, Flora seems to have enjoyed a good relationship with the soldiers, recalling an incident when she served an unpopular pudding: *'...then I heard questions as to what it was. At last someone said 'Why Sister, you have given us chicken meal. Then some funny things were said (no grumbles, although scarce one ate it)... When I entered again, there sat several of them on the back of their chairs on perches & the whole lot started to crow. Oh, the noise & how silly they looked...'*

The rare appearance of eggs on the menu just two days later led to a

168

Nurse Scott after Serbia

predictable revival of the joke about chickens...

One soldier in particular, liked to give Charlie Chaplin impressions and Flora's brother-in-law, Neil, had donated an old hat, collar and tie to enhance the performance. Somewhat ungratefully, the soldier had frightened Flora nearly to death by pretending to fall down the stairs and break his leg. Bed time was also a particular problem for Flora:

'I turn them all out of sitting rooms, billiard room etc at 9, give 10 minutes to get into bed. The minute I open a door (generally see pillows etc going) there is a great scuffle, shirts are flung off & often they hop into bed half dressed. Oh, there is such laughing & shouting. I make them come out & undress properly then just put their light out. Sometimes I find a bed upside down with man, sheets, blankets, mattress then bed with legs in the air. Needless to say, bed clothes are often torn, also pillows. They are just children, real babies, I tell them...'

Such behaviour apparently escaped the Colonel's attention and the soldiers enjoyed a good social life, despite their hijinks. On most Mondays and Wednesday evenings, there was a *'good entertainment'* of an unspecified nature and on Fridays, there was the inevitable whist drive. Every man was given a pass for the first house of The Empire on a Tuesday evening and tickets for the pictures every Tuesday and Friday afternoons. Even on a Saturday there was a good tea, billiards or cards from 2.30 until 7.

Food here was not quite as good as that enjoyed at Welbeck Abbey:

'Of course, food is scarce, but the men get plenty, the staff also gets meat once a day. The bread is horrid, really one can scarcely fancy it: great lumps of potatoes & patches of black stuff, very dark coloured & so stodgy. Toast is horrid, sugar, the staff allowed ½ lb weekly, tea 1 ½ oz. Of course we never see butter, but I don't in the least mind, for we generally have plenty of good dripping & I have always had a great weakness for that you remember. The men also have it, milk, we generally have plenty...'

Nursing in Serbia with Lady Paget in 1915

Enjoyable though the post may have been, Flora did not stay in Nottingham very long. On 2nd March 1918, Flora took up her post as the new matron of Leicester Frith Home of Recovery. As the *Leicester Pioneer* reported on 18th March 1918, the new hospital had admitted its first seventeen patients on 1st February but the first matron had resigned only twenty seven days later , not having found the work *'congenial'.*[182]

Leicester Frith Neurasthenic Hospital

'One of the many painful effects of the war has been the large number of cases where men have been so shaken by shell shock and other causes that reason has been temporarily unsettled from its throne. These cases are even more distressing than those where bodily injury has been sustained, for the brain is an organ that cannot be operated on in the same way as other parts of the body. With patience and good special treatment, however, much good can be done, and in this direction the Leicester Frith Home of Recovery is likely to play a prominent part...' Leicester Pioneer 5th Oct 1917

In June 1917, the Mayor of Leicester, Jonathan North , had proposed to employ the funds he had raised in support of 'Disabled Warriors' in the provision of a 'home of recovery' for the treatment of neurasthenic cases.[183] In the company of Dr Astley Clarke, a Colonel serving as Assistant Director of Medical Services for the Territorial North Midland Division and, incidentally, a neighbour of Flora's in Victoria Road, North had visited such a 'Home of Recovery' at Golders Green and been greatly impressed:

'There is no patriotic work which has been supported in Leicester during the war that is more pressing than this effort on behalf of neurasthenic soldiers. One has only to see these men to have one's sympathies touched and to realise that no time should be lost in applying remedial measures.'[184]

These *'neurasthenic cases'* , literally cases of 'weak nerves', also known as sufferers of shell shock, would today receive a lot more understanding as sufferers of 'post trauma stress disorder' . However, as laudable as

Nurse Scott after Serbia

the Mayor's intentions were in 1917, it is clear that understanding was often fairly limited. The Mayor went on :

'We were impressed at Golder's Green with the arrangements made for training men in new industries, not so much that they would follow the employment in after life, but as the means of stimulating their interest in diverting their thoughts from their real or supposed ailments...' The remedy which North and the medical men of Leicester who advised him had in mind, was the provision of a hospital where patients could receive massage and electrical treatment alongside training in workshops or gardens where it was hoped they would rediscover *'the brighter outlook on life'*.

When the Ministry of Pensions made it clear that they welcomed the offer of capital from the Mayor's fund and were willing to bear the cost of treatment and maintenance, the project was agreed and a public

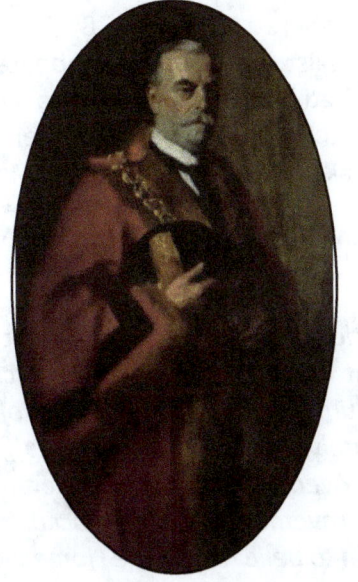 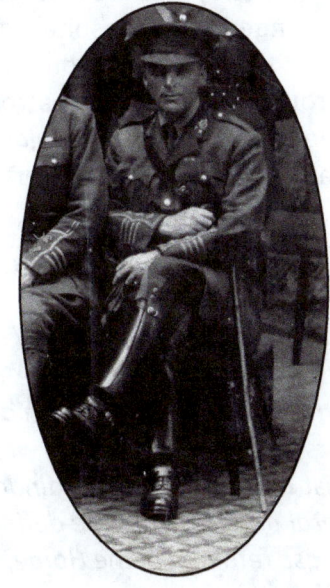

Jonathan North, Mayor of Leicester (left) and Dr Astley Clarke (right)

Nursing in Serbia with Lady Paget in 1915

appeal for funds as well as practical help in fitting out the building was launched. By October 1917, work had commenced on converting and enlarging a large house, known as Leicester Frith House, into a hospital of one hundred beds. The building still stands today and is part of the Glenfield Hospital. Dr Astley Clarke had agreed to act as medical director with two doctors resident at the Home as well as regular visits from consulting neurologists from London and other centres. Although it was intended to have the hospital open by the end of the year, progress was slow and it was not until 1st February 1918 that the first seventeen patients were admitted.

Work was still proceeding on the conversion of outhouses into workshops and the addition of a new wing. There must also have been some misgivings about the hospital, because the other seventeen patients who had been recommended for treatment had failed to appear. According to Colonel Astley Clarke's first monthly report in March 1918, every case recommended to the hospital had been offered a place by 28th February and there were no names on the waiting list. There had also apparently been trouble with the first matron who had had very little time to decide that the work was *'uncongenial'* but had nonetheless resigned on 22nd February. The new matron, Flora, had taken up her duties on 2nd March.

Dr Astley Clarke remained undeterred and the *Leicester Pioneer* reported his declaration with enthusiasm:

'The early days of opening new institutions are always difficult, but one expected them to be still more difficult in the case of a Home such as this, where it was a venture on almost untrodden paths. The type of the patients and their disabilities were entirely new to most of the staff, but the past month the extraordinary improvement which had taken place in several patients, and the definite improvement which had occurred in every case retained in the Home, led him to believe that the Home would more than justify its creation, and would be of great national utility.'[185]

As early as April, the *Illustrated Leicester Chronicle* had included on its front page a group picture of *'first patients, doctors and officials'* showing a relaxed Flora seated in place of honour as Matron beside Dr

Nurse Scott after Serbia

Astley Clarke and Dr McMillan, the Resident Medical Officer under the title *'Fine Work at Leicester Frith'.*[186] By the time of the official opening of the Leicester Frith Home of Recovery (neurasthenics) by the Right Honourable John Hodge MP, Minister of Pensions on 25th July 1918, all was apparently going well. Photographs depict the pension minister *'radiating geniality'* as he mingled with patients who appreciated the *'skilled and attentive'* treatment which they were receiving.[187]

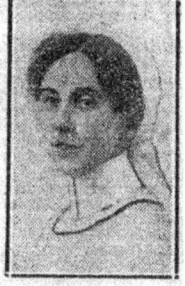

Here you have a photograph of the matron of this splendid institution. Miss Scott, in the earlier days of the war, spent a considerable time in Serbia nursing the wounded soldiers, and a very wonderful time she had. She was particularly impressed with the patience and kindly manners of the Serbian soldiers. After the terrible retreat of the Army she came back to England, and after an interval tried hard to get back to South Russia and Rumania to be with the Serbian troops again.

―o―

Many difficulties cropped up, and she was obliged to give up her desire, but obtained immediately the post of matron-in-charge of the Duchess of Portland's Hospital in Welbeck Abbey, and, later, of a V.A.D. Hospital outside Nottingham. While serving there she was appointed, two years ago, to her present post.

An untitled newscutting, amongst Flora's papers, dated around 1920, records in glowing terms the work of Flora at the Leicester Frith *'where shell-shock men are being brought back to complete health.'* The article points out that Leicester enjoyed the distinction of having started the first hospital for shell-shock cases outside London and *'one of the most successful too'.* Alongside a photograph of Flora, looking suspiciously young, the report continues:

'Miss Scott finds the work at the Leicester Frith exceedingly interesting, and can tell of some remarkable cures. One man who came in a presentation bath chair, never expecting to use his legs again, left the Frith at the end of three months able to do a walk of four or five miles, and is now back at his pre-war work. Other men who have been absolutely dumb for many months have left the Frith able to speak and laugh and sing as well as anybody. The fame of the Frith has spread throughout the land, for there is always a long list of men waiting to be admitted.'

Since no records survive relating to this period in the history of what was later known as Glen Frith Hospital, it is necessary to rely on newscuttings

Nursing in Serbia with Lady Paget in 1915

amongst Flora's own papers in order to establish the length of Flora's stay. An undated report headed *'Resignation of Miss Scott'* records that Flora had handed in her resignation and regretted that she would not remain as matron until the closing of the Home. This suggests a date around 1921, when the Ministry of Pensions had announced that they were no longer willing to fund the hospital and Leicester Borough Council was negotiating to take it over for mental health purposes.

The tone of regret suggests that Flora's departure was precipitate but the article is very complimentary about her time there:

'[Miss Scott] has proved herself remarkably efficient in caring for inmates. Not only has she been a kind friend to those who had to seek treatment afforded by the Home, devoting the best of her nursing skill and experience to their service, but she has also proved invaluable in looking after the recreation and material comfort of the patients. Only as recently as last Tuesday evening she organised a fancy dress dance, for which she secured a number of prizes from friends, the dance proving a great success...'

Another cutting, this time from *'Women's World'* also relates to Flora's time at Glenfrith:

'Miss Scott, Matron of the Leicester Frith Home, had a delightful surprise packet by post the other morning in the shape of a decoration sent by King Peter of Serbia in recognition of the valuable services she rendered his distraught countrymen in the time of their bitter trial.

The cross which is a replica of the one issued after the last Serbian War, is in the form of a Maltese Cross, and is beautifully produced in silver and blue enamel, with the Serbian coat of arms worked in, the whole being surmounted by a crown. Miss Scott is naturally as proud as she is pleased with her beautiful decoration.'

A letter amongst Flora's papers suggests that Flora requested a translation of the Cyrillic lettering on the front of the St Sava decoration from the Secretary of the The Serbian Relief Fund, Marjory L Biggs. Miss

Nurse Scott after Serbia

Biggs' letter in response, addressed to her as Matron at Leicester Frith Home of Recovery and dated 29th April 1920, explained –misleadingly- that the phrase translated as 'With His Work He Achieved Everything'. A more modern translation of 'One's own work achieves all' makes rather more sense.

The order of St Sava had first been awarded by the King of Serbia in 1883 as a medal for civilians for meritorious conduct. It was divided in to five classes with the highest, the Grand Cross, bestowed on leading figures amongst the English medical units, such as Elsie Inglis, James Berry and Lady Paget. Presumably, Flora like many other members of the units in Serbia, received the fifth class. Later, she would also receive a medal from the War Office for women's service commemorating her work as a Nursing Sister with the Serbian Relief Fund but since all members of the Serbian Relief Fund and other bodies like the Scottish Women's Hospitals qualified for this medal, it cannot have been as pleasing as her St Sava decoration.

After her sudden departure from Glen Frith, perhaps reflecting her frustration at the imminent change of purpose for the hospital, Flora apparently disappears from Leicester. She does not resurface again until 1933, when surprisingly, she is to be found working as matron of The Dunraven Nursing Home at 25 Trinity Street, Ryde in the Isle of Wight. Flora had evidently returned to her first calling, running a nursing home for medical, convalescent and chronic cases but in doing so, had left behind her Leicester roots for good. By 1935, she had moved to be matron of Home Hospital, Eastridge Court, Bellevue Road in Ryde. It was here that she would spend the rest of her life.[188]

Where was Flora between 1921 and 1933? It is tempting to think that she went to visit her family in Canada but there is no trace of her name in surviving passenger lists. Her brother Sydney was by now the Treasurer of an Anglican School in Montreal and Gertrude was working as a secretary at the Ritz Carlton Hotel in the same city. She was the first to pay a home visit between July and September in 1920. Did she persuade Flora to join her in Canada? Gertrude again visited England in October 1924, this time on a visit paid for by her brother, in order to recover from illness.

Nursing in Serbia with Lady Paget in 1915

Her brother Sydney and his wife did not visit England again until 1933 by which time Flora was apparently settled in the Isle of Wight. Gertrude it seems, did not remain in Canada, for by 29th September 1939, when a national emergency register of civilians was compiled, she was working as a secretary for Flora in Ryde.

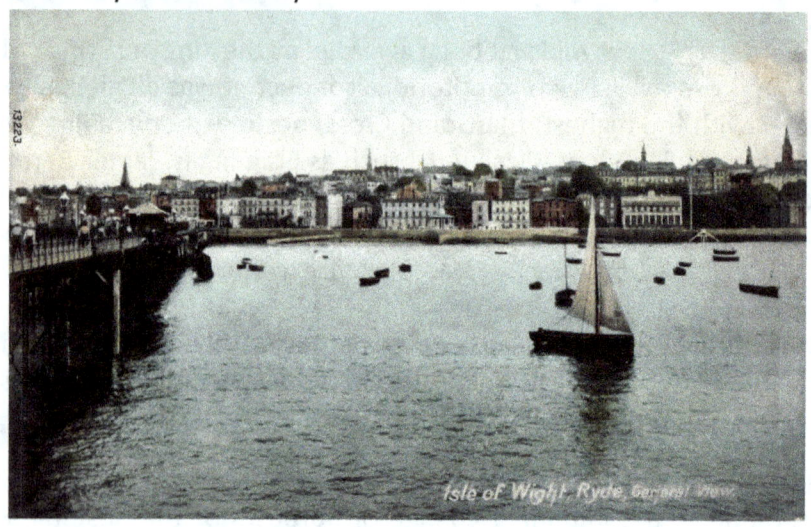

Postcard of Ryde Pier, 1915

It is not difficult to understand why Flora chose the Island as a site for her Nursing Home. The clement climate there seems to hold a particular attraction for Midlanders and during the First World War Sir Arthur Hazlerigg had even offered a house in the Isle of Wight, rent free for the duration of the war, to the Mayor of Leicester for use by disabled soldiers, although the offer was politely declined.[189] The site of Eastridge Court, a large Villa much like the former nursing home in Victoria Road, has now been replaced by modern apartments but the appeal of the site, conveniently close to the centre of the town, with fine views over the Solent to Southsea and Portsmouth, is very obvious.

There is no record of Flora's time in Ryde. When her sister Gertrude died at the Home Hospital – a name recalling Miss Pell's establishment in Leicester all those years ago- on 14 April 1953, Flora was an executor with her sisters Constance Annie Scott-Roy, a widow and Mrs Agnes

Nurse Scott after Serbia

Morwood Stewart. She left an estate of £5887.0s11d. Flora died at her Home Hospital just over a year later on 19th May 1954 and her effects of £8936.17s 10d went to the Bank for payment of debts. Like her sister before her, Flora was cremated at Southampton Crematorium, there being no crematorium on the Island at this date.[190]

Presumably, it was at this point that a family member decided to present her surviving papers to the Imperial War Museum. Aunt Tod's trip to Serbia was by then a very distant memory...

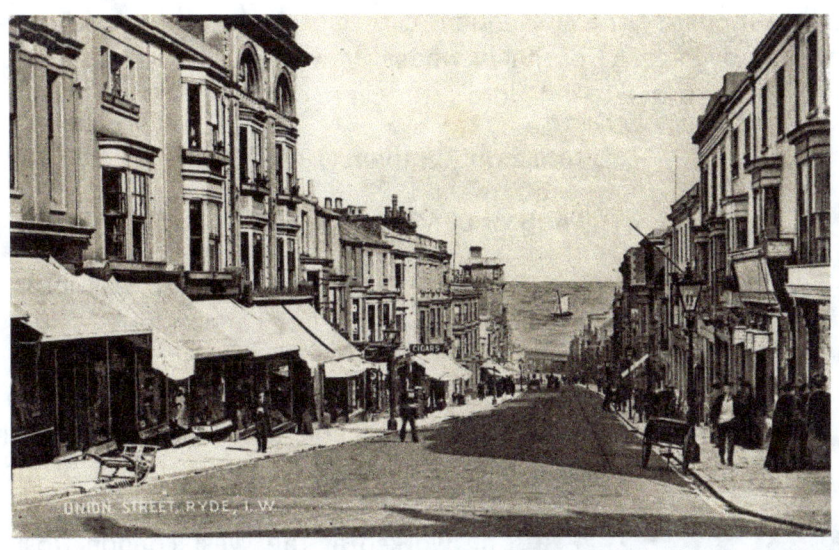

Postcard of Union Street, Ryde, c. 1924

Nursing in Serbia with Lady Paget in 1915

Chapter 9

The Cast of Characters

It proved impossible to tell Flora's story without a wider explanation of Lady Paget's mission to Serbia and the background of British humanitarian efforts in that country during the First World War. In doing so, I encountered so many characters that deserve a book in themselves, that I could not conclude the tale without acknowledging at least a few of those who played such an important part. The following biographical notes summarise the subsequent career of some of those who were part of Lady Paget's Hospital or whose eyewitness accounts of events in Serbia have helped to put Flora's story in to context.

Dr J Johnston Abraham (1876-1963)

Author of *My Balkan Log*

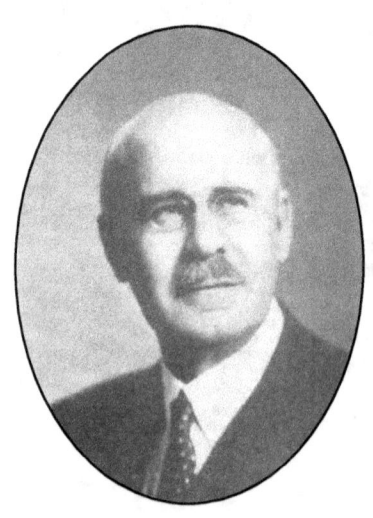

James Johnston Abraham was born in Coleraine, County Londonderry on 16 Aug 1876. He was the eldest son of William Abraham JP, a tea merchant.[191] He was educated at Coleraine Academical Institute, University of Dublin and the London Hospital. After qualification as a doctor, he worked at the West London Hospital as a house surgeon from 1901 until 1906. Having spent a year as a ship's surgeon in 1907, he published a book about his experiences entitled 'The Surgeon's Log' in 1911 . Other books about his medical experiences followed, including 'My Balkan Log' in 1922 which recounted his time as a medical officer with the British Red Cross in Skoplje, from October 1914 to March 1915.

Finally, Abraham broke down in health and as his contract and those of his colleagues with the British Red Cross had expired, the unit accepted

The Cast of Characters

an offer from the Wimborne Unit to relieve them of their work :

'The end came quite quietly, and yet suddenly. There was hardly a word from anyone. We just melted away like passengers from a ship after a long voyage.'[192]

His colleague Dr Banks accepted command of the British Red Cross unit in Vrintski and took with him two doctors, but Dr Abrahams departed for Salonika in the company of two nurses from the Paget unit, Sister Fry and her brother. Abraham later joined the RAMC and served with distinction in Portugal and Egypt, rising to the rank of Lieutenant Colonel. He received several awards for his war service, earning the Serbian Order of St Sava in 1915, the DSO in 1918, and CBE in 1919.

The Doctor seemed loath to use real names in his memoirs and consistently recorded the Russian Doctor, Esther Kadisch, as 'The Little Red Woman' in a reference to her red hair. His colleague Dr Banks, was likewise always 'Barclay' in his memoirs and Dr Holmes was inevitably 'Sherlock'. Accordingly, Sister Fry was named as Sister Rowntree thoughout, in a deliberate confusion of names of chocolate manufacturers.

In 1920, Abraham married Lilian Angela Francis of London. His medical career had included terms as resident medical officer in London Lock Hospital, and Assistant surgeon at Princess Beatrix Hospital but he finished his career in general practice in County Clare.

In the epilogue to *My Balkan Log*, Abraham described a chance meeting in Egypt with the former leader of the British Red Cross unit in Skoplje, Dr Mclaren, a Canadian Scotsman always referred to as 'the Chief':

'A tall thin man, with a slight stoop, wearing the South African ribbons and that of the order of St Sava entered... Instead of the dazzling sunshine of Egypt outside... I saw the mud and rain of Uscub, the horrible pesthouse hospital, heard the song of the dead played by a Serbian band in the distance, felt that if I turned my head and went outside I should smell the sickly odour of dead and dying Austrians in the straw. I found that in spite of my tight tunic and the sweltering heat I was shivering;

Nursing in Serbia with Lady Paget in 1915

for somehow at the sight of him the whole incredible nightmare of it all came back to me, as vividly as if it had happened on the previous day..'[193]

Edward Beric Alabaster (1893-1971)

Dresser with Lady Paget's Unit

Edward was the fifth son of Arthur Alabaster, a goldsmith and later manufacturer of jewellery, and his wife Catherine Birch. He was born at Park Hill, Mosely in Birmingham on 14 April 1893 and educated at King Edward VI School.[194] From there, he followed his older brother George Herbert to commence medical studies at Birmingham University in January 1912.

In October 1914, he left his studies to join Morrison's party with Lady Paget's unit. Morrison wrote later :

'My four dressers – Mr E B Alabaster, Mr H W Hall, Mr Frank Newey and Mr Cloudesley Smith – were indispensable, for on them fell the brunt of dressing noisome wounds all day long. Mr Newey was my house surgeon and right hand man...'[195]

Alabaster returned with the unit in April 1915 and resumed his studies, qualifying in 1916. He immediately joined the Royal Army Medical Corps and was posted to Mesopotamia rising to the rank of Captain. In addition to the victory medals awarded by the British Army he was awarded the Serbian White Eagle Cross.

On demobilisation he resolved to specialise in ophthalmology and qualified at Oxford in 1921. The following year, he was appointed as surgeon to the Birmingham Eye Hospital where he was to continue serving for thirty six years. There followed a distinguished career in ophthalmology, culminating with his election as a Fellow of the Royal College of Surgeons in 1948. The extent of his influence is clear in Kelly's trade directory for 1937 which listed him as Hon. Surgeon to Birmingham and Midland Eye Hospital; Hon. Opthalmic Surgeon to the Children's Hospital, Birmingham; Opthalmic Surgeon to the City of Birmingham Mental Hospital; Oculist to Worcestershire County Council

The Cast of Characters

and ophthalmic specialist to the Ministry of Pensions.

He married Margaret Verrinder Sydenham at Edgbaston on 2 July 1924. He and his family were resident at The Highlands, Marlborough Avenue in Bromsgrove in 1939 with his elderly mother, when he was serving as a Quartermaster in the Emergency Medical Service.

In later life, Alabaster struggled with diabetes. In 1946, ill health forced him to relinquish his appointment at the Children's Hospital but he continued at the Eye Hospital until 1958.[196] He died on 13 July 1971.

Dr Fergus Armstrong (1887-1976)

Surgeon

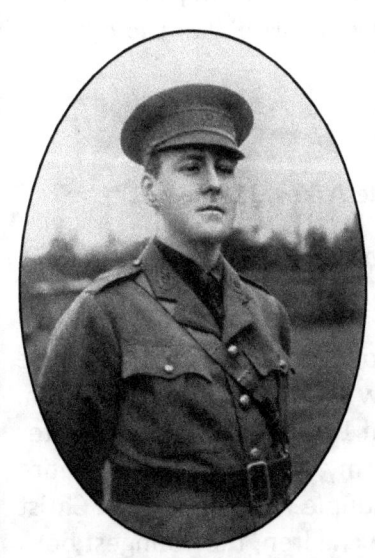

Born on 9th December 1887 at Llanfair Talhaiarn, a village a few miles south of Abergele in the County of Denbigh, Fergus was the youngest of the seven children of Charles and Janet Armstrong. Although, Charles and his wife were both originally from Scotland, and two of the oldest children were born in Newcastle, the family by this stage had settled into farming in Wales. Fergus qualified as a Doctor at Edinburgh University in 1909 and subsequently became a Fellow of the Royal College of Surgeons in 1913.

He first appeared in Skoplje when he was surgeon with the First British Field Hospital under Dr Hartnell-Beavis, which spent six weeks helping out at Lady Paget's Hospital in April 1915. Claude Askew who accompanied the unit, said of Armstrong: *'Our chief surgeon was Mr Fergus Armstrong FRCS who had given up an important post to join us, and a more able operator or pleasant companion could not have been desired...'*[197]

Nursing in Serbia with Lady Paget in 1915

Armstrong accompanied the Serbian Army on an expedition into Albania which led to the occupation of Durazzo but once his contract with the First British Field Hospital had expired, agreed to serve as Surgeon in Chief to Lady Paget's Hospital in Skoplje. He remained in Skoplje and was repatriated with the rest of the party in February 1916. He would recall years later, how on the journey home, he had met Queen Marie of Romania and worked in her hospital.[198]

Once back in England, Armstrong joined the Royal Army Medical Corps and was posted to Netley Hospital near Southampton with the rank of Captain.

After the war, he appears to have established a practice in Treorchy in the Rhondda Valley, residing at 'Gilnockie', 65 Dyfodwy Street. He died there on 5 November 1976 and was buried at St Michael's Lutheran Church Cemetery. He remained a close friend of Dr Thomas Gwynn Maitland, a fellow Welshman, who had served with him in Skoplje at Lady Paget's Hospital.

Alice Askew (1874-1917) and Claude Askew (1865-1917)

Writers and authors of *The Stricken Land Serbia as we saw it*, pub.1916

Claude Askew was born in Kensington, on 27 November 1865, the youngest child of the Reverend John Askew and was educated at Eton. Alice Jane de Courcy was born in London on 18 June 1874, the daughter of Henry Leake, a captain in the British army who was later to retire with the honorary rank of Lt-Colonel. The couple were married at Christ Church, London in July 1900 and had three children, the youngest born in July 1916. It was shortly after their marriage that they collaborated on their first novel *'The Shulamite'* which was published in 1904 under their joint names. It was the first of some ninety novels.

At the beginning of the First World War, the pair volunteered with Dr Hector Munro's Red Cross Ambulance Corps at Furnes in Belgium which

The Cast of Characters

enabled them to write several novels set against the background of Red Cross work. It must have been during this period, that they made

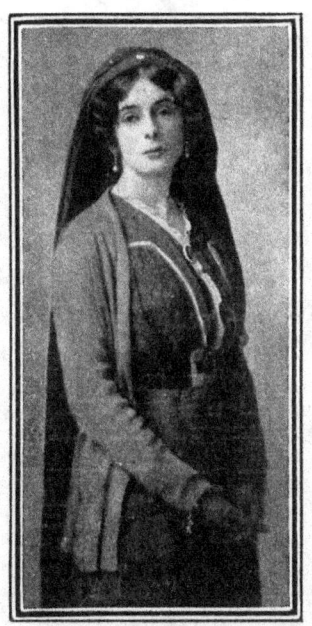
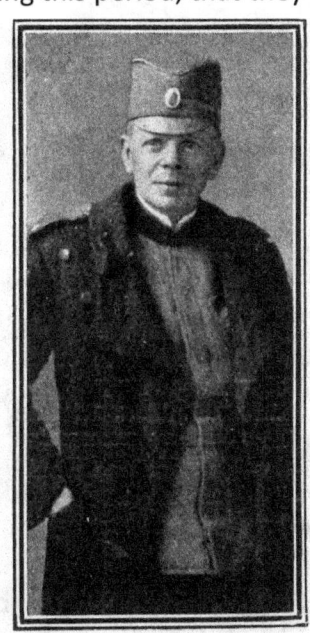

Mr and Mrs Askew (from The Great War*, VI, p. 113, 1916)*

the acquaintance of Dr Hartnell Beavis who worked closely with the Corps. In April 1915, they travelled to Serbia as part of a relief effort with the British Field Hospital under Dr Hartnell Beavis, acting as Special Correspondents for the *Daily Express*. After a visit to Skoplje, they accompanied the Serbian army and were part of its famous 'Great Retreat' across the mountains of Albania during the winter of 1915/16. Their account of the experience '*The Stricken Land*' was published on their return to England. Claude was given an honorary commission of major in the Serbian army.

By October 1916, Alice had joined her husband in Corfu where most of the Serbian army had been evacuated and worked there for the Serbian Red Cross. On the night of 5th October 1917, after a visit to Rome, the couple were returning to Corfu aboard the Italian steamer *Citta di Bari* when the ship was hit by a German torpedo and sunk. Both Alice and

Nursing in Serbia with Lady Paget in 1915

Claude were drowned. Alice was buried on 30 October 1917 at Porto Karboni on the island of Korcula. Claude's body was never recovered.

Ada Ann Barlow(1880-1953)

Auxiliary worker

Born on 6 Dec 1880 in Runcorn, in Cheshire, Ada Ann Shallcross was the daughter of a waterman. By the time of the 1901 census, she was a servant working in Salford although by then she had probably already met her future husband Henry Barlow, a house decorator. The couple were married in the summer of that year and went on to have two sons: Henry in 1903 and Stanley in 1905, both baptised in Weaste in Salford.

When Dr Abrahams encountered Ada working in a hospital in Nish, he described her in unnecessarily harsh terms as *'an unwanted woman'* but something of her personal tragedy can be gleaned from the census for 1911. By this time, poor Ada was boarding in Salford and earning her living as a packer. Her husband however, was also living in Salford with his new 'wife' Minnie, an Irish girl from Middleton in County Cork, his two sons by Ada and two more children aged two and six months.

There is no record of Mrs Barlow having any formal training as a nurse but it is likely that she had some experience of hospitals, perhaps as a VAD. Somehow, this indomitable woman found herself part of the group of women who left London for Serbia on 12 August 1914 under the auspices of the Serbian Red Cross. This rather odd group had been hastily assembled by Mabel Grujic, the beautiful forty-one year old American wife of Slavo Grujic, the Serbian Under-secretary of foreign affairs. With her were Flora Sandes, another American Miss Emily Simmonds and four other 'nurses': Miss O'Brien, Mrs Hartney, Miss McEwan and Miss Mann.

After travelling through France and Italy, they sailed from Brindisi to Salonika and arrived at a military hospital in Kragujevatz at the beginning of September. It was here that the correspondent of the *Daily Chronicle*

The Cast of Characters

encountered Mrs Barlow and the four other nurses labouring under appalling conditions in December. By this stage Flora Sandes had returned to England to raise funds and Emily Simmonds had departed for America with the same intention.[199] The correspondent found the women full of praise for their Serbian patients, but also noted:

'Anything more unlike the environment in a hospital at home than their surroundings, it is impossible to conceive. Primitive is too mild a term for it. But these women make light of difficulties and discomforts, and do not spare themselves in their efforts to secure a measure of comfort for those committed to their charge.'[200]

Mrs Barlow told the correspondent that they had also just admitted Austrian wounded for the first time. She had talked to them in German and found that they were glad to be prisoners:

'Altogether some 2,000 patients have passed through the hospital and there have been remarkably few deaths – not more than 50 I think- and very few amputations...'

A day later, the correspondent returned to the hospital but found it dismantled. He was told that the English nurses had been transferred to a hospital at Nish. He hoped that this was untrue and that the women had proceeded to Lady Paget's hospital at Skoplje: '*...for there they will find better quarters and adequate equipment. They have encountered and overcome difficulties with such an indomitable spirit that one is proud to think they are one's countrywomen.*'

It was at Nish, that the British Red Cross found Mrs Barlow, by now working on alone. They eventually brought her back to their hospital in Skoplje where in a by now familiar pattern, she found herself labouring alone once again, after the British Red Cross had withdrawn. Dr Kadisch also refused to leave the patients at this stage and it is possible that Mrs Barlow and the Russian Doctor were the *'two suffragettes'* to whom Mabel Dearmer referred when she recalled a speech by Sir Thomas Lipton:

Nursing in Serbia with Lady Paget in 1915

'He said that there were, when he left, some three hundred deaths a day at the hospital at Skoplje. One place that he described had no doctors and no nurses; the dead and dying were tended only by two suffragettes. He did not seem to realise the enormous compliment he was paying to the pioneers of that women's movement.'[201]

There is no record of Mrs Barlow's opinion about women's suffrage but she would certainly have more cause than most to resent the unequal status of women.

As the Bulgarians closed in on Skoplje in October 1915, Lady Paget found Mrs Barlow alone, nursing over a hundred wounded, after the Serbian staff had fled. She joined Lady Paget's Hospital at this point and became a prisoner of the Bulgarians with the rest of the staff.

After repatriation in February 1916, this dedicated woman went on to work with Serbian refugees in Corsica. Once home again she devoted herself to fund raising for the Serbs, organising amongst other things the Mayor's Fund for Serbia in Manchester. The local newspapers for Burnley in 1918, contain several reports of Mrs Barlow addressing meetings with patriotic fervour, retelling her experiences as a prisoner of the Bulgarians and urging local women to serve as auxiliary workers.

After the war, like Flora, she returned to her previous existence and obscurity. She was to spend the rest of her life in Salford and the surrounding area, still using her married name.

James Berry (1860-1946)

Surgeon

Berry was born on 4th February 1860 at Kingston, Ontario, the eldest son of Edward Berry, a solicitor and shipowner who had originated from Leicester but at this stage, seems to have divided his time between Croydon and Canada. James was born with a cleft palate and a short leg but did not allow such disabilities to confine his ambitions. He was

The Cast of Characters

educated at Whitgift School in Croydon and St Bartholomew's Hospital.

From 1885, he served as surgeon to the Alexandra Hospital for Diseases of the Hip and earned a respected reputation as a surgeon and teacher. It was for his work on cleft palates and goitre, that he would earn most distinction.

In 1891, he was elected surgeon at the Royal Free Hospital in London.

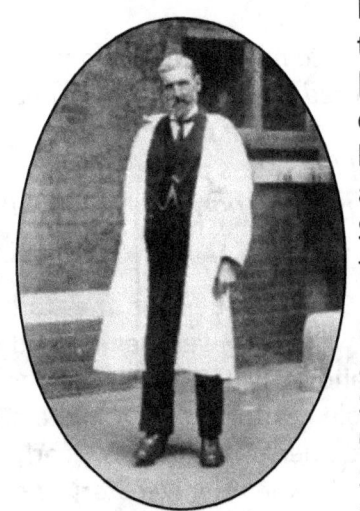

He proceeded to marry the anaesthetist at the Royal Free, Dr Frances May Dickinson [qv] in the same year. The couple worked closely together and spent their holidays bicycling round southern Europe, acquiring a fluency in French, German, Magyar and Serbian that would set them in good stead for their coming adventures.

In December 1914, the couple were inspired at a meeting held in aid of Serbia at the Steinway Hall, to offer their help to Madame Grujic, the ubiquitous American wife of the Serbian Under-Secretary for Foreign Affairs. She urged them to assemble a hospital unit whilst she secured approval from the Serbian Government. The couple proceeded to gather personnel and supplies, drawing largely upon the staff and resources of the Royal Free Hospital. Although the Berrys attended a meeting of the Serbian Relief Fund on 7th Jan 1915, Berry declined to join the Wimborne Unit as surgeon in charge under Mr Graham and judged it wiser to preserve the independence of their unit.[202] In the end, Berry and his wife went out as joint leaders of the unit, with funding of £1000 from the Serbian Relief Fund, and further support from the British Red Cross Society. Although they had aspired to be known as the Royal Free Hospital Unit, this was opposed by the Hospital Board and the unit eventually sailed under *'the colourless title of Anglo-Serbian Hospital',* a name which was fairly swiftly forgotten. Instead, the unit was universally known as 'The Berry Mission'.[203]

Nursing in Serbia with Lady Paget in 1915

Flora met the ebullient James Berry aboard the SS Dilwara and evidently enjoyed his company. When the Berry unit was firmly established at Vrnjatchka Banja, a former health spa in Northern Serbia, it enjoyed a considerable reputation not only for its medical facilities but also for the musical evenings enjoyed there. Elsie Corbett who was nursing with the British Red Cross unit which was also based in the town, attended a musical evening at 'Tirapia', the hydropathic establishment taken over as a hospital by the Berry unit:

'We sat on the terrace outside the big self-contained building and were fed upon delicious fruit and cakes, illuminated by gentle lighting and regaled by song... The artist, Jan Gordon, and his wife played and sang to the banjo; an Austrian prisoner and one of the sisters played the violin and two Sisters sang. A prisoner orderly played the native gusla and a Serbian officer sang to it, quaint little tunes...'[204]

The Berry hospital fell to the Austrians on 9th November and the staff remained prisoners until 18th February 1916 when they were repatriated via Belgrade, Budapest, Vienna and Switzerland, arriving home in March. A highly entertaining account of the whole venture, with chapters contributed by Berry, his wife and other members of what was clearly a very happy unit, was published in 1916, under the title *'The Story of a Red Cross Unit in Serbia'*.

Undeterred by this adventure, the intrepid couple went on to lead a Red Cross unit in Rumania and serve with the Serbian Army again at Odessa in Southern Russia 1916-1917. For these feats, Berry was awarded the Order of St Sava, the Star of Rumania and the Order of St Anna of Russia.

In 1917, Berry returned once more to his medical career serving as honorary military surgeon at the military hospitals at Napsbury and Bermondsey. He retired in 1927, having received a knighthood two years earlier. The couple spent their last years together at their country house 'Bramblebury' at Dunsmure, Wendover near Aylesbury.

A year after his wife's death in 1934, Berry married Mabel Marian Ingram, a fellow surgeon who had joined the Berry Unit as a dresser and

The Cast of Characters

radiographer in May 1915, later also accompanying them to Rumania and Southern Russia. The couple settled at Kirby Gate, Westmead, Roehampton and the new Lady Berry continued to practise in the district. Berry died on 17 March 1946 at the age of eight six.[205]

The Honourable Richard Cecil Frederick Chichester (1889-1915)

First secretary to Lady Paget

Chichester was the youngest son of Arthur Henry Chichester 3rd Lord Templemore and his second wife, Alice Dawkins of Dunbrody Park, Arthurstown, Co Wexford. His great grandfather had been created a peer in 1831 after serving as an MP and at court. His family's relationship to the Paget family was complex. The 1st Lord Templemore had married Lady Augusta Paget, daughter of Henry Paget, 1st Marquess of Anglesey (also the great grandfather of Lady Paget). His son, Chichester's grandfather, very unhelpfully complicated matters further, when he married his first cousin once removed, Laura Caroline Paget, the daughter of Sir Arthur Paget (a cousin of his mother, Lady Augusta).

Chichester was educated at Harrow and University College, Oxford, graduating in 1910.

At the beginning of the war, having been judged medically unfit, Chichester joined his 'cousin' Lady Paget to serve as her secretary in Serbia. Like other leading men in the unit, he was awarded the honorary title of Captain in the Serbian Army. His efficiency seems to have impressed all who met him. Flora certainly enjoyed his humour and Lady Muriel Herbert socialised with him happily, trekking with him to Novi Bazar.

At the end of June, when the Wimborne unit broke up, Chichester joined up with Lady Herbert and her friend Elia Lindon and started to plan a scheme of relief for the many families left destitute after the departure of the men to war. Occupying *'a funny little house outside Skoplje'*[206] called the Villa Velika which they rechristened *'The Nest'* because of the

Nursing in Serbia with Lady Paget in 1915

abundant wildlife, the party did all their own cooking and relied on the one soldier posted to them for the washing up . Here they entertained royally before starting on *'our great trek'* round Southern Macedonia. Lady Herbert later wrote that they were *'wonderfully happy'* and recalled 'Dick Chichester' as she termed him, spontaneously striking up *'Now Thank we all our God',* which they all sang together as they trotted down a stony road.[207]

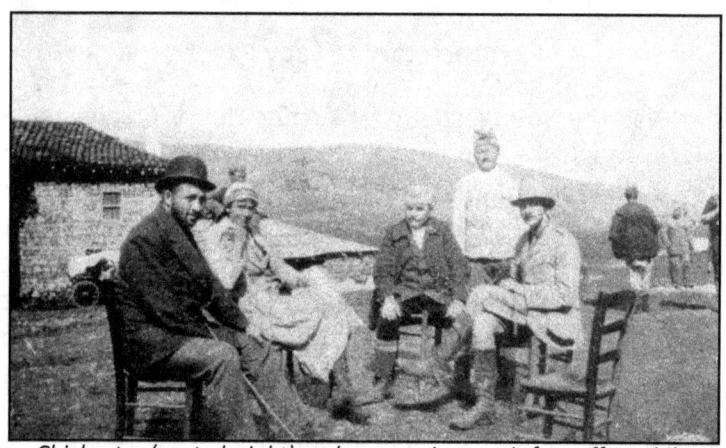

Chichester (seated, right) and companions wait for coffee whilst trekking. From Serbia and the Serbians *by Lady Herbert, 1915*

After three weeks on horseback, often sleeping out under the stars, the happy threesome returned to Skoplje and iced beers at Zurinsky's where most of the English community who could afford it, used to congregate: *'If the previous journey to Novi Bazar had been almost perfection, this one has proved to be its equal... And we proved again that three was by no means a bad number to make a travelling party of, in spite of all old adages.'*[208]

Chichester died on 31st July 1915 having contracted a virulent form of typhoid fever whilst he continued to distribute aid to destitute families .

His parents, Lord and Lady Templemore, who visited Lady Paget in Skoplje in August, probably took some comfort at least from the fact that their son was so happy during his last days in Serbia.[209] Amongst many tributes paid to him by Serbs, including even their Prime Minister, was

The Cast of Characters

this telegram received by Lady Paget from a member of the municipality of Novi Bazar:

'In the name of the citizens of Novi Bazar, I beg you to accept my deepest sympathy, learning the news of the sudden death of our young and noble Richard Chichester, who came to Serbia under pressure of his love for right, and far away from his own country left his life on the field of duty'[210]

Helen Marion Coleman (1867-1956)

Nurse with Lady Paget

Helen was born on 16 October 1867 at Sulgrave in Northamptonshire. She was the daughter of a farmer, William Goodwin Coleman and his wife Frances, the sixth of their eight children. Although her father was from Greatworth in Northamptonshire, her mother had been born in Amersham in Buckinghamshire and the young Helen spent time with her mother's sisters Annie and Sarah Fowler, who had settled in Banbury.

At the time of the 1891 census, Helen was working as a governess in Lewisham but evidently abandoned this career when she enrolled at the Queen's Hospital in Birmingham in January 1893 to train as a nurse. She was registered as a nurse in October 1895 and worked as a staff nurse at Queen's before turning to private nursing. In 1905, she was living in Erdington, Birmingham, when she made one of many Atlantic crossings to visit her brother in Covington, Virginia. The *Leicester Daily Post* would later describe her as *'a lady of culture'* who had travelled *'a great deal and lived for a number of years in America.'*

Helen was one of the large contingent of Birmingham nurses who were recruited by Mr Morrison and joined Lady Paget's Unit in October 1914. She claimed an association with Leicester as the niece of Alderman G T Coleman, a Leicester magistrate and her letter to friends there was published in the *Leicester Chronicle and Leicestershire Mercury* on 20 February 1915 under the headline *'Life in a Serbian Hospital whither Leicester Nurses have Gone'*. The wide ranging letter chronicled the

Nursing in Serbia with Lady Paget in 1915

early difficulties of the hospital when they took over the school buildings but also the charm of Skoplje and the evident pleasure in haggling with the Turkish shopkeepers : '...*if he will not come down enough, you can walk out of the shop, say 'scoop' (too much) and he will watch for your return and hand it over promptly at your own price. There is a wonderful outdoor market every Tuesday, where country folk, Serbs, Albanians, Turks, Macedonians and others bring their wares and sell. We have bought some very nice things there...'*[211]

The letter also described some of the health problems encountered by members of the unit:

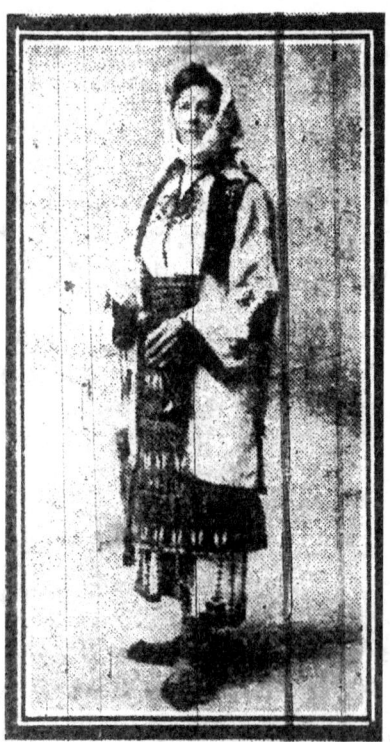

Coleman in Serbian costume, pictured in the Leicester Daily Post *on her return from the Balkans, 19 June 1915*

'I am thankful to say I have kept well so far except for bad throats from the smells but most of our party have been ill, four with scarlet fever, several with a kind of malarial fever and one sister died on Christmas Day from blood poisoning. She had never been well since we came out

The Cast of Characters

here. *She was buried in the Serbian cemetery near an English doctor who died two years ago, and had a very big funeral. Four Serbian priests in gorgeous robes took part in it but our burial service, or part of it, was read by the British Vice-Consul who attended in full uniform, and his flag covered the coffin. It was very sad, and we all felt it very much...'*

Helen returned to England with the main unit in April 1915, determined to raise funds which she planned to distribute on her return to Serbia. In June, she was in Leicester, posing for photographs dressed in Serbian costume and offering 'little talks' about her recent experiences as a nurse in the country. She had organised an exhibition of Serbian artefacts at St Peter's Parish Room and at the Robert Hall Memorial in Narborough Road and an interview with her was published on the front page of the *Leicester Daily Post* of 18th June 1915. Under the eye-catching headlines of *'Soldiers Whose Limbs Dropped off'* and *'Atrocities by Magyars'*, she recounted once more the horrors of the recent war and the typhus epidemic. She had been in Nish, the seat of the Serbian Government, in order to nurse the unit's interpreter and recalled the shortage of food there:

'Serbia is in urgent need of money for food and clothing. The crops last year were destroyed by the Austrians and there is such a shortage of bread that the government are issuing only a certain quantity each day. Miss Coleman actually saw the Minister of Finance coming away from a place where bread is handed out with a loaf under his arm...'[212]

Despite her plans to return to Serbia, by July 1915 , she was bound for Egypt with the Queen Alexandra's Imperial Military Nursing Service. However, she remained only a short time before ill health forced her to return in November. Evidently her *'bad throats'* were still a problem. She was posted to the hospital at Bramshott but after an operation on her tonsils, was still deemed unfit for duty in December . She finally resigned from her post at the 1st Southern General Hospital in Birmingham on 29 November 1916.

A medal card at the National Archives records that Helen eventually returned to Serbia with the Australian Serbian Canteens.[213] This was an

Nursing in Serbia with Lady Paget in 1915

organisation set up in October 1918 by Olive King, an Australian who had served as a driver with the Scottish Women's Hospitals and later with the Serbian Army. (She had on the way earned a medal for bravery for her part in the great fire at Salonika). Aided by a rich father, Kelso King, and funds he managed to raise from the people of Sydney, Olive set up canteens across Serbia to serve the Serbian soldiers as they reconquered their country. Coleman was one of the three salaried helpers whom Olive hired initially to help in the canteens at a rate of £2.2.0 per week.[214]

In April 1919, Olive found Coleman in charge of a flourishing canteen in a ruined hotel opposite the fortress in Belgrade and was agreeably surprised by the encounter:

'After much searching, I ran her to earth, & was quite touched by the warmth of her welcome. I had expected something quite different, from the tales I heard... She was certainly most awfully kind...'[215]

In June, Coleman was helping Olive at a new canteen in Kragujevatz although she was troubled once more by ill health and in need of a holiday. She was still working there at the end of the year.[216] Dr Katherine MacPhail also encountered her in Belgrade in 1919 and benefitted from her fundraising skills:

'Miss Coleman, attached to some other mission, and two Serbian ladies, got up a concert for us and we had a most delightful evening in a hall in Belgrade, which was a cinema...'[217]

When the canteens were finally wound up in 1920, the remaining funds were divided between Belgrade University and Dr MacPhail's hospital for tubercular children near Belgrade.[218]

After her return from Serbia, Helen continued to live with her sister at 24 Hillaris Road, Gravelly Hill, in Birmingham but made regular trips to America. By 1939, she was living at 108 Banbury Road, Stratford on Avon describing herself as a trained nurse, supervising a First Aid Post in Stratford. She died on 29 August 1956 in Banbury, leaving effects of

The Cast of Characters

£1793.9s to her two unmarried sisters.

Letitia Louisa Cluley (1887-1980)

Nurse with Flora Scott

Letitia was the eldest girl of eight children born to John Cluley, a commercial traveller in boots, and his wife, Louisa. She was born on 12th Mar 1887 in Leicester, but the family moved shortly afterwards to Blaby.

Letitia worked as a hatband maker before she joined North Evington Poor Law Infirmary [later the General Hospital] at the age of twenty two, to train as a nurse.[219] She entered the Hospital on 25 April 1910 and passed her qualifying exam, three years later. Although she stayed on to qualify as a midwife on 28th April 1914,[220] she left the Hospital to enter Miss Scott's Nursing Home on 30th June 1914. She had not therefore been working with Flora very long before she agreed to accompany her to Serbia.

Details from Letitia's letter home to her mother Mrs J Clully [sic] at 3 Lansdowne Road, in Leicester, describing the journey to Malta and alluding obliquely to her trials in the Bay of Biscay, were published in the *Leicester Daily Post* of 4th February. A further letter, published on 8th April, under the headline *'Nursing Serbian Wounded. Leicester Lady's Experiences'* quoted extracts from her letter describing the horror of the typhus epidemic. The article concluded:

'Miss Cluley adds 'I think I told you about the young boy who had his leg off. He had been wounded four times. He is only 21, and married. He's improving wonderfully and I'm so proud of him. Every morning when I go on duty he calls me to shake hands and say 'Dobrolutre' or 'Good morning'.[221]

In June 1915, when Flora was safely back in Leicester, it was stated that Nurse Pickering had returned home but that Nurse Cluley was still in the surgical hospital in Skoplje.[222] Since she is not listed as a member of staff

Nursing in Serbia with Lady Paget in 1915

in Lady Paget's second report, she presumably returned in July.

Letitia was baptised as an adult at Christ Church in Leicester on 7 March 1917 and was apparently back living with her parents at 3 Lansdowne Road by this stage. In June of the same year, Letitia joined the Territorial Force Nursing Service and served as a staff nurse in the 5th Northern General Hospital in Leicester, both in Swain Street Military Hospital (in part of the workhouse) and the North Evington War Hospital (formerly the Poor Law Infirmary), until May 1919.[223] The register of nurses for Evington Poor Law Infirmary recorded that she returned as a ward sister, although there is no date given and this may refer to her time wartime service.

After the war, Letitia continued to work as a midwife and nurse in Leicester, registered in the Midwives Rolls and Registers of Nurses at various addresses: 97 Princess Road in 1926, 9 De Montfort Square and 101 Clarendon Park Road in 1931. At the outbreak of the Second World War, Letitia was living at 260 Queens Road in Leicester with her eighty one year old mother, Louisa Cluley. She gave her occupation as state registered nurse with the Territorial Forces. In 1946, there was an entry for her in the Register of Nurses at the same address.

Letitia died at Fakenham in Norfolk in January 1980, aged ninety two.

Dr Elsie Jean Dalyell (1881-1948)

'The Lady Doctor'

Elsie Dalyell was born in Newtown, Sydney, Australia on 13 Dec 1881. She was educated at Sydney Girls High School and started working life as a pupil teacher before entering The Women's College in 1909. She graduated in 1910 and first worked as the female resident Medical Officer at the Royal Prince Alfred Hospital in Sydney. In December 1912, she took up a fellowship at the Lister Institute of Preventative Medicine in London. Dr Dalyell arrived in Skoplje with the Wimborne unit and served as a bacteriologist under Dr G T Maitland at the Typhus Colony

The Cast of Characters

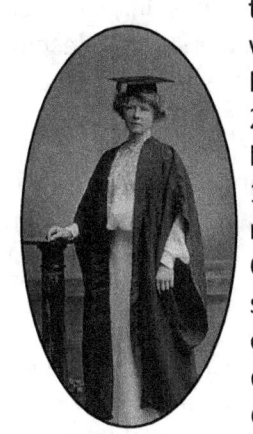

from March to April 1915. She went on to work as a bacteriologist with the Scottish Women's Hospitals – an organisation with close ties to the Serbian Relief Fund- at Royaumont Abbey near Paris from 2 May 1916 until 2 Oct 1916, serving latterly as Medical Officer at Hopital Auxiliare Asnieres sur Oise. On 20 October 1916, she embarked for Malta, as part of a women's medical unit attached to the Royal Army Medical Corps and served in Malta until 1 June 1917 when she moved with her unit to Salonika. In the early part of 1919 she moved to Constantinople to aid efforts during the cholera outbreak. She was mentioned in despatches twice [London Gazette 28 Nov 1917and 5 Jun 1919] and was awarded the Order of the British Empire. She returned to England in July 1919 and worked in Vienna on a committee appointed by the Medical Research Council and Lister Institute investigating the effect of vitamin deficiencies amongst the malnourished from 1919 until 1922.

Dr Dalyell finally returned to Australia in March 1923. After an attempt to set up a private practice failed due to financial problems, she was appointed an assistant microbiologist with the Department of Health in January 1924. From 1925 until 1935, she served on the committee of the Rachel Forster Hospital for Women in Sydney, a hospital set up in the aftermath of the First World War and staffed exclusively by women. She died on 1 Nov 1948.

Mabel Dearmer (1872-1815)

Novelist, dramatist, children book illustrator and orderly with Mrs Stobart's Unit

Mabel was born Jessie Mabel Pritchard White on 22nd March 1872 and was the daughter of Surgeon-Major William White and Selina Taylor Pritchard. In 1891, at the age of eighteen, she entered Hubert von Herkomer's Art School at Bushey and it was as an artist that she first distinguished herself, contributing her work to literary and fine art

Nursing in Serbia with Lady Paget in 1915

periodicals like *The Yellow Book* and *The Savoy*. She progressed from this to illustrating children's books and, eventually, publishing her own fiction and drama for children and adults. She achieved all this despite marrying at the tender age of nineteen and giving birth to her second son before her twenty second birthday.

Her marriage to the socialist and liturgist priest Percy Dearmer (1867-1936) led her at the last minute, to join the Third Serbian Relief Unit, under Mrs St Clair Stobart. She had attended the farewell service arranged for the all women unit, under the auspices of the Church League for Women's Suffrage, without any knowledge that her husband, who was presiding, had just been appointed Chaplain to the British Units working in Serbia and would be accompanying them:

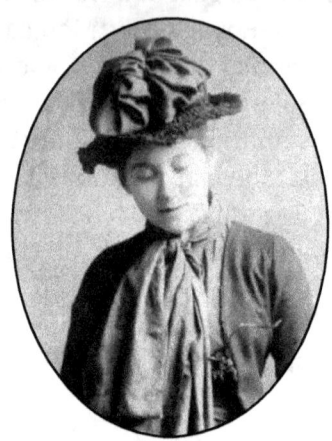

'I had only heard of Serbia as a country penetrated by disease that brought death to those who went to minister to it, and I wondered as I looked at them how many would return at the end of the expedition...'

Startled by this discovery of her husband's plans, she at once persuaded a sceptical Mrs Stobart to allow her to join the unit as a hospital orderly. Her account of the journey out to Serbia in April 1915 and her life there, which was published posthumously in 1916 as *'Letters from a Field Hospital'*, is a sensitive and revealing account of the experience.

Despite her initial misgivings, even the redoubtable Mrs Stobart came to appreciate Mrs Dearmer:

'I could not see much of her, as I never allowed myself the privilege of individual friendships, but as I passed to and fro about the camp, I loved to meet her, and to hear her humorous accounts of various little troubles. I would often stop her and ask hopefully, 'Any grievances today?' just to have the fun of a chat with her . I grew to love her, and looked forward

The Cast of Characters

to the time, when in happier days in England, I could hope to count her amongst my real friends.'[224]

Despite the obvious difficulties encountered as a lowly orderly, with frequent sickness and often chaotic organisation, Mabel endured all with good humour and had just resolved to stay on beyond her three month contract, when she fell ill with typhoid .After a brief rally, she died on 11 July 1915, aged only forty three. She was buried in Kragujevayz beside Sister Lorna Ferris who had died earlier that month and Dr Elizabeth Ross who had died from typhus in February.

Despite all she had endured, Mabel remained convinced of the futility of war:

'This war will not bring peace – no war will bring peace- only love and mercy and terrific virtues such as loving one's enemy can bring a terrific thing like peace...'

She is commemorated with her youngest son, Christopher, who died at Gallipoli a few months later, on the war memorial fountain in Oakridge Lynch near Stroud in Gloucestershire where the Dearmer family had a country cottage. Her name also appears on St Mary's Primrose Hill memorial in London.

Dr Frances May Dickinson (1857-1934)

Joint leader of the Berry Unit

Frances May Dickinson was baptised at Painswick in Gloucestershire on 21st May 1857. She was the eldest child of Sebastian Stewart Dickinson a barrister and later, Liberal MP for Stroud from 1868 to 1874. Her father had been born in Bombay, the son of Major General Thomas Dickinson of the East India Company. Her mother Frances Stephana was the daughter of William Henry Hyett of Painswick House. Her brother Willoughby Hyett Dickinson was a Liberal MP for St Pancras North from 1906 to 1918, during which time he campaigned steadfastly for women's suffrage.

Nursing in Serbia with Lady Paget in 1915

Thereafter, he was an active figure in the London County Council, raised to the peerage as Baron Dickinson in 1930.

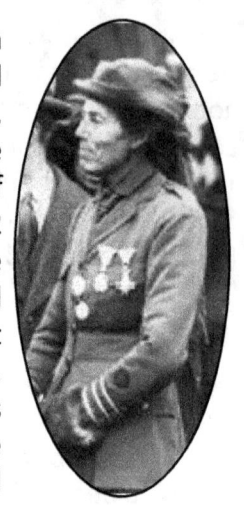

Frances, unable to follow the straightforward path of privilege so readily open to her brother, attended Bedford College in London in 1884 to study physics, chemistry, botany, biology and physiology. She went on to study medicine at the University of London, qualifying as a doctor of medicine in 1892 and surgery in 1895, before proceeding to practise in various London Hospitals. She met her husband James Berry [qv] whilst serving as the anaesthetist at the Royal Free Hospital and they married in 1891. She was a joint leader of the Berry Unit but seems rather unfairly to have remained very much in the shadow of her husband, although she accompanied him throughout the war. Her sister, Annie Dickinson joined the Berry Unit as an orderly in May 1915 and was captured with the rest of the Unit in November.

Frances served as assistant medical officer (education) to the London County Council, President of the Association of Medical Women and Honorary Secretary of the section of anaesthetists at the Royal Society of Medicine.

When she died on 15 April 1934 at the age of seventy six, she left £500 each to the Royal Free Hospital and its school of medicine for women and £1000 to a fund for medical scholarships for Serbian girls.[225]

Walter Musgrave Eaton MD (1863- c1940)

Surgeon

Eaton was born on 12 March 1863 at Wynberg in the Cape Colony. He trained at Edinburgh University qualifying as a surgeon in 1885. On 5 May 1898, at Reading in Berkshire, he married Margaret Emily Ibbetson,

The Cast of Characters

an Australian teacher who had studied at Bedford College in London, 1896-1897.

According to the biographical index for South Africa, Eaton practised in Capetown, Port Elizabeth and Basutoland before being appointed Assistant Medical Director of the Public Health Department for Southern Rhodesia c1911. Early medical directories list him as resident at Drooge Obi, Malmesbury, Cape of Good Hope.

Eaton joined Lady Paget's unit in October 1914, whilst on furlough and remained until February. Morrison spoke warmly of his colleague:

'It was a happy chance that associated me with such competent surgeons and staunch comrades as Mr Eaton, director of Bulawayo Hospital who spent his furlough from near the tropics in strenuous work for the Serbians through a Balkan winter...'[226]

Eaton returned to his posts as Assistant Medical Director and Medical Superintendent at Ingutsheni Mental Hospital in Bulawayo and was awarded the OBE for his services in 1924. His second son Sir John Willson Musgrave Eaton (1902-1981) had a distinguished career in the Royal Navy.

Ernest Frederic Eliot MD (1862-1936)

Surgeon

Eliot was baptised at Minchinhampton in Gloucestershire, where his father was serving as Curate, on 20 April 1862. His father, William Eliot, from Weymouth, went on to occupy livings in Compton Abbas in Dorset and Bristol before becoming Vicar of Aston near Birmingham. His mother Barbara was a British subject born in Madras in India. Eliot qualified as a Doctor at Edinburgh in 1884 and became a Fellow of the Royal College of Surgeons in 1898. He married Ivy Katharine Thomson, a Southsea girl, in 1890 and the couple moved to East Park Terrace in Southampton where Eliot established a medical practice. By the time of the 1901 census, the

Nursing in Serbia with Lady Paget in 1915

family were resident at 20 Cumberland Terrace and Eliot was describing himself as a surgeon and Justice of the Peace.

In January 1915, Eliot resolved to leave his wife and children and sign a three month contract with the Serbian Relief Fund to serve as a relief surgeon at Lady Paget's Hospital. He travelled out to Skoplje with Flora, apparently sustaining all his charges on a diet of champagne and cigarettes. When he arrived, the orderly Henry Squire was clearly impressed and wrote home to his parents: '... *another doctor apparently a keen humorous man with a physiognomy like a prize fighter'.*[227]

Morrison, in his account of his experiences in Serbia recorded his thanks to Mr Eliot *'who joined the staff when Mr Eaton returned in February, and is now on active service as a Major in the Royal Army Medical Corps at Malta. The loyal friendship and unfailing help of these gentlemen are entwined in all my memories of the work in Skoplje...'*[228]

When Morrison departed in February to tour Serbian hospitals, Eliott took charge in his absence.

By the time of his daughter's marriage in May 1919, Eliot was a Lieutenant Colonel in the Royal Army Medical Corps and he and his family were resident at 'The Lammas', Minchinhampton, apparently having returned to his birthplace. He died in July 1936.

Frances Ann Fry (1871- 1947)

Matron with Lady Paget's 1st Unit

Frances was born in Timsbury in Somerset on 15th February 1871, one of nine children born to John Lovell Fry and his wife Lucy Ann. At the time of her birth, her father was a brewer and farmer although in later life he moved to Stapleton in Gloucestershire to work in the wholesale stationary trade.

By the age of twenty, Frances was working as a nurse at the small cottage

The Cast of Characters

hospital in Shepton Mallet. She subsequently qualified as a midwife in 1898, and worked at the West London Hospital. It may have been here that she first met Dr Abraham, who she later encountered working with the British Red Cross in Skoplje.

By 1911, Frances, now aged forty, was working as the superintendent sick nurse in a 'surgical home' at 6 Beaumont St. in Marylebone. In October 1914, she and her brother James Duncan Fry who was five years younger, volunteered to join Lady Paget's hospital unit. Frances was appointed matron and her brother served as an orderly.

In his account of the British Red Cross work in Skoplje, Dr Abraham made frequent mention of Frances, always referring to her as 'Miss Rowntree'. In December 1914, when Abraham described his unit as *'almost at our wits' end'* as they struggled to cope with the endless stream of wounded, Frances visited the hospital to see him: *'Even though she was an old hospital sister of mine , I could give her only an occasional word, time was so precious.'*

Frances was clearly appalled as she followed Abraham *'down the dirty ward, littered with the refuse of two or three days, picking her steps with raised skirts. "But this is awful" she said. "None of these beds seem ever to have been made". "They haven't " I answered. "We have no sheets to put on them, and no nightshirts to change the men out of their dirty uniforms. I wish I had you and twenty nurses."*[229]

Frances, whom Abraham described as *' a first class theatre sister,'* was keen to help but succumbed to 'relapsing fever' on the following day, so was unable to do anything more. However, once recovered, she obtained permission to help out the British Red Cross in the afternoons and in January decided to work there full time since there was so little surgical work at Lady Paget's hospital by this time.[230]

As fears of a typhus epidemic began to mount, Frances asked to join the British Red Cross unit permanently. Abraham felt it incumbent upon him to explain all the risks to her and recalled the conversation:

Nursing in Serbia with Lady Paget in 1915

"Now you can keep out of it quite easily. You came for three months. Your time is up. You can go home to England to your work there with an absolutely clear conscience. If you join us, you are doing so at a risk we have no right to ask you to accept. I don't advise you to join us. What do you think?"

I have ceased marvelling at the things the English nurse is capable of doing. It isn't as if it were one woman. They seem all to be alike.

"I'll come" she said quietly.

"Knowing the risk?"

"Certainly"

And that settled it."[231]

When, in February, Dr Holmes fell ill with typhus, Frances insisted on nursing him. Abraham was pathetically grateful: *'Our one and only nurse, remained smiling through it all. She looked after all our people - our three typhus, one diphtheria and the doubtful case.'*[232]

In March, the British Red Cross unit in Skoplje decided to disband and Frances elected to return home with her brother, to her work in London. Abraham remained in contact and wrote in 1922, that he had seen her only a few weeks ago *'looking as if she had never heard of Serbia or typhus.'*[223]

In retirement, Frances lived with an unmarried sister in Bath and later moved to Weston super Mare where she died on 7th December 1947. She left her effects of £1197.12.1 to her brother John Duncan Fry, a retired physicist.

The Cast of Characters

Jan Gordon (1882-1944) and Cora Gordon(1879-1950)

Artists, travel writers and members of the Berry Mission

Born in Finchampstead, Berkshire, on 11 March 1882, Jan was the eldest son of Alexander Gordon, clerk in holy orders and his wife Juliette Blanche Gabville Gordon. As his father moved between curacies in Berkshire, Wiltshire and Dorset, the young family moved with him. Jan's full name was actually Godfrey Jervis Gordon but he always styled himself as 'Jan', also at times, writing under the pseudonym 'John Salis'.

Jan was educated at Marlborough College and then attended Truro School of Mines. He even spent a little time in the Malay States as a mining engineer before firmly deciding that he preferred to be an artist. He duly returned to London to attend the Kensington School of Art. In 1906, he moved to Paris where he met his future wife Cora. The couple shared a love of art and music. Whilst he was a keen banjo player, Cora was an accomplished pianist, violinist and singer of madrigals.

Born in Buxton, Derbyshire, on 9 March 1879, Cora was the daughter of Frederick Turner, a general medical practitioner and surgeon and his wife Sarah of Grafton House, Fairfield. Although her father, when he became a widower, was keen for his youngest daughter to remain at home and keep house for him, Cora had other ideas .She attended Slade School of Art before moving to Paris.

Jan and Cora were married in Chelsea on 7th July 1909 and back in Paris, rented a studio in the heart of the artist district of Montparnasse, which they were to retain until 1932. When war broke out in 1914, the couple returned to London and according to their own account, persuaded Mr and Mrs Berry to include them in their unit as engineer and VAD, solely because of their musical skills. The couple's joint account of their service in Serbia with the Berry mission was published in 1916 under the title *'The Luck of Thirteen'*. A second edition, dedicated to Sir James Berry, was published in 1939, under the new title of *'Two Vagabonds in Serbia and Montenegro'* .

Nursing in Serbia with Lady Paget in 1915

In October 1915, as the scale of Serbia's defeat became clear, Sir Ralph Paget advised that all men of military age who were not qualified doctors, should escape and avoid the risk of internment. Whilst most of the Berry Unit remained in Vrnjatchka Banja, Jan and Cora, gathering a small group of fellow fugitives as they went, escaped by a little known route over the mountains of Montenegro, arriving back in London on 6th December, well ahead of other British Hospital Units.

Once back in England, Jan worked making aircraft components for Rolls Royce at Derby and then designing Naval camouflage at the Royal Academy of Art. He also briefly joined the Royal Naval Volunteer Reserve, serving as a war artist for the Navy's medical section. Several of his paintings are held at the Imperial War Museum.

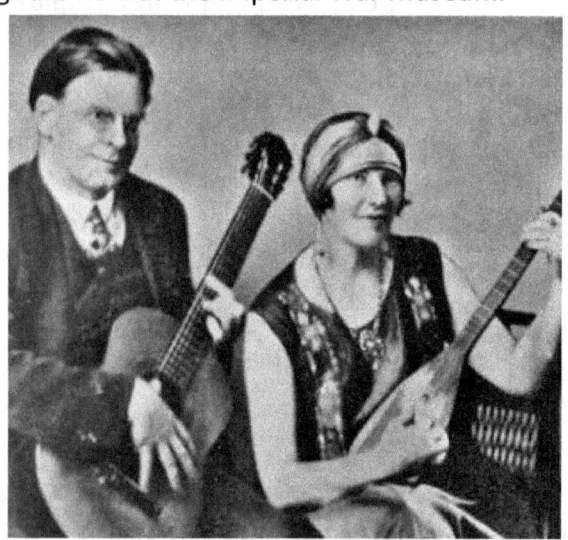

Between the wars, the couple returned to their two enthusiasms of art and travel and the first of a long series of popular travel books 'Poor Folk in Spain' appeared in 1922. In all, the couple wrote twenty seven books, as well as numerous magazine articles.

After a series of heart attacks, Jan died at the age of sixty one on 2 February 1944. Cora lived on in their Bayswater home at 48d Clanricarde Gardens, until her death on 1 July 1950.

The Cast of Characters

Dr John Douglas Wilson Hartnell-Beavis (1874-1942)
Leader of the First British Field Hospital for Serbia

John Douglas Wilson Hartnell [widely known as Dr Beavis] was born on 28th September 1874 at Kirkdale in Lancashire. He was the son of Samuel Tanner Hartnell, a master mariner and his wife Eliza Henrietta [née Holland], the daughter of a doctor. Samuel died in 1877 when his son was only three and there seems no evidence that Eliza ever remarried. At the time of the 1881 census, the widowed mother and her children were living at Minchinhampton in Gloucestershire. 'Beavis' went on to study at Bristol and Guy's Hospital in London, qualifying as a doctor in 1897. By the time of the 1901 census, the whole family appear to have added the name Beavis to their surname but the reason for this is unclear. At her marriage in 1903, Beavis' sister Henrietta Grace not only gave her surname as Hartnell-Beavis but also ascribed the same surname to her deceased father, Samuel Tanner. There is no evidence that he ever used the name 'Beavis'.

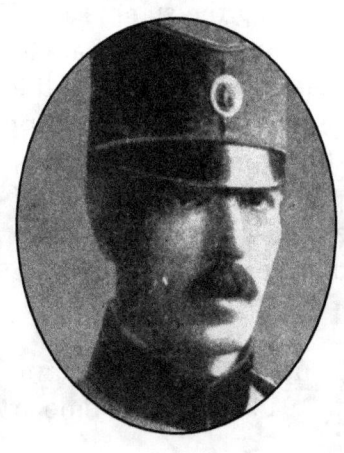

On the outbreak of war, Beavis seized the opportunity to serve as director of a British Field Hospital for Belgium. The unit, consisting of eight doctors, twenty nurses and five dressers initially set up a well equipped hospital of one hundred and fifty beds, in Antwerp.[234] Over the first five weeks they admitted five hundred Belgians and seventy British. On 8th October, as the Germans occupied Antwerp, the unit successfully evacuated all its wounded in seven motor buses. After a week in London refitting, the unit returned to Belgium, this time setting up a hospital in the large Episcopal college of St Joseph in Furnes, five or eight miles behind the front line, which served as the official field hospital of the Belgian army. The hospital had around one

Nursing in Serbia with Lady Paget in 1915

hundred beds and patients were quickly moved on from there to Calais or Dunkirk, working in conjunction with Dr Munro's Ambulance Corps.

By March 1915 the unit had been disbanded and Beavis turned to a new project, undertaking the formation of the 1st British Field Hospital for Serbia, attached to the 2nd Serbian Army. The unit reached Salonika on 15th April expecting to be sent to the front line but instead were directed to assist Lady Paget in Skoplje. The unit which also included the writers Claude and Alice Akew, consisted of twenty six individuals including dressers, orderlies, chauffeurs, nurses, a cook, washerwoman and interpreter. Gerard Sim, who had been a chauffeur in Belgium remained as Beavis' *'right hand man'* and the chief surgeon was Mr Fergus Armstrong, who later joined Lady Paget's Hospital *'during the slack period that preceded the Bulgarian occupation'*.[235] Dr G Landsborough Findlay served as physician and his wife Lady Sybil served as *'an indefatigable nurse'*, both having great experience of foreign travel.

The 'Beavis Unit' as it was usually termed, remained in Skoplje for six weeks before moving on to Mladenovatz, where the Second Army was quartered. In September they moved on with the Army to Pirot on the Bulgarian frontier. There had been little work during the summer, and several of the surgeons and dressers, like Armstrong, had drifted back to work at Lady Paget's Hospital. Dr Beavis himself took advantage of the lull to return to England to collect fresh stores and, incidentally, marry the Unit's matron, Miss Ethel Mary Long.[236] Having married in London, the couple dutifully returned to Salonika, only to find themselves cut off from their Unit by the Bulgarian invasion. It fell to Gerald Sim to assume command and lead the Unit home through hardships and horrors of the Serbian retreat.

Beavis was awarded the Honorary rank of Colonel in the Serbian Army and the Order of St Slava. He also received the 1914 Star for his time in Belgium.

After posts as junior house surgeon at the District Hospital in West Bromwich, and house surgeon at the General Hospital in Stroud, Beavis and his family retired to Little Tors in Combe Martin in Devon. He was

The Cast of Characters

killed with eight other civilians during an air raid on Gloster Aircraft Company's car park in Hucclecote in Gloucestershire on 4th April 1942.[237]

Lady Muriel Herbert (1883-1951)

Orderly with 2nd Serbian Relief Unit and author of 'Serbia and the Serbians'

Born in Marleybone on 29th April 1883, Muriel Katherine Herbert was the daughter of Sidney Herbert 14th Earl of Pembroke and 11th Earl of Montgomery, of Wilton House in Wiltshire.

Muriel served as an orderly with the Wimborne Unit which arrived in Skoplje in March 1915. She seems to have been largely concerning with ordering the stores. The letters which she wrote home to her sister Lady Beatrix Wilkinson Countess of Wicklow describing this time, were published privately in aid of the Waifs and Strays Society in 1915.

Muriel's friend, Elia Lindon, of Portuguese extraction, joined her at the end of April and the pair clearly socialised with doctors and nurses from all the British units. She celebrated her birthday with a dinner of sardines and potted meats attended by Doctors Sinclair, Dalyell and Bellingham and *'possibly Maitland from Paget'* but also spent considerable time with Richard Chichester, dining with him and other dignitaries at Zurinsky's, the one restaurant in Skoplje . Whilst Chichester returned briefly to England in April, she took over his position as treasurer of the Refugee Rice Committee.

In the beginning of June, at the end of the typhus crisis, she and her friend Elia joined Chichester trekking through the surrounding countryside and distributing maize to destitute families. Plans to set up local relief committees were presumably thwarted by Chichester's death at the end of July.

Muriel must have returned home with rest of the Wimborne unit but this was not to be the end of her association with Serbia. On 21st June, Dr Isobel Emslie, the lively and talented doctor who was to lead the Newnham and Girton Unit of the Scottish Women's Hospitals, met her

Nursing in Serbia with Lady Paget in 1915

on board the SS Mossoul as it travelled from Marseilles to Salonika:

'*Three khaki clad women on board, all have been out in Serbia before and have told us much of what happened in those early months of 1915. All have short hair, which is the envy of our unit, all of whom are still unshorn... They are Lady Muriel Herbert, Miss Linden and Dolly Miles...*'[238]

Emslie described Muriel as '*tall, dark and slim with great tragic eyes and a lovely face*' whilst Elia had '*a great shock of hair*' and '*prominent, china-blue eyes, a wonderful carriage and much assurance*'. On 31 October as the ship left Piraeus, Lady Muriel conveyed news to her fellow passengers from the Serbian minister '*that things were very bad in Serbia, and that it was feared that Lady Ralph Paget and her hospital at Uskub have been captured by the Bulgars...*'[239]

On 15th November, Emslie again encountered Lady Muriel and her friends when they arrived in Ghevgeli, having been evacuated from Monastir as the Serbs retreated. Now they went to work in the French evacuation hospital: '*...which had been arranged in some barns at the station, and which was overcrowded, very cold and dark, and lacking in equipment of every kind. They were quite untrained, but did excellent work, although their methods would have shocked and indeed did shock our English sisters; they however, made up in intelligence and courage what they lacked in training...*'[240]

Emslie recalled that the intrepid trio made a curious sight each morning as they trudged passed her hospital on the way to their own:

'*Miss Linden, immaculate in French nurse's uniform, with white robe and white veil, looked most professional. Lady Muriel wore the somewhat unusual garb of chamois-leather breeches, leather jerkin and apron. Dolly Miles was draped in a sort of overall with many jerseys piled one on top of the other, and all buttoned up awry and gaping...*'

There is little information about Lady Muriel's subsequent nursing career but In 1920, she married Dr Arthur John Jex-Blake (1873-1957), whom she had met and worked with in Boulogne whilst he was serving as a

The Cast of Characters

Major in the RAMC.[241]

Jex-Blake came from a distinguished family of scholars which included one sister who was Principal of Lady Margaret Hall in Oxford and another who was mistress at Girton College Cambridge. His aunt was the Sophia Jex-Blake who had played such a prominent role in the campaign to admit women to the medical profession. Now however, he gave up his consultancy as a physician at St George's Hospital and the newly weds set off for Kenya. There they purchased a coffee plantation named 'Kyuna' where they established a private botanical garden.[242]

Lady Muriel gave birth to a daughter, Daphne Marian in 1923, the same year that she co-founded the Kenya Horticultural Society. She went on to publish several books on the flora of Kenya. She died in Nairobi on 13 February 1951, aged sixty eight.

Rex [Reginald] William Jackson (1893-1965)

Medical Orderly with Lady Paget

Jackson, was born in Sidcup, Kent on 9th April 1893, the son of John Jackson of Kinniside, Dale Road, Purley in Surrey, the secretary to a Mission to Lepers.[243] After education at Oak House College in Bexley and Taunton School, Rex commenced his medical training at Sidney Sussex College, Cambridge in October 1912 but left his studies to join Lady Paget's expedition in October 1914. His letters home were published in the *Cambridge Magazine* in 1915 and several letters also survive amongst the papers of his fellow medical student Henry Squire at the Imperial War Museum.

In a letter home, dated 27th December, he gave an account of the funeral of Nellie Clark:

'Yesterday (Boxing Day) we had the funeral, and I was honoured by being one of the bearers. It was to me most impressive. We had a simple

Nursing in Serbia with Lady Paget in 1915

English Service here, read by the Consul in court dress, and Dr Morrison, and then went in procession to a Greek Church, and the Service there was magnificent. Then we went slowly to the cemetery—a long way off. There the rest of the English Service was read. All Uscub turned out to do reverence to 'Sister Clark,' from the Governor, who is Commander-in-Chief for this part of Serbia, with eight Greek or Roman Priests, in bright-coloured robes, down to the little street arabs, crossing themselves as the hearse passed. We were preceded by a Serbian military band and the music in the Greek Church was perfectly lovely. It was very sad—but also grand!'[244]

In letters home to his parents, which were published in the *Cambridge Magazine*, Jackson described doing night shifts with Sister Marianne Hall, caring for the wounded in eight wards in the main building from nine at night until nine in the morning. Besides details of the awful wounds of his patients, he also gave details of the lighter side of life such as celebrations for the New Year:

'...most of us went with Lady Paget to a cinema. The best cinema—the one to which we went—is the only decent restaurant of the town. The other one is now in use as a hospital, I believe. The pictures were quite good, and we came home and had a sing-song after it, and punch was served a little before twelve. Then we drank the usual toasts and all joined hands and sang 'Auld Lang Syne.' This was quite novel under the existing conditions. It was so different from the times we had sung it before. It was a thoroughly enjoyable evening, and on Friday evening we again had the Red Cross doctors to dinner, and had turkey and Christmas pudding again, with lighted brandy sauce.'

In January 1915, Squire wrote home to say that he and Jackson were isolated with suspected scarlet fever. Whilst they both recovered, Squire suffered further health problems and went home at the beginning of February. Jackson wrote to his friend assuring him that there was no dishonour in leaving and saying that Lady Paget had spoken of his departure as a *'tragedy'*. The pair, had been known to entertain 'Lady P' at impromptu tea parties and were apparently known as *'The Heavenly*

The Cast of Characters

Twins'. Squire clearly approved of the title, proudly confiding to his parents: *'even Lady Paget calls us that'*.

In a letter written from 'The Cottage', dated 11th March, Jackson thanked Squire for his letter written aboard the Erin and posted in Athens, which Chichester had brought up to the Hospital. He reported that Lady Paget had developed typhus four or five days ago but was believed to have only a *'slight attack'* and that Dr Knobel had caught it two days later: *'As I expect you know they and Maitland have been doing administrating work and running a typhus hospital in the town. We are very well here indeed and very rarely do we have a case of typhus. Of course it is sent out when it does occur...'*[245]

At this point, he proposed to stay on with Dr Eliot *'who is exceedingly nice'* until mid April: *'If the Serbian Relief Committee approve we shall stay on with a smaller staff after 31st* [March]*and Greeve and I will take Newey and Alabaster's places* [as dressers] *which of course would be ripping...'*

A further letter, dated 29 August 1915, gave his address as *'c/o Colonel Beavis Mladenovatz'* but it is evident from a letter published in the *Cambridge Magazine* that he had returned home in the intervening period and that he sailed out to join the Beavis unit aboard the SS Abbassieh in June 1915. Camped with the Second Serbian Army, he was enjoying the beautiful countryside and the opportunity to ride every day, but expected to return to Skoplje and take over the Citadel Hospital at The Grad. Others, intended to join Lady Paget during the lull in fighting: *'When there is fighting we'll return and reform this field hospital unit.'* Ominously, he also reported that he was having trouble with his digestion in the hot weather, not at all enjoying a diet of unremitting stews from the English cook.

In October, his last letter published in the *Cambridge Magazine* was written from the Czech Hospital in Nish where Jackson was relishing the surgical experience he was gaining. A note appended to the letter, reported receipt by his parents of a cable, dated 27th October, from Colonel Beavis which stated that the hospital was now *'safe'* with the

Nursing in Serbia with Lady Paget in 1915

Second Army.

Jackson never returned to his studies but was allowed a BA degree by 'special grace of the senate' based upon his preliminary examination results in natural science. He subsequently served as a Lieutenant in the Royal Field Artillery and as an honorary lieutenant in the newly formed RAF as an observer.

After the war, Jackson worked for the Burmah Oil Company in Rangoon for two years and then moved to Calcutta in 1923. He remained there until 1954 when he retired to Tedburn St Mary near Exeter. He died on 16 November 1965 leaving effects of £5323 to his wife Elizabeth Fairbairn.

Dr Esther Kadisch (b1890)

Russian Doctor at British Red Cross Hospital in Skoplje

Esther Kadisch was born at Friedrichstadt [modern Jaunjelgava], a town eighty kilometres south east of Riga, in Latvia on 12 May 1890.[246]

Mr Morrison, the surgeon at Lady Paget's Hospital was a great admirer of *'this courageous member of our profession'* and added a few *'fragmentary notes'* about her to his account of his time with Lady Paget:

'When a girl in her teens she visited relatives in Dublin and gained a modern languages scholarship in Trinity College. Her medical course, which began in Paris (where she concurrently passed examinations in French law), was continued in Russia, Germany and England, and completed by graduation in a Russian and in a German University. I first met Miss Kadisch in 1913, when she was a student at the Queen's Hospital, Birmingham, and strangely enough, next met her in Skoplje as a member of staff of the Serbian hospital to which my unit succeeded. I learned that on the outbreak of war she had been arrested in Berlin as an alien enemy and detained in a cell on prison fare for several days until released by the intervention of a Socialist member of the Reichstag. She then became associated with a Russian Grand Duke in collecting a party

The Cast of Characters

of refugees, whom she piloted across to Finland and thence to Petrograd. A short visit to her home in Riga was followed by an adventurous journey to Serbia, by way of Bucharest and the Danube (her boat being under Austrian fire) to Belgrade. At the close of her two months' work in the Gymnasium Hospital, Dr Kadisch joined the staff of the British unit which presently became installed in the factory, and proved an invaluable colleague as a doctor and interpreter.'[247]

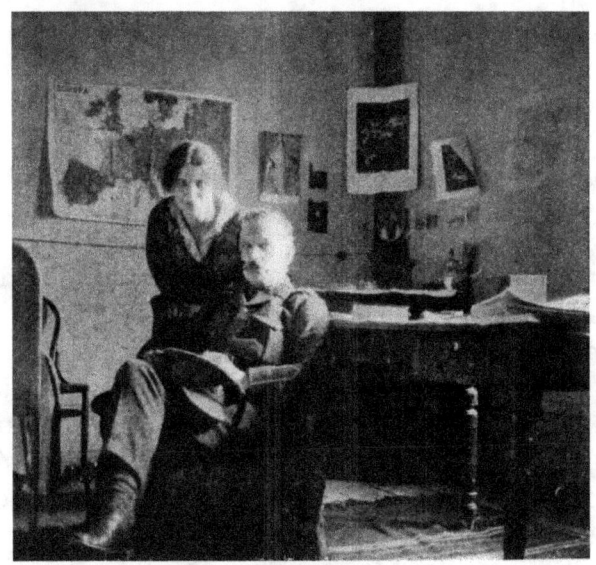

Dr Kadisch and Dr Banks (from My Balkan Log by J Johnston Abraham, 1922)

When the British Red Cross withdrew from Skoplje, *'nothing would induce her to vacate the post'*:

'Toiling night and day in a desperate effort to rescue a few among the forlorn crowd of miserables dying from typhus and septicaemia, this accomplished and heroic lady nearly gave her life as the price of her devotion... It was my privilege on her recovery to introduce her to the Prime Minister, M Pachitch, and to witness His Excellency's emotion in thanking her for the noble services rendered to his people. Dr Kadisch's departure brought a grateful concourse of Serbians and Austrians to the

Nursing in Serbia with Lady Paget in 1915

station, including some who were indebted to her for their life. I had the pleasure of hearing of her safe arrival at Riga by telegram from her father, and I have since heard she was working at Petrograd.'

Dr Kadisch or 'The Little Red Woman' as she was named by her colleagues, similarly made a great impression upon the British Red Cross doctors when they first found her working in the hospital to which they had been posted:

"That little red-headed woman is a marvel" said Barclay. "The way she handles the awful crowd is wonderful. She's been at it since eight this morning. She's been up twice in the night. She's going to carry on all afternoon. And do you know what's worrying her most? You'd never guess. She's afraid we'll take the place from her..."[248]

Dr Johnston Abraham recorded not only the important role which Dr Kadisch played within their hospital as a doctor but also a moving occasion when her Austrian patients showed their own appreciation of her kindness. *'With her warm over-flowing heart'* she had realised that Christmas eve was an important event for the Austrian prisoners who were patients in the hospital and had persuaded the Commandant of the hospital to provide them with a special dinner. At the close of the meal, the Russian doctor was toasted with enthusiasm and responded with a *'little halting speech in German'* thanking them and hoping that next year they would all enjoy Christmas in their own homes *'when the cruelties of war would be over'*. As she ceased speaking and prepared to depart, a young Austrian, apparently *'a leading star in the Conservatoire in Prague'* in happier days, led the orchestra assembled for the occasion in a solemn rendition of the Russian National Anthem amidst much emotion. *'It seems a shame we have to fight the Austrian'* commented one of the Doctors.

When Dr Johnston Abraham published his memoirs in 1922, he recorded that he had heard from Dr Kadisch at intervals from places as far afield as Moscow, Riga and finally Georgia: *'always keen, always active, always working in the most impossible places.'* He had not then heard from her for two years and was apprehensive about her fate.

The Cast of Characters

Dr William Bernard Knobel (1875-1951)

Surgeon

Knobel was born on 14th January 1875 in Stapenhill, a village on the outskirts of Burton on Trent, in Staffordshire. His baptism didn't occur until 1891 when the family were away from their home in Bocking, Essex, staying in Swindon. His father, Edward Bell Knobel, at the time of the 1881 census, was the manager of a textile factory owned by Courtaulds in Bocking, near Braintree, in Essex but by 1901 was the director of a photographic plate company at 32 Tavistock Square, London and the family retained the two addresses in later directory entries. The entry for his son in the register of Cambridge Alumni also recorded Knobel senior as a Fellow of the Royal Astronomical Society. His wife Margaret, like him, was a Londoner.

William Knobel was educated at Sherborne and Trinity College, Cambridge before pursuing his medical studies at University College, London and St Bartholomew's Hospital. He qualified as a doctor in 1905, working first as assistant medical officer at the London County Asylum. In 1910, he moved to be superintendent at the Midland Open Air Sanatorium at Bourne Castle in Belbroughton near Stourbridge in Worcestershire.

Knobel joined Lady Paget's expedition when it left in October 1914 and presumably returned home, with the main unit on 31st March 1915. Mr Morrison acknowledged his help in his account of the experience: *'Dr W B Knobel and Dr T G Maitland rendered valuable services in their domain, and voluntarily came to the rescue when the surgical demands were excessive..'*[249]

An unnamed correspondent in the Birmingham Post went further in praise of the pair:

'A British surgeon, chief of another British unit, has said of them that he has been more impressed by them than by any other doctors there, for while others have planned and discussed, these two have gone down into the fight in hourly danger of their lives, Dr Knobel personally undertaking

Nursing in Serbia with Lady Paget in 1915

the examination and separation of all typhus cases in the town, both civil and military, and Dr Maitland taking charge of the typhus hospital and supervising the treatment of cases. It is natural that they should have been the two to undertake the practical work, as they were the physicians attached to the unit; and it is because they performed their work unsparingly and unflinchingly that they have earned the undying respect of all the British and Serbians here. These are the two who, after Lady Paget, have borne the chief brunt of the fight and made the great sacrifice...'[250]

Although he returned to his duties at the sanatorium at Bourne Castle, Knobel subsequently served in the Royal Army Medical Corps as a Captain. In May 1915, he sold his X-Ray equipment to the Serbian Relief Fund for £125.

After the war he was appointed as Divisional Medical Officer and later Senior Medical Officer for London County Council. In 1940, he retired to Spear Hill, in Ashington near Pulborough in Sussex where he died on 17 Sep. 1951. His effects of £16734.18 went to his widow Ellen.

Knobel was married twice. In 1905, he married Gladys Maude Ommaney in Hatfield, Hertfordshire. The marriage was dissolved and he married Ellen Rintoul in St Pancras, London in 1924.

Sir Thomas Johnstone Lipton (1848-1931)

Owner of the steam yacht 'Erin'

Lipton was born on 10 May 1848 in Glasgow, the son of Thomas Lipton and his wife Frances [née Johnstone]. His parents were Ulster small holders, forced to emigrate by the potato famine. In the 1860s, his parents established a small grocery in the Gorbals area of Glasgow. Lipton, the only child to survive infancy, left school at thirteen to find various employments including printer's errand boy and cabin boy on

The Cast of Characters

a steamer running to Belfast. After this, he spent five years travelling around America, earning his living in places which varied from a tobacco plantation to a New York grocery.

In 1870, Lipton returned to Glasgow and helped his parents briefly before setting up his first grocery – Lipton's Market. This small provisions shop was to be the foundation of an empire which would go on to include groceries throughout Britain. In 1888, he entered the tea trade, eventually purchasing his own plantations. He prospered by being able to sell tea at low prices to the poor working class markets, boasting that the secret of his success was selling the best goods at the cheapest prices - and good advertising.

Besides his numerous business interests, he also had a passion for yachting and he seems to have littered the world with trophies in his name, in addition to the famous brand of 'Lipton Tea' which still exists today.

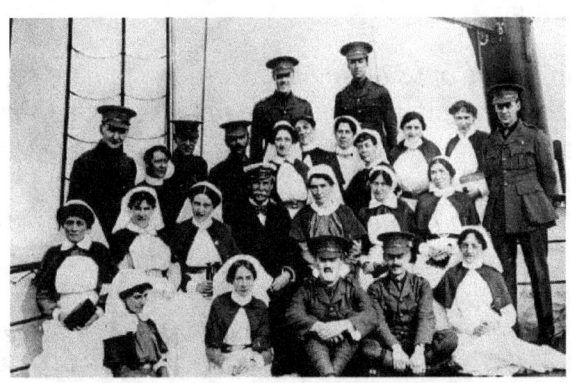

Sir Thomas Lipton (centre) with passengers aborad the Erin

At the outbreak of war, Lipton offered to help transport personnel and goods to Serbia in his luxury steam yacht 'Erin'. The British Red Cross took up the offer and Lipton personally escorted several groups from Marseilles to Salonika.

Interesting traffic went both ways. On 1 March 1915, H Fremlin Squire, an orderly with Lady Paget who was being sent home due to sickness,

Nursing in Serbia with Lady Paget in 1915

wrote to his colleague Rex W Jackson who was still at the Hospital, that he was having *'a great trip'* travelling home in Sir Thomas Lipton's private yacht via Euboea, Chalcis, Aigina, Corinth Canal and Naples. Also aboard was a Serbian Prince *'quite a nut'* and *'quite near the throne'* who was returning to Oxford.[251]

In May 1915, Elsie Corbett who was part of a British Red Cross Unit, boarded Sir Thomas Lipton's large steam yacht in Marseilles and embarked on a luxury cruise of the Mediterranean:

'As well as our Unit of nineteen we had Sir Thomas Lipton himself on board, along with his considerable staff; also a very stately Times correspondent called Robinson and an eager young cub reporter...'[252]

The yacht put in at several ports too small for the larger steamers and passed through the Corinth Canal, reaching Athens in good time. She was impressed with Sir Thomas who obviously involved himself deeply in the plight of Serbia:

'... Sir Thomas took some of us up to his stateroom, to hear copies of the letters of condolence he had written to the families of the previous Unit he had taken out and who had died of typhus; large tears rolled down his cheeks as he read them. He was a great 'character' boasting that he was 'born in two rooms and a kitchen' and full of elaborate practical jokes: receiving false telegrams that the Unit had been recalled; or posing groups to be photographed with great elaboration, and when at last everything seemed right and the button was pressed, a large snake on springs sprang out of the camera. He had his dead fox terrier, stuffed, in his stateroom...'[253]

It was after this voyage that Lipton entertained Flora to tea and then set off on a tour of Serbia. He lunched with Sir Ralph Paget at Nish with Mrs Stobart and paid a visit to the Stobart camp at the beginning of June, arriving at Kragujevatz station at 5.17 am. Mrs Stobart recalled meeting the honoured guest:

'I hope we gave him porridge, but I've forgotten. But we showed him

The Cast of Characters

the camp; then he lunched at the officers' mess, inspected the arsenal in the afternoon and came back to us for tea and supper. In the evening in his honour, we gave a little supper party, which included Colonels Guentchitch and Popovitch and Captain Yovannovitch of the Intelligence Department, Mr Robinson of The Times and Mr Stanley Naylor of The Daily Chronicle. Sir Thomas seemed to like the cheery, homely atmosphere of the corporate supper table, at which all members of our unit... messed as always together...'[254]

Dr Katherine MacPhail who was serving in Kragujevatz with the Scottish Women's Hospital unit, also recalled a grand reception held in Lipton's honour in the dining room of an old hunting lodge which had belonged to a former Serbian Prince:

'The reception was very amusing... the orchestra of the Royal Guard played for us. When Sir Thomas entered the room, the orchestra greeted him with a loud cheer. He was very interested in us, and our work, and he was pleased to meet someone from Glasgow. We had a good chat, and as the night got on he got very cheery and he began to crack jokes. I must say I was very pleased the Serbs could not make out some of his jokes...'[255]

Sir Thomas evidently enjoyed his royal progress around Serbia, being photographed extensively and, incidentally, collecting an honorary citizenship at Nish. He afterwards wrote several articles on the plight of Serbia. In a letter to the editor of the *Morning Post*, under the headline 'Serbia's Great Need', he described the typhus epidemic in dramatic terms:

'The country has been attacked by disease as, I think, no country has ever been attacked before. It is a plague such as the world has seldom known, and all the benevolence of humanity will be required to deal with it...What I have seen convinces me, however, that the efforts of the Red Cross, splendid as they are, must prove inadequate. The whole of the resources of humanity must be organised to fight this epidemic in such a way that full force can be brought to bear upon the entire stricken districts, and thus save the Serbian people from a fate even more terrible

Nursing in Serbia with Lady Paget in 1915

than annihilation by the enemy...'[256]

After the fall of Serbia, Lipton must have sold the yacht, for it was sunk by a mine in the Mediterranean in May 1916, less than a year later, bearing its former name of 'Aegusa' once again.[257]

Sir Thomas died at his home 'Osidge' in Southgate, London on 2nd October 1931. He left most of his extensive fortune to the city of Glasgow.

Dr Katherine S MacPhail OBE (1887-1974)

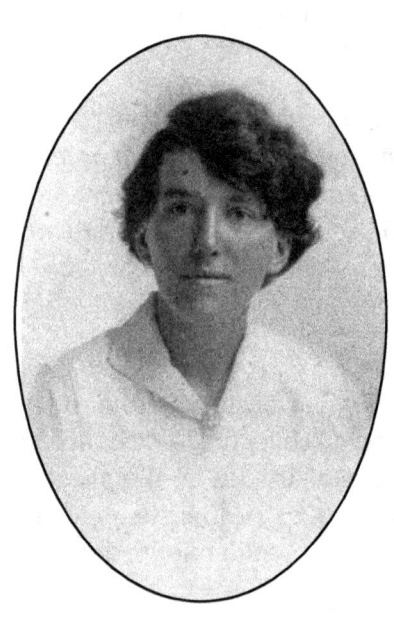

Katherine was born on 30th October 1887, the third daughter of Dr Donald MacPhail and his wife Jessie (neé Mitchell) whom he had met when she was a probationer nurse at Glasgow Western Infirmary. The family with their four daughters settled at Coatbridge, twelve miles east of Glasgow. The girls attended school in Glasgow, staying with their grandmother during the week. Against the advice of her father, Katherine enrolled at Glasgow University to study medicine in 1906. Having qualified in 1911, she worked for a period at Glasgow Royal Infirmary before joining her father at his practice in Coatbridge.

At the beginning of the war, Katherine, finding herself unwanted by the War Office, joined the first unit of the Scottish Women's Hospital sent to Serbia, under Dr Eleanor Soltau. Anna Christitch, a young journalist of Serbian Irish origin, left her job with the *Daily Express*, to accompany the unit as a translator and teacher of Serbian.

After Christmas in Malta, the unit arrived in Salonika on 1st January 1915 and was then sent to Kragugjevatz where the Serbian army and

The Cast of Characters

medical service was stationed. At Skoplje railway station, they were met and greeted by Lady Paget who warned them of the difficulties to come. During the typhus epidemic, the unit suffered particularly badly losing two nurses, Sister Jordan and Sister Minishull and Madge Neill Fraser, a health worker from Glasgow who drove one of the cars and was incidentally a renowned golfer.

In the Spring, as work became quieter, Katherine visited Skoplje and also tended a sick doctor, Dr V A Haig who had arrived in Palanka only three weeks earlier. Nearly at the end of her contract, she and her friend Dr Adeline Campbell asked Dr Soltau for leave to move somewhere where they would be more useful. With her agreement, they approached the Serbian Army Medical Corps and were sent to Belgrade to take over the infectious diseases section of the military hospital. When Dr Elsie Inglis, founder of the Scottish Women's Hospital, arrived on the scene at the end of May, she interviewed Katherine and her colleague and urged them to join her new unit at Valjevo. However, she failed to persuade the young doctors, who felt that they were more useful in their present post.

In June, Katherine herself fell seriously ill with typhus and was looked after by Dr James Ryan of the American Red Cross. In September 1915, she returned to Scotland to recuperate. When she applied to rejoin the Scottish Women's Hospitals, she was dismayed to have her application refused and from then on she resolved to act independently. She spent the autumn giving talks and raising money for the Serbian Relief Fund. A photograph which she had taken of young boy she had met a Kragujevatz, was sold around local schools to raise funds for the Childrens' Fund of the Serbian Relief Committee.

At the beginning of 1916, Katherine was working with the Society of Friends at a maternity hospital at Châlons-sur-Marne in France, when Lady Grogan of the Serbian Relief Fund invited her to join the work in Corsica. She spent around six weeks working at Bastia under Kathleen Courtney, before returning to France to work amongst French refugees.

In early 1917, Katherine was invited by the head of the Medical Corps

Nursing in Serbia with Lady Paget in 1915

of the Serbian Army to work at their newly established Crown Prince Alexander's Hospital in Salonika. Whilst she awaited final completion of the hospital, she worked once more for the Serbian Relief Fund at their hospital in Sorović . Living under canvas, in the mountains, she helped to care for civilian casualties injured during the bombardment of Monastir, running a mobile dispensary and providing inoculations in the hope of preventing further epidemics. When the Serbian Relief Fund moved their hospital to Germijan, she continued her work assisting the population of the local villages.

In August 1918, Katherine and her younger sister Isabel who was by then, also working at the Hospital in Salonika, returned to Scotland to help their father who was struggling to cope with the recent influenza epidemic. It was not until November that Katherine was able to make her way back by a circuitous route to Belgrade. Here, amidst the post war chaos and confusion when so many foreign missions competed for scarce resources, Katherine succeeded in establishing the first children's hospital in Belgrade, later to be known as the Anglo-Serbian Children's Hospital.

Aided by donations from her former colleagues and friends, and often employing ex-nurses from the war time missions, who could not bring themselves to return home, Katherine seized every opportunity she could to keep the hospital afloat financially. When the Serbian Relief Fund established a charitable kitchen for a local school, she arranged for them also to supply food to her hospital. She was also helped by her old friend Admiral Troubridge and his marines who were now stationed close by once more.

Despite all the many challenges, the hospital prospered and eventually moved to larger premises before finally opening as a new hospital at Sremska Kamenica in the region of Novi Sad, close to the Danube, in 1934. Under Katherine's directorship, the hospital specialised largely in tubercular patients. The hospital, envisaged by Katherine as a symbolic memorial to the British women who had worked in Serbia during and after the war, flourished until 1941 when the German invasion forced the staff to flee. Katherine was captured by the Italians and interned in

The Cast of Characters

Central Italy for five weeks before being repatriated. Although after the war, she returned to Yugoslavia and attempted to restore the hospital, her efforts were thwarted by the new state of Yugoslavia's hostility to foreign missions. In 1947, Katherine returned home to Scotland and retired to St Andrews.

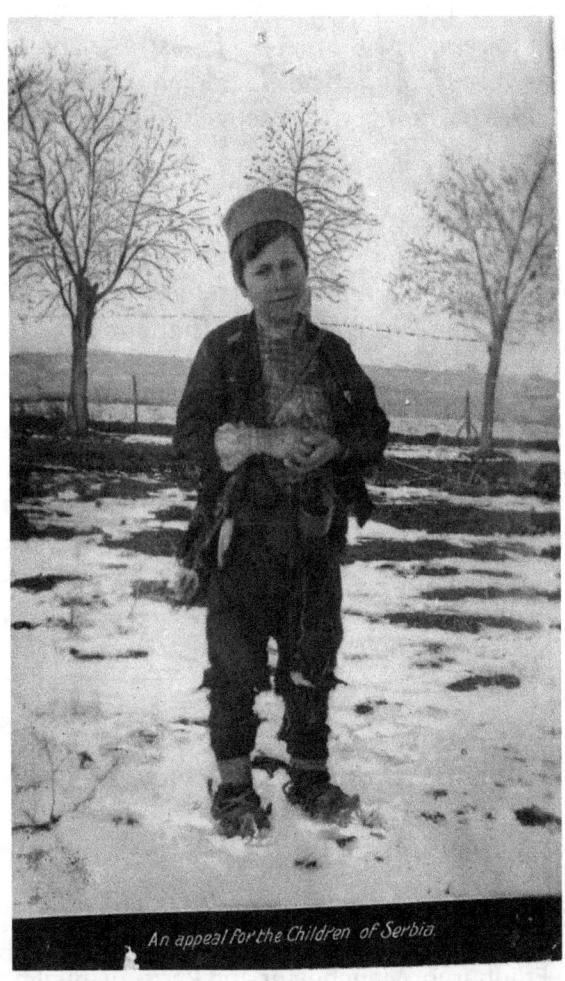

Photograph taken by MacPhail and sold as a postcard in aid of the Children's Fund of the Serbian Relief Committee, c. 1916

Nursing in Serbia with Lady Paget in 1915

Her enormous efforts to help the children of Serbia had resulted in several honours. During the war, she had received the Order of St Sava (4th class) and the medal of the Serbian Red Cross and in 1926 she also received a medal from the Russian Red Cross for her work amongst the children of Russian émigrés. In a rare example of recognition by the British government for work in this sphere, she was awarded the Order of the British Empire in 1928. In later life, as restrictions in Yugoslavia relaxed, she was very pleased to be elected an honorary member of the Serbian Medical Association, finally recognised as 'a noble benefactor of our people'.

Katherine died on 21st September 1974 just a few days before a meeting of the Yugoslav Orthopaedic and Traumatological Association elected her as an honorary member and awarded her the Order of the Yugoslav Flag with a Golden Star, in recognition of her contribution to the relief of suffering caused by two brutal wars.

In 1969, Katherine took part with Francesca Wilson and Anna Christitch, in a BBC documentary by Jean Bray, entitled 'Yesterday's Witness. Mission to Serbia'. An impressive account of her life, drawn from her letters home to her family was written by Professor Želimar Mikić, a specialist in orthodpaedic surgery in Novi Sad in 1998. An English translation was published under the title *'Ever Yours Sincerely. The Life and Work of Dr Katherine S MacPhail'* in 2007.

Dr Thomas Gwynne Maitland (c1876-1948)

Director of the Typhus Colony, Skoplje

Thomas Gwynne Maitland was born at Merthyr Tydfil in South Wales on 19th May 1875 and educated at University College School and the Universities of Edinburgh, Manchester and Paris. He qualified as a doctor at Edinburgh University in 1908 and received a doctorate in philosophy from Manchester University in 1911.[258] He married Clarissa Gwendoline Radcliffe, the daughter of the Cardiff shipowner, Henry Radcliffe, in

The Cast of Characters

Newport, Monmouthshire in April 1910.

His career at different times involved serving as a demonstrator in physiology at the University of Manchester; assistant lecturer in physiology at Cardiff University College; house surgeon at Dumfries and Galloway Royal Infirmary and honorary physician to Walsall General Hospital. He also served as a lecturer of psychology at Birmingham Medical Institute. However, by the time of the 1911 census he appears to have been settled as a physician and surgeon at Kenmare House, 55 Bridge Street in Walsall, Staffordshire.

He was a member of the medical and surgical staff that went out with Lady Paget in October 1914 and played a leading role as director of the Typhus Colony, obtaining the honorary rank of Lieutenant-Colonel in the Serbian Army. With his colleague Dr Knobel [qv], he was greatly praised for his work during the typhus epidemic.

Amongst many articles for medical and psychological journals, he wrote an account of the typhus epidemic in Serbia with his own observations on the disease, which was published in the *British Journal of Nursing* in August 1915. Maitland served again with Lady Paget as her Medical Director when the unit was reformed in July 1915. Fergus Armstrong who had come out with Dr Hartnell-Beavis, served with him as surgeon in chief. Both were repatriated with Lady Paget in February 1916.

On his return from Serbia, Maitland resumed his medical career working for the Royal Army Medical Service and becoming a Fellow of the Royal College of Physicians in August 1916.[259]

His career took a new and unusual direction in November 1920, when he was registered as a merchant seaman, serving as the surgeon on the Cunard Line ship *Elysia*.[260] In 1926, he was appointed medical superintendent for the Cunard White Star Company and made it his aim to improve working conditions for merchant seamen. Before retirement in September 1946, he had undertaken much important work in the field of occupational health and had become an international authority on workmen's compensation.

Nursing in Serbia with Lady Paget in 1915

The obituary which appeared in *the British Journal of Independent Medicine* spoke warmly of Maitland's capacity for making and retaining lifelong friendships and his modesty:

'He was modest to a fault and abhorred publicity... his most appealing asset was his sense of humour...'

When Maitland died suddenly at his home, Hatchmere Wood, Norley in Cheshire on 10 August 1948, he left his effects to Fergus Armstrong, the surgeon who had worked with him all those years ago in Skoplje.

Dr Caroline Matthews (1878-1927)

Doctor and author of *A Woman Doctor in Serbia* (1916)

Much mystery seems to surround the life of this intrepid woman. Her medals and some of her medical equipment survive at the Science Museum in London and are the main source of information about her.

She graduated from Edinburgh Medical College for Women in 1903 and seems to have spent most of her life working abroad. In 1905, she published *'Hints by a Lady Doctor'* and three years later was serving with the Italian Red Cross during the earthquake at Messina. For her service there, she received a medal from Victor Emmanuel, King of Italy.

During the Balkan Wars, Matthews acted as correspondent for *The Sphere* and held the rank of surgeon in the Montenegro army, receiving another medal for her trouble.

In April 1915, pursuing her customary independent course, Matthews travelled out to Serbia on the *Ceramic,* in the company of the Scottish Women's Hospital Unit led by Alice Hutchinson. She had been assured by the Serbian Legation in London that she could work with a Serbian Field Army Unit under the Red Cross but was deeply disappointed on arriving in Nish, to learn that no woman would be permitted to serve at the front. Instead, she was sent to a large military hospital at Skoplje.

The Cast of Characters

Later, she moved to a unit under canvas at Valjevo and spent the summer working amongst the civilian population. From here she moved to a large military hospital at Uzsitsi on the Bosnian border. When the order came to evacuate, she preferred to remain with her patients and was captured by the Austrians. There followed a difficult time of illness and imprisonment when Matthews believed herself *'the only Britisher left in Serbia'*.[261] She was imprisoned in Belgrade for espionage and endured many adventures before arriving at a police station in Hungary. Here, she was delighted to encounter once more, Dr Alice Hutchinson, who had been interned there with her Unit, for three months: *'The sound of her cheery 'How are you Twiggie? ' took my breath away. It was a rare and unexpected pleasure to grasp her hand again!'*[262]

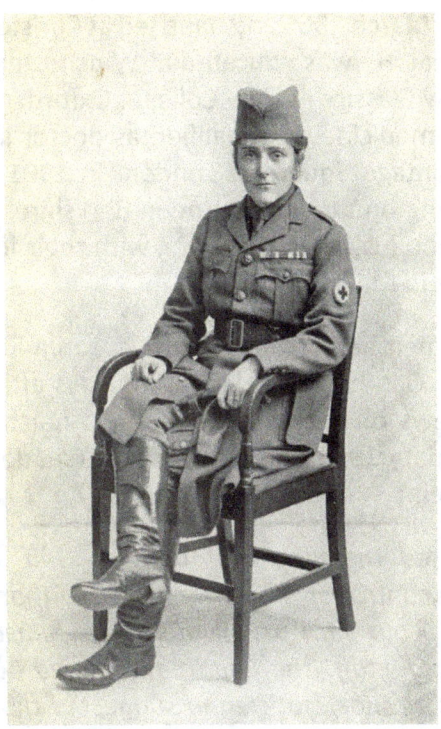

Dr Caroline Matthews (from her book Experiences of a Woman Doctor in Serbia, c. 1916

Nursing in Serbia with Lady Paget in 1915

Matthews remained with the Scottish Women's Hospital Unit and was eventually repatriated *'with other oddments'* who had strayed from the Stobart Unit, via Budapast, Vienna and Zurich.

She is thought to have spent the rest of her life travelling in India.

Robert Oswald Moon (1865-1953)

Physician with Lady Paget

Moon was the third son of Robert Moon a barrister at law, born in Liverpool, and his wife Mary Jane who was born in Rio Janeiro in Brazil. He was born on 17 March 1865 and baptised at Christchurch, Paddington on 19 May that year. He was educated at Winchester College and went on in 1884 to study Classics at New College, Oxford, graduating in 1890, before turning to medicine. He qualified as doctor in 1896 and set up practice at 62 Montagu Square in London. In 1901, he married Ethel Rose Grant Waddington at Pangbourne in Berkshire. At the time of the 1911 census, he and his wife were living with their four young children at 45 Green Street in Mayfair.

Moon became a member of the Executive Committee of the Serbian Relief Fund, on 1st October 1914 just a few days after it had been first formed. When news of the typhus epidemic reached London at the beginning of February 1915, Moon tried to persuade the committee to send him out to help:

'Dr Moon expressed the idea that another Unit should be started entirely under the control of the committee and that he would himself [be] willing to take out such a unit and make himself responsible for securing the medical staff. The Chairman pointed out the difficulty of securing surgeons at short notice and suggested that Dr Moon should make enquiries and report progress. It was ultimately decided that the Chairman should see Mrs Stobart and also Dr Moon in consultation...'[263]

The ensuing negotiations are not recorded but two weeks later on 18th

The Cast of Characters

February, the Chairman announced that Dr Moon would be leaving the following week with two nurses *'with the object of giving assistance to Lady Paget's Unit and advising on a site for a future unit.'* They would take the quickest route overland to Brindisi on the east coast of Italy and then sail from there.

Morrison, incorrectly ascribing to Moon *'the dangerous post of superintendent of the fever hospital'*, recorded:

'Dr R O Moon arrived in March. Besides adding distinction to the staff, he strengthened our hands most acceptably by his good counsel and firm support. ...both he and Dr Knobel passed through perilous attacks of typhus...'[264]

Moon did not remain with Lady Paget after the summer and presumably returned to his practice at 21 Wimpole Street in London. He retired to Winchester and died at Wallingford and District Hospital on 28 July 1953. He left effects amounting to £128,854.1s.9d to Arthur Frances Evelyn Gott, architect.

James Thomas Jackman Morrison (1856-1933)

Surgeon and Medical Officer of Lady Paget's Hospital

Born in Okehampton on 8th December 1856, Morrison was the eldest son of James Morrison, and Elizabeth Jackman. His father, an Irishman, served as a Quarter Master Sergeant with the Army Service Corps, subsequently obtaining a commission in the Royal Artillery. At the time of the 1871 census, James Morrison senior was resident with his family at Woolwich dockyard. Judging from the varied places of birth of Morrison's siblings, the family had moved between Okehampton, Woolwich and New Zealand. His grandmother Ann Jackman, who was living with them in 1871, was a former housekeeper.

Morrison's early education is unclear but he commenced his medical studies first at Guy's Hospital in London (1875-1879) before proceeding

Nursing in Serbia with Lady Paget in 1915

to study natural sciences at Christ's College, Cambridge, 1881-1883.[265]

The early years of a distinguished medical career involved service as a house surgeon at Guy's and senior assistant demonstrator of anatomy at Cambridge University. In 1886, he went to Birmingham as house surgeon at Queen's Hospital and was appointed a casualty surgeon there a year later. In 1895, he was elected Assistant to the Chair of Surgery at Mason University, Birmingham where he remained until 1899, when he was appointed Professor of Forensic Medicine at the University of Birmingham. He was to hold this chair for thirty two years.

In 1908, when the Territorial Force was first formed, Morrison was commissioned a Major in the 1st Southern General Hospital, a unit of the Royal Army Medical Corps and he went on to rise to the rank of Lieutenant- Colonel. At the outbreak of war, however, he turned to the St John Ambulance Association, of which he was an honorary associate, to organise a hospital unit for Serbia, with himself at the head. To what must have been his considerable annoyance, it was decided for financial reasons to amalgamate with the Serbian Relief Fund's unit under Lady Paget. The seeds of dissension were thus sewn at an early stage. It is probably no accident that the biographical entry in *Plarr's Lives of the Fellows* of the Royal College of Surgeons records quite incorrectly that *'he organised a British Hospital unit in Serbia acting as surgeon in chief for about two years.'* The same entry also conceded that he was *'a man of high aim and undeviating rectitude, whose inflexibility sometimes brought him unpopularity.'*

Edward Alabaster, a dresser with Lady Paget's unit, recalled that Morrison left the unit once the numbers of wounded had declined:

'In the middle of February, Professor Morrison was commissioned by the Serbian Government to report upon the hospitals of the country, and left the party to travel to the various hospitals, Dr Eliott taking charge in his absence. The hospital was not so crowded then, as there had been no fighting for some time, and they were able to takes eighty cases from other hospitals...'[267]

The Cast of Characters

In his own account of his time in Serbia, published in *The Lancet,* Morrison acknowledged by name all the doctors, dressers and the five medical students who served as orderlies.[268] However, with an arrogance which was perhaps typical of his privileged class, there was no mention of any other member of the unit. In recognition of his service he received the Serbian Order of the White Eagle and the Order of St Sava.

In 1914, Morrison was appointed a magistrate for the City of Birmingham where he also served as Police Surgeon for thirty five years.

In 1889, he married Edith the daughter of J W Titterton and niece of Sir Charles Soame .There were no children from the marriage.

Morrison died at Southfield, 48 Church Road, Edgbaston on 10 May 1933 and was buried at Brandwood End Cemetery. He left a personal estate of £23,433.17.9

Sir Ralph Paget (1864-1940) and Lady Leila Paget (1881-1958)

Ralph Spencer Paget was born on 26 November 1864 at the British Legation in Copenhagen where his father Sir Augustus Paget was serving as minister to Denmark. He was educated at Eton, where he excelled at German and rowing and afterwards studied abroad becoming proficient in Arabic and Turkish.[269] In April 1888, he served with his father, then Ambassador to Austria-Hungary, in Vienna as an attaché in the Foreign Office. Postings followed in Egypt, Zanzibar, Washington, Tokyo and Guatamala. In September 1902, he was promoted and appointed chargé d'affaires at the Bangkok legation in Siam and served there, from 1904 as Envoy Extraordinary and Minister Plenipotentiary, until 1909.

On 28 October 1907, he married his third cousin once removed, Louise Margaret Leila Wemyss Paget. She was born at 3 Halkin Street West, Belgravia, London on 9 October 1881, the only daughter and second of four children of Sir Arthur Henry Fitzroy Paget (1851-1928), an army officer and his wife Mary Fiske (Minnie) Stevens (d1919). The couple had no children.

Nursing in Serbia with Lady Paget in 1915

In recognition of his services in Siam, Paget was knighted in 1909 and his wife became Lady Paget. Although considered, for the post of Ambassador to the German Empire, he was instead despatched to Munich to become Minister Resident in the Kingdoms of Bavaria and Wurttemberg. In July 1910, Paget was appointed Envoy Extraordinary and Minister Plenipotentiary to the Kingdom of Serbia. He remained until 1913, when he was recalled to London and appointed an Assistant Under-Secretary of State for Foreign Affairs in charge of the American Department. He was serving in this post when he agreed in March 1915 to become British Commissioner acting on behalf of the Serbian Relief Fund and British Red Cross Society in Serbia. Sir Ralph played an important and probably vital role in assisting all the British Units in Serbia and yet the post is seldom mentioned amidst his long list of prestigious diplomatic appointments.

Sir Ralph Paget joined other members of the British units who retreated across the mountains of Albania. His safe arrival back in London was reported to the executive committee of the Serbian Relief Fund on 23 December 1915. For a brief period, Sir Ralph agreed to act as the representative of the Serbian Relief Fund in Rome and in February he attended a conference in Paris as their representative. However, by then a large camp of Serbian refugees had been established in Corsica and it was thought inadvisable to open any further camps in Italy. With the safe return of his wife in February, Sir Ralph's involvement with the work in Serbia seems to have come to an end.

By 1917, the couple had moved to Copenhagen where Sir Ralph served as British Minister from 1916 to 1918.[270] On 26th September 1918, Sir Ralph reached the pinnacle of his career when he was appointed British Ambassador to Brazil. Before taking up this post, however, he was employed first as a permanent official of the British delegation to the Paris Peace Conference, with responsibility for the Balkans. In this role he was to play a crucial role in the reorganisation of Central and Eastern Europe out of which eventually the longed for pan-Slavonic alliance of the Kingdom of Serbs, Croats and Slovenes (from 1929 Yugoslavia) would be created. It was not until 1919 that Sir Ralph finally took up his post in

The Cast of Characters

Rio de Janeiro and the couple remained only for a year, before retiring to Sittingbourne in Kent. Recurring bad health and a bout of depression had finally put paid to Sir Ralph's diplomatic career.

In 1929, this well travelled couple moved to Lady Paget's father's house, Warren House, in Kingston Hill, Surrey. Here Lady Paget enjoyed breeding birds and flowers but also kept in contact with all her Serbian friends, proving a strong supporter of the new nation of Yugoslavia. When in October1934, the Yugoslav King was assassinated, Lady Paget attended his funeral in Belgrade. It was her last visit to Serbia. Her husband Sir Ralph died on 11th May 1940 in Saint-Raphael, France.

During the Second World War, Lady Paget turned her home in to a Convalescent Home for soldiers and when the Germans invaded Yugoslavia in 1941, she offered her support once more to the Government in Exile. After the war, she devoted herself to helping the ten thousand or more Serbs who found themselves 'displaced persons' in Britain and her home became a meeting place for Serbian political refugees. She is said to have spent a fortune in supporting a large number of students amongst them, through higher education and she also helped to finance both the Serbian Club and the Serbian Church of St Sava in London. The church which opened in 1952, still has today a Lady Paget room.

Lady Paget died at her final home, Soames House, Coombe Hill Road, Kingston upon Thames on 24th September 1958.[271] A memorial service for her, held at the Church of St Sava was attended by members of the Yugoslav Royal family but it is clear that many ordinary Serbs had equal cause to remember her with affection. After her death a memorial to her entitled 'Spomenica Ledi Pedžet' was published in Serbia. Even sixty years after her death she was still remembered by the Serbian community with a special service.

The highest honours awarded to Lady Paget in her life time were the Dame Grand Cross of the Most Excellent Order of the British Empire and the Serbian Order of St Sava but perhaps she would have been most pleased with the use of her name for a street in Belgrade. She is often recalled as saying: *'Should it happen that everyone forgets me, I wouldn't*

Nursing in Serbia with Lady Paget in 1915

care! But I would not take it lightly should my Serbs forget me!'.

Ivy Grace Pickering (1889-1961)

Nurse with Flora Scott at Lady Paget's Hospital

Ivy was born in Rodeheath near Congleton in Cheshire on 22 October 1899. She was the daughter of Clement W Pickering 'a dealer in table salt' and his wife, Frances. By the time of the 1911 census, her family had moved to 19 Parry Street in Leicester, but Ivy herself was resident at the Nurses' Home run by Flora's sister, Jessie, at 31 Highfield Street.

Her medal card records that she served with the Serbian Relief Fund from January to July 1915 as a VAD nurse and she does not appear to have had formal training as a nurse.[272]

On 19 January 1918, she married Archibald Harry Tollemache, a Captain with the King's Own (Royal Lancaster) Regiment at St Michael's, Ramsey in Essex. Ivy gave birth to a daughter Joyce Ramsay in June 1919 but by this time her husband had been forced to resign his commission owing to ill health caused by his wounds.[273] He died in December 1930, aged only thirty five.

Ivy and her mother settled at 2 Newfield Square, off the Narborough Road in Leicester where she died on 27th July 1961.

Henry Fremlin Squire (1893-1961)

Medical Orderly with Lady Paget

Born on 10 August 1893, Squire was the son of Leonard Harding Squire, Vicar of All Saints, Kenley in Surrey and his wife Alice Mary Brooker. He was educated at St Laurence College, Ramsgate and went up to Gonville and Caius College, Cambridge to study medicine in 1912. With the outbreak of war, he left his studies to serve as a Red Cross volunteer

The Cast of Characters

with Lady Paget.

A rough diary which Squire kept from 15 Nov 1914 to 7 Feb 1915 and his letters home to his parents, which survive at the Imperial War Museum chronicle the early days of the hospital.[274] Typical is the entry for Sunday 15th November:

'We hope to disembark at Salonika tonight as everyone is sick of this pokey smelly little boat. Arrive about 6. Can't land owing to various ceremonies to be performed by the port authorities. Fed in resignation but were cheered to find that the combined pressure of the Serbian & British consuls stirred up the sleepy port & we got on shore into a decent hotel. Mon 16th Saw Salonika. In morning found a priceless cake shop which provided cakes better than any Cambridge: 'Deadly'. Helped oversee the disembarking of bales & bathed on the quay drying in the sun as we had no impedimenta therefore. Ghastly news. We have to get up at 4.30 am tomorrow. Lost our way in several Turkish bazaars & alleys...'

On 17th January, Squire wrote home enthusiastically, that the unit would be staying until 31st March and that he hoped to be home mid-April for a brief holiday before taking *'promised jobs as dressers with the St John's Ambulance Society in France'*. Professor Morrison, the Chief Surgeon, was obviously being relied upon to use his influence to secure the posts. By the end of January, he had changed his mind and liked the idea of serving with the Berry unit which had just arrived, but was reluctant to leave Lady Paget whilst she was so understaffed. In the event, ill health forced him to abandon all these ambitions and on 22nd February he reported to his parents that he was coming home in Sir Thomas Lipton's private yacht. He was eventually discharged from the Red Cross with a Silver War Badge in 1917

Back in England Squire returned to his medical studies at Cambridge and St Bartholomew's Hospital in London, serving briefly as a house surgeon there. He contributed a letter on 'Serbia's Crying Need' to the *Cambridge Magazine* in February 1918.

Nursing in Serbia with Lady Paget in 1915

Once qualified, Squire joined his brother in the newly formed Royal Air Force. He was appointed a Lieutenant in the RAF Medical Service on 18 June 1918 and promoted to Captain a year later.

Demobilised in 1922, Squire returned to general practice, firstly in Huddersfield and then in Henfield in Sussex. He went on to serve as District Medical Officer for Steyning in Sussex where he had married his wife Dorothy I V Walter in June 1918.

Squire's career in the RAF, however, continued as a member of the RAF Volunteer Reserve and he held a commission as a Flight Lieutenant in the medical branch with effect from 27 December 1937.[275] In 1939, he was appointed full time Medical Officer at RAF Tangmere and in 1940, despite his age, persuaded his superiors to post him to RAF Heliopolis in Egypt. From there he went on to serve in the Western Desert, Greece, Cyprus and Malta. During the evacuation of Greece he was pleased to find he still remembered a little Serbian as he helped with the reception of refugees from Yugoslavia. Squire returned in time to serve in France from July to October 1944, before resigning his commission with effect from 14 December 1944. He retained the rank of Squadron Leader.

Squire's memoirs of this period were published in 1997 by his son David under the title *'Middle East Scrapbook by RAFMO'* and included transcriptions of a selection of his letters home whilst serving with Lady Paget.

Squire died on 5th February 1961, aged sixty seven at Batts, Henfield, leaving effects of £33,620.12.10 to his son Dr John Walter Squire.

Monica Marie Stanley (1878-1972)

Head Cook with Mrs Stobart's Unit

Monica was born at Marple in Cheshire, the daughter of Dane Stanley and his wife, Flora Middleton. Her father described himself in the 1881 census as a civil and mining engineer involved in cotton transportation

The Cast of Characters

as well as a farmer of fifteen acres at Godley in Cheshire. Apparently these various ventures prospered, for ten years later he was living on his own means and the family were resident in Llandrillo yn Rhos near Conway in Denbighshire.

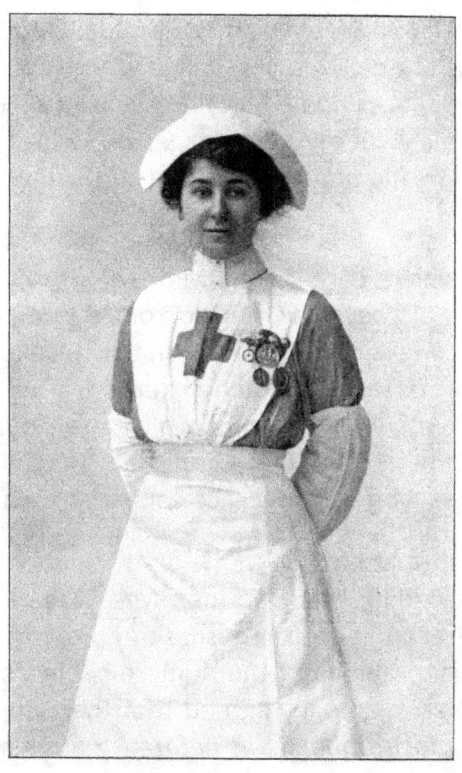

Monica M Stanley (from her book My Diary in Serbia, *c. 1916)*

Monica left home to study domestic science in London, living with her aunt Elizabeth Stanley at 35 Albert Mansions in Battersea. Having trained at Battersea Polytechnic Domestic Science Training Department, she was able to list attainments in cookery, high class cookery, needle work, laundry work, dress making, housewifery, millinery and hygiene. When she registered as a teacher on 1st August 1914, she was employed as head cookery mistress at Wandsworth Technical Institute and had worked there since 1905.

Nursing in Serbia with Lady Paget in 1915

In April 1915, the governors of the Wandsworth Institute generously granted Monica leave so that she could serve as head cook with Mrs Stobart's unit. In July, they granted her a three months extension. On 1 April 1915, Monica departed from Liverpool aboard SS Saidieh, equipped with the permitted one cabin trunk and a hold-all. It was a boat crowded with units on their way to Serbia, and Monica delighted – once the sea was calm- in the social side, enjoying bridge with Claude Askew and his wife, the delights of dances and a fancy dress party which she attended as a mattress, as well as learning two pages of Serbian a day with Mrs Stobart: *'We are all such a happy party, and all the units on board have been so friendly...'* [276]

The unit once assembled, consisted of Mrs Stobart, Mr J H Greenhalgh the treasurer, a secretary, seven women doctors, eighteen trained nurses, four trained cooks, one dispenser, one sanitary inspector, the English chaplain Percy Dearmer and fourteen orderlies, of which some were chauffeurs together with a field hospital which was *'perfectly equipped'*. They also took with them over £300 of food stuff. The unit established its hospital under canvas a on a former race course at Kragujevatz.

In June, the unit was struck down by typhoid with twelve members of the unit off sick, including Mrs Dearmer. Mrs Stobart, Monica and a doctor had a conference about the disease and debated the cause of the outbreak. Suspicion fell upon the numerous flies, and even eating *'raw salad'* but it was eventually agreed that the camp itself was the problem: *'This was most probable, as before we arrived this camp was covered with refugees from all parts; and with the very dry weather and then the heavy rains, most of the doctors think it is due to this...'* [277]

Amidst the misfortunes of a hurricane and an air raid, Monica herself fell ill and she was eventually sent to convalesce with the Berry unit. Here she delighted in learning Serbian dishes down in the kitchen. Whilst there she heard of the first death of a member of her unit – Nurse Lorna Ferris: *'...a strong healthy girl of twenty-five years of age. She was to be married in September. She was taken ill just about a week before me with typhoid. It does not say much for inoculation. Nurse Ferris was a good nurse; she had a bright, cheerful manner and was always the same. She*

The Cast of Characters

knew Serbian better than anyone in the camp, and could sing the Serbian anthem...' [278]

On 9th July Monica returned to the Stobart camp just before the death of Mrs Dearmer. She made a wreath for the funeral in the shape of a cross, using wild flowers and acacia and clematis and described the funeral in detail.

As Monica was still subject to fevers, she was sent to the British Fever Hospital in Belgrade and also spent a week with Lady Paget at Skoplje before returning to work at Kragujevatz at the end of August. News reached the camp at this time that Nurse Vivyan Berry *'a beautiful girl and a splendid nurse'*, who had nursed Monica when she first became ill, had died on arriving home in England.[279]

Monica continued to suffer ill health and, much to her annoyance, was advised that she should not work in the kitchen departments for six months. As her leave of absence was running out, she was wisely fearful that it might be *'rather difficult later on to get away',*[280] and obtained permission to return home in October 1915. She was asked on the journey, to look after an orderly from the second Farmer's unit who had just recovered from typhoid and was also returning home. On their way down to Salonika amongst large crowds of refugees from the bombardment of Belgrade, they found a brief haven at the rest station at Nish which Sir Ralph and Lady Paget provided for staff of the English units. Monica was still in Salonika on 17th October when Lady Paget arrived with five nurses from Admiral Troubridge's unit, on her way to try to persuade the Allied generals to save Serbia.

Monica boarded SS Sydney bound for Marseilles on Tuesday 19th October. With her also travelled one of the doctors from Lady Paget's hospital, two nurses from Admiral Troubridge, six Scottish Women's Hospital nurses from Valjevo, two French doctors and an English lady who had been teaching in Bulgaria for six years.[281] She reached Boulogne on the last day of October.

Monica returned to work at the Wandsworth Institute and her account

Nursing in Serbia with Lady Paget in 1915

of her recent experiences *'My Diary in Serbia'* was published in February 1916, dedicated to her *'very dear aunt'* Elizabeth Stanley.

In June 1927, Monica married Leon Daviel, an artist who was a close neighbour at Albert Mansions, at St Mary Le Park Chapel of Ease in Battersea. She was forty eight and he was a widower, fifteen years older. Leon, a portrait painter, wood engraver and illustrator had moved to London from his native France in 1891. The couple lived together at Stanley House, 16 Glebe Place in Chelsea until Leon's death, aged sixty seven in June 1932.

In January 1938, Monica, apparently alone and describing herself as a domestic science teacher, embarked for Columbo in Sri Lanka. She may well have remained there during the war, since there is no further record of her in England until she disembarked at Southampton at the end of 1959. She died on 25th July 1972 at St Luke's Hospital in London, leaving effects of £3,556.

Mrs St Clair Stobart (1862-1954)

Administrator of the Serbian Relief Fund's 3rd Unit

Mabel Annie Boulton, was born on 3rd February 1862 at Woolwich in Kent. She was the second daughter of Samuel Bagster Boulton, a continental timber merchant and his wife Sophia of Charlton, Greenwich. In 1905, in recognition of his services to British commerce, Boulton was made a Baronet and in later life settled at Copped Hall, Fotherbridge in Hertfordshire, where he no doubt enjoyed his role as Lord of the Manor of Totteridge, Justice of the Peace and Deputy Lieutenant of Hertfordshire.

On 16 July 1884, his lively and adventurous daughter married St Clair Kelburn Mulholland Stobart. At the time of the 1891 census, the couple were settled with their two sons at Penmorvah in Budock, Cornwall where Stobart was working as a stone granite merchant. The granite business was obviously lucrative for the family were at this time served

The Cast of Characters

by a governess, cook, three maids, a gardener and a coachman. The couple shared a love of fly fishing and had the time and money to enjoy fishing in countries which ranged from Finland and Northern Sweden to Corsica.[282] By 1901, they were resident at 11 Chelsea Gardens in London but Stobart declared no occupation on his census return.

In 1903, in the wake of financial misfortune, the family moved out to South Africa where they trekked over the Karoo and established a farm and trading station. The enterprise was not wholly successful and in 1907, Mrs Stobart returned to England. Her husband, following her home a year later, died at sea on 9th April 1908.

Although she always retained her first married name, Mrs Stobart remarried in early 1911. Her new husband was John Herbert Greenhalgh, a retired barrister, originally from Mansfield in Nottinghamshire and the newly weds settled at 3, Reynolds Close in Hampstead Garden Suburb. The couple took the unusual step of using their combined surnames.

So far, it had been an eventful life full of adventure which would have been quite sufficient for most, but now Mrs Stobart and her compliant husband embarked on the greatest adventure yet. On her

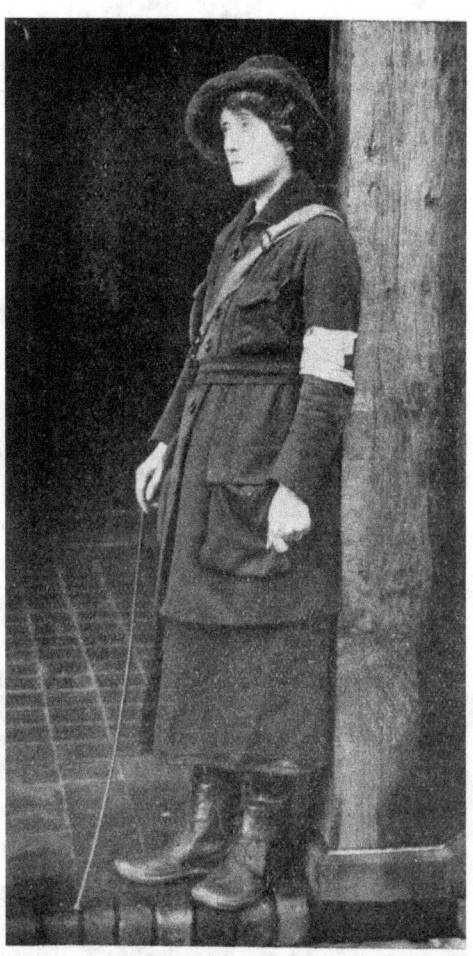

Mrs St Clair Stobart (from Women of the War *by Barbara McLaren, 1917)*

243

Nursing in Serbia with Lady Paget in 1915

return to England, Mrs Stobart had become interested in the struggle for women's suffrage, regularly attending meetings of the National Union of Women's Suffrage Societies. She saw a clear need to prove that women were worthy of the same opportunities as men. To this end, in 1912, she founded the Women's Sick and Wounded Convoy Corps, a medical unit staffed by women including three 'lady doctors', and six nurses, and proceeded to lead them out to Bulgaria during the First Balkan War. There the unit successfully established a surgical hospital at Kirk Kilisse close to the front line and for the first time female doctors and surgeons tended to men wounded in battle. It was a gruelling and appalling experience, but the important point had been made that women doctors exposed to the horrors of war were just as skilful as their male counterparts. The unit served for five weeks until the armistice and Mrs Stobart wrote an account of the experience entitled *'War and Women from Experience in the Balkans and Elsewhere'.*

It was natural, at the outbreak of war, that Mrs Stobart should want to be involved. As the Corps which she had founded had, much to her annoyance, resolved to amalgamate with the British Red Cross, she had resigned her membership. Now with the assistance of The St John's Ambulance Association and the Women's Imperial Service League, she assembled a new Women's unit and offered its services to the Belgian Red Cross. With her husband in tow once more as treasurer, Mrs Stobart now set about establishing a hospital at the Summer Concert Hall in Antwerp.

The hospital functioned for three weeks before the bombardment of Antwerp and German occupation, forced them to evacuate. Amidst the chaos and horror, the unit gallantly saved their wounded but lost all the equipment. Aided once more by the St John's Ambulance Association and the Women's Imperial Service League in conjunction with the British Red Cross, the unit was reequipped and invited by the French Red Cross to establish a new hospital at Tourlaville near Cherbourg.

Mrs Stobart had been at Cherbourg for four months when she first read that an epidemic of typhus had broken out in Serbia: *'... that the hospitals were overcrowded with sick and wounded; that one third of*

The Cast of Characters

the Serbian doctors had died, either of typhus, or at the front, and that nursing and medical help were badly needed. I knew from the moment when I read that report, that I should go...'[283]

On 4th February 1915, Mrs Stobart first proposed to the Serbian Relief Fund that she should organise a Women's Hospital Unit for Serbia.[284] The Executive Committee agreed to give £2000 towards the project. On 1st April, a group of forty nine, including seven women doctors, eighteen trained nurses and an extensive support staff of cooks, orderlies, chauffeurs and interpreters travelled in two parties to Salonika, with the redoubtable Mrs Stobart at its head and her no doubt long suffering husband as treasurer. This 3rd Serbian Relief Unit, usually referred to as the Stobart Unit, was in many ways the least successful of the Serbian Relief undertakings and it certainly suffered the most casualties. However, its later fame was assured by the high visibility of its often controversial leader.

A hospital of three hundred beds was established under canvas at Kragujevatz on a large area which had formerly served as a race course. The site was flat and did not drain well but more disastrously still had recently housed large crowds of refugees and their livestock, a fact which probably accounts for all the sickness suffered by the staff there and the high casualty rate.

However, the hospital impressed many and in September, Mrs Stobart was honoured to be asked by the Serbians to lead a flying field hospital, delighted to receive the temporary rank of Major in the Serbian army. With a detachment of eighteen from her unit and sixty Serbian soldiers, Mrs Stobart left her hospital and entrained for Pirot. The new corps was to be known as the First Serbian-English Field Hospital but had little time to operate before being swept up in the retreat across the mountains of Montenegro and Albania. The rest of her former unit was also involved in the long trek across the mountains and reached home with only one casualty. Nurse 'Ginger' Clifton was accidentally shot by two Serbs quarrelling over a gun. She was seriously wounded and a doctor and two nurses from the unit remained behind to nurse her and were captured by the Austrians. All were eventually safely repatriated.

Nursing in Serbia with Lady Paget in 1915

Mrs Stobart published a vivid account of her exploits in Belgium, Serbia and the tragic retreat of the Serbian Army during which, with typical flamboyance, she led her unit astride a black charger. Sir Ralph Paget, for one, was intensely irritated by her activities since he was not kept informed of developments and it is clear that there was tension between Mrs Stobart and her medical staff. Mrs Stobart's unit eventually caught the last boat out of San Giovanni di Madeua on 23rd December and travelled home via Brindisi and Rome. In London, to her chagrin, she met a frosty reception, being reprimanded by the Chairman of the Serbian Relief Committee for having exceeded her instructions and led her unit to unnecessary risks in accompanying the army to the front.[285]

Mrs Stobart later departed to America for a lecture tour. After the war she became interested in spiritualism and she and her husband retired to Studland in Dorset. Her husband John Greenhalgh died on 2nd March 1928. Mrs Stobart took command briefly for a last time when she served, as a presumably rather formidable, air raid warden in Hendon and died at Bournemouth on 7th December 1954. She is buried with her second husband in St Nicholas Church, Studland.

James William Wiles (1877-c1950)

Interpreter

Wiles was born in Cambridge, the son of James Wiles, a marble mason and erstwhile insurance agent and his wife Harriet. Although in the 1891 census, he was the clerk in a grocery, Wiles' fortunes apparently changed dramatically for by 1901, he was a 'college student'. In 1911, he was a school master at King Edward VI School in Birmingham. He had also been married that year to Louisa Duncana McPherson.

It must have been in Birmingham that Wiles made the acquaintance of the surgeon Mr Morrison who described him as *'an old friend'*.[286] In 1913, Wiles went out to Serbia to take up a position as reader in English at Belgrade University but presumably returned to England on the outbreak of hostilities. Morrison recruited him as the interpreter for Lady Paget's hospital unit and he seems to have spent most of his

The Cast of Characters

time serving as secretary-interpreter to Morrison. In Skoplje, he was quartered with Morrison and the four dressers in a villa placed at their disposal by the Italian Consul.

Towards the end of January 1915, Morrison was convalescent after typhus and paid a visit to Nish where the Prime Minister asked him to make inspections of several hospitals as part of the Typhus Commission. Wiles clearly accompanied him on this tour and himself fell ill with typhus. Helen M Coleman, a nurse with Lady Paget told the *Leicester Daily Post* that she was *'a month in Nish helping to nurse our interpreter who taught us some Serbian and phrases on the outward journey. These proved very helpful to us in our work...'*[287]

Dr Abraham of the British Red Cross also recalled Wiles as *'a large, blond man, loosely built, carelessly dressed and full of enthusiasm'*. In early March 1915, he was returning from a visit to the Berry unit at Vrnjacka Banja to Nish when he was delighted to be *'hailed by a friendly voice from a passing fiacre, asking if I wanted a lift.'*[288]

Wiles or *Professor Wiles* as Abraham termed him, seemed to be wandering round the country on his own and was returning to Nish that day:

'The Professor, after his agglutinative manner, had picked up another companion, an odd looking little waiter from one of the hotels, whose only baggage seemed to be an atomiser filled with some antiseptic fluid with which he continually sprayed himself and wished to spray us also... The Professor, talking fluent Serbian, collected everyone within hearing distance round him by his kindly enthusiastic aura. With such a companion one's journey was a sort of Royal progress. We talked and laughed and ate each other's luncheons- the inevitable bread, salt boiled bacon and red wine- seated in a cattle truck labelled 'Cheveaux 10 hommes 40'...'

The happy pair eventually reached Stallash to find there was no train until the next day and resolved to sleep under the stars until deterred by a sentry and distracted by attending to his sick wife. At Nish, the pair

Nursing in Serbia with Lady Paget in 1915

took breakfast at the 'Ruski Tzar' amidst English and French newspaper correspondents and then dined at one at 'The Colunna' where Colonel Hunter and his second in command were dining with representatives of Dr Clemow's mission:

'Altogether some thirty British doctors, with Sir Charles Des Gras our Minister, Colonel Harrison, the military attaché, several Serbian War Office officials and Professor Wiles made up a large and cheery company...'

Abraham clearly enjoyed the experience and was briefly distracted from the horrors of the typhus epidemic.

Wiles must have returned to England with Morrison when the first unit withdrew on 31st March. There are few clues as to his later career but in 1930 he was appointed the first English lector in the newly founded Department of English in the University of Belgrade and published an English translation of *'the Mountain Wreath of PP Nyegosh, prince bishop of Montenegro'*.

Wiles subsequently appears to have left the academic world to serve as head of the British and Foreign Bible Society for South Eastern Europe. In 1939, he was in Gislingham, in Suffolk, recently widowed and describing his occupation as *'Secretary to the British and Foreign Bible Society in Yugoslavia'.*

Lady Cornelia Wimborne (1847-1927)

Founder of the Wimborne Unit

Lady Cornelia Henrietta Maria Spencer Churchill was born in 1847, the daughter of the 7th Duke of Marlborough. As the sister of Lord Randolph Churchill she would later become the Aunt to a certain Winston Churchill but, more importantly still, in 1868, at the tender age of twenty years, she became the bride of Sir Ivor Bertie Guest. Guest was the heir to the vast iron works at Dowlais in Glamorgan and, amongst other properties, an estate which his parents had purchased at Canford Manor near Poole in Dorset. The first of their nine children was born in 1869.

The Cast of Characters

The couple enjoyed a life of great opulence but Cornelia also found time to indulge her interests in philanthropy, sponsoring the building of local schools and cottages for their tenants. When her husband was raised to a peerage in 1880, she became Lady Wimborne. She was known as a great public speaker and a local Mayor once observed not altogether kindly that she *'had an irresistible means of getting her own way which should cause any man that did not agree with her to fly to the uttermost ends of the earth.'*[289]

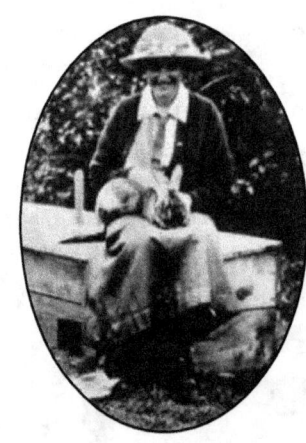

Another field of interest was medical health and she at first established a small surgery in Poole before, In 1890, she bought an old mansion house there and set up a hospital of thirty beds, known thereafter as the Cornelia Hospital. She threw herself in to fund raising, as in all things, with enormous energy and given the interest of so many titled ladies in the cause, it was natural that she should look to the Serbian Relief Fund as a channel for her energies. The minutes of the Executive Committee record that she and Lady Rodney were added to the Committee on 7th January 1915, on the same day that she gave notice of her proposed hospital unit. She funded the Wimborne Unit and played a full part as a member of the committee despite having recently been widowed.

When she died in 1927, an obituary recalled her as a *'great force of character'* who, had she been born a few years later *'might have figured as prominently in politics as her brother or nephew...'*

Nursing in Serbia with Lady Paget in 1915

Appendix 1

The Serbian Relief Fund 1914-1920

The outstanding achievement of the Serbian Relief Fund [SRF] was its success in raising money. Through letters in the Press and the organisation of 'Flag Days' and other fund raising events and aided, no doubt, by the stout resistance of the Serbian nation to the Austrian hordes, the committee was able to raise an astonishing amount of money. Subscriptions received by 1st October 1914 amounted to £1750 and by the beginning of December had increased to £14, 487.16.5.[290] Crucially, the success of their publicity was also able to attract the support of wealthy patrons. By February 1915, the organisation was sufficiently well established to be able to boast of Queen Mary as Patroness and political figures such as the Prime Minister Herbert Asquith, Andrew Bonar Law, Samuel Herbert, Winston Churchill and Austen Chamberlain as Vice Presidents.

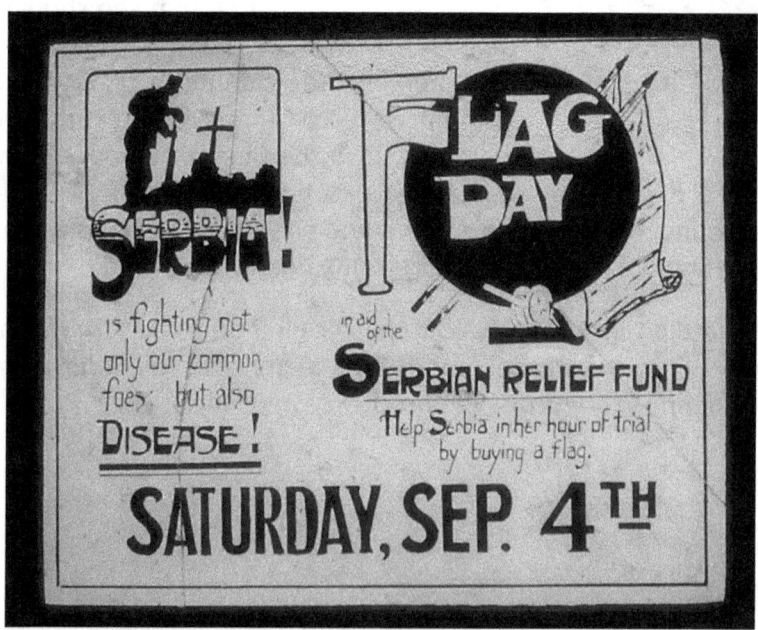

Glass lantern-slide issued by the Serbian Relief Fund for fund-raising, c. 1915

Serbian Relief Fund

The Fund which had initially set out with the modest aim of supplying Red Cross aid to Serbia, was able to equip and maintain four hospital units:

1st Serbian Relief Unit: Formed by the St John Ambulance Association in conjunction with the Serbian Relief Fund, the first hospital unit of fifty six members under Lady Paget, set out for Serbia aboard the SS Dongola on 29th October 1914. Although the Serbian Government undertook to supply rations, the Serbian Relief Fund provided all stores and equipment. In December, £8000 was reserved for the maintenance and equipment of the hospital in Skoplje. A further £1000 was sent at the beginning of March *'in view of the serious sanitary condition existing'*. The unit was recalled at the end of March 1915 although several supplementary members who had joined the unit later stayed on after this period.

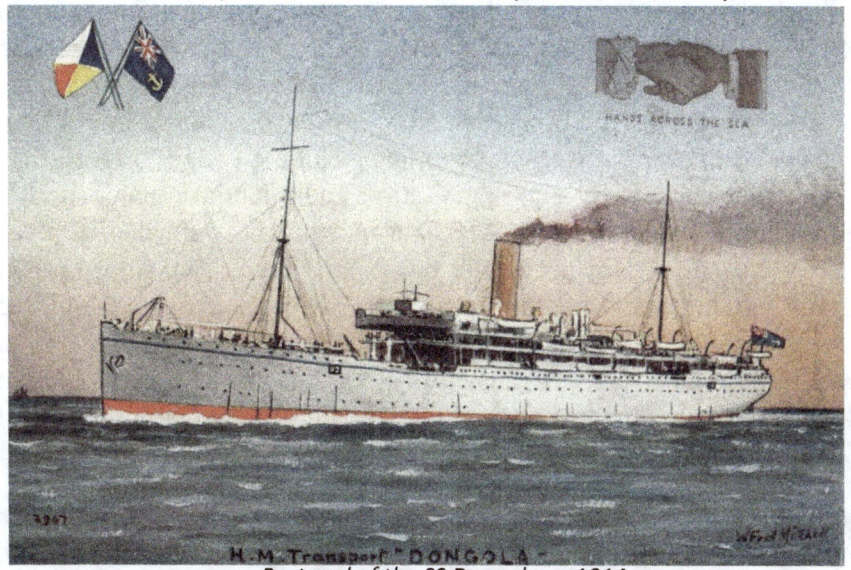
Postcard of the SS Dongola, c. 1914

In July 1915, Lady Paget established a second unit, drawing upon British personnel who were already working in Serbia as well as many of the fever nurses who joined the Typhus Colony in April 1915. Doctors and nursing staff from America and Denmark also joined this unit, as well as three Dutch nurses and a solitary French nurse. In September, a special

Nursing in Serbia with Lady Paget in 1915

grant of £2000 was made at the request of Lady Paget *'in view of the situation'*. The unit was captured by the Bulgarians and repatriated in February 1916.

A full list of personnel for both units, extracted from Lady Paget's reports, is given in appendix 2.

2nd Serbian Relief Unit: A second hospital unit of forty five members, funded by Lady Wimborne and under the leadership of W P G Graham was sent out in February 1915. The Serbian Relief Fund, contributed a grant of £2000. Miss Monsie Scott, sister of the famous Polar explorer acted as principal assistant and the surgeon in chief was Mr Barrington Ward. The assistant surgeons were Mr G H Sinclair and Mr Edmund B Jones and the physician was Dr Bellingham Smith. Dr J Dalyell 'the lady doctor' served as bacteriologist and anaesthetist and the matron was Miss Eveline Roberts. Nurses were Miss M G Davies; Miss Eleanor Davies; Miss Atkinson; Miss Bishop; Miss Frost; Miss Sinclair; Miss Davidson; Miss Sketchley; Miss Thompson and Miss Ethel Thompson.[291] There were in addition nine women orderlies including Lady Muriel Herbert; twelve male orderlies; a cook; assistant cook; laundry-maid; assistant laundry maid; dispenser and quartermaster. The unit was furnished with X-Ray equipment presented by a Mrs Aitken. Their hospital was established in the old fortress known as 'the Grad' in Skoplje and took over Lady Paget's hospital from 31st March. In March 1915, Mr Graham was authorised to carry out measures for the sanitation of Nish and Skoplje up to an initial expense of £5000. The sum was later modified to £2000. The unit was withdrawn in June 1915.

Details of the Unit appear in *'Serbia and the Serbians. Letters from Lady Muriel Herbert who was with the Second Serbian Relief Unit'* published by her sister Lady Beatrix Wilkinson in 1915

3rd Serbian Relief Unit: Organised by the Women's Imperial Service League under the directorship of Mrs St Clair Stobart [qv], the unit received a grant of £2000 from the Serbian Relief Fund. Mrs Stobart and nineteen of the unit of forty nine members, left Liverpool on 1st April 1915 on SS Saidieh. Also aboard were members of the British Farmers' Unit;

Serbian Relief Fund

Dr Beavis' unit, the Wounded Allies Relief Fund and Admiral Troubridge's unit, as well as *'a Russian one'*. The remaining thirty members travelled to Salonika via Folkstone, Boulogne and Marseilles.

Stores including sixty three tents – the large ones sufficient to hold fifteen to twenty patients- three hundred beds, hospital equipment and £300 worth of food stuff had already been despatched on the Admiralty transport SS Torcello.

Surgical and medical staff for the main unit were Mrs King-May Atkinson; Miss Beatice Coxon; Miss Helen Hanson; Miss Mabel Eliza King-May; Miss Edith Maude Marsden; Miss Catherine Payne and Miss Isabel Tate. Mrs Stobart's husband acted as treasurer and the Reverend Dr Percy Dearmer served as chaplain.

Planned to be under canvas so as to be 'free of infection', the hospital was erected on a former racecourse at Kragujevatz and subsequently set up roadside dispensaries for the civilian population. Unit members accompanied the Serbian army on its disastrous retreat across the mountains of Montenegro and Albania in November 1915 and reached London in December.

A full list of personnel including nursing sisters, women orderlies, men orderlies and chauffeurs for the main unit and the dispensaries' staff is to be found at the end of Mrs Stobart's account of the expedition: *'The Flaming Sword in Serbia and elsewhere'* published in 1917 [See also p. 292 below]. Vivid descriptions of camp life at Kragujevatz appear in *'Letters from a Field Hospital with a memoir of the author by Stephen Gwynn'* by Mabel Dearmer, published in 1916 and *'My Diary in Serbia April 1915-November 1 1915'* by Monica M Stanley(the unit's cook) published in February 1916.

4th **Serbian Relief Unit:** Known as the British Farmers' Hospital because it was partly funded by the British Farmer Red Cross Fund, this unit was equipped as a fever hospital under the directorship of Mr L M Wynch with Mrs Arthur Moore acting as secretary. The unit included four medical men [Dr Fabian First; Mr A J Beadel; Dr R M Morison and Dr J Wilman[292]],

Nursing in Serbia with Lady Paget in 1915

a matron [Miss Mozley], a dispenser, fifteen nursing sisters [Mrs Bailey; Mrs Wilman; Misses Helena Bird; E Burgess; KM Coaling; I R Hudson; H M Jackson; E B Mellis; E L Pybus; Roodhouse; E Scammel; P Searle; F M Shoring; M Terry and L Trendell[293]], thirteen women orderlies and four male orderlies. One of the latter was Hugh Watts Taylor, a medical student of 47 St Stephens Road, Leicester who had already served with the Belgians in Antwerp and Flanders.[294] The majority of the nurses had received training in dealing with fevers and many of them already had experience of typhus and other fevers abroad. Several subsequently joined Lady Paget's second unit.

On its departure from Liverpool on 1st April 1915 aboard the same ship as Mrs Stobart, T G Howe, organising secretary of the Fund, declared to the Daily Chronicle: *'In every way Unit no 4 is the finest we have yet dispatched to Serbia. We are particularly proud of the completeness of the scientific bacteriological and sanitary equipment of the hospital.'*[295]

The unit established itself in Belgrade and staffed the British Fever Hospital which was widely admired and used by other units. Monica Stanley, when she fell ill with typhoid, was sent to the hospital and was pleased to know many of the Farmers' unit already, having travelled out with them: *'This hospital faces the Danube and is most interesting ... This is a lovely hospital, it will hold over 500 beds; it was an university before the war; the art rooms on the top floor are splendid...'*[296]

On 21st July 1915, the executive committee of the SRF resolved to maintain Unit 4 after 10th August as a nucleus hospital and a requisition of £900 for the unit was agreed. Mrs Moore was further authorised, so far as the hospital permitted, to establish a temporary orphanage in consultation and conformity with the general scheme initiated by Madame Pashitch. On 18th August it was further agreed that Mrs Moore should be permitted to have a staff of four and a hundred beds from the No 4 unit, whilst Mrs Moore herself agreed to pay the salary of the matron. This temporary orphanage was designed *'to meet the needs of the present'* until Madame Pasitch was able to organise her planned institution. A third of the stores recently consigned to Unit 4 were diverted to the use of Mrs Moore.

Serbian Relief Fund

A second British Farmer's unit of forty five people under Mr Parsons was sent out to relieve the unit in June 1915 and was posted initially to a Serbian military hospital at Posharevatz eight miles from the Austrian frontier. It was at first planned that this unit would take over in Belgrade at the end of October when the six month contracts of the staff there was due to expire. However, with the renewal of war, the group was overtaken by events. The last members of the 2nd Farmers' unit reached Belgrade at the beginning of October.

It is clear that some members of the 1st Farmers' unit did make it home before Belgrade fell. On 8th October, Monica Stanley, on her way home from the Stobart camp because of ill health, met some three or four of the 1st Farmers' unit at Lapovo, amongst a crowd of refugees from Belgrade:

'They all looked very ill and were covered with mud. They had left Belgrade at 6 o'clock the night before, and had had to walk many miles before they could get the train, and had left everything behind them, only having the clothes they stood up in...' [298]

Mr Wynch had returned to London by 27th October, when he received a vote of thanks from the committee of the Serbian Relief Fund.

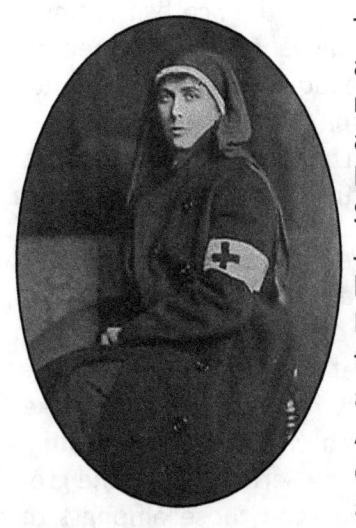

The writer Ellen Chivers Davies who was an orderly with the 2nd Farmers' unit wrote movingly of the bombardment of Belgrade and the evacuation of the hospital, first to Mladenovatz where they were aided by the Scottish Women's hospital staff and then to Jagodina where they nursed briefly before being moved to the spa town of Vrngatchka Banya. Here they were captured along side the British Red Cross unit and the Berry unit and a small contingent of the Wounded Allies Relief Fund. They remained prisoners of the Austrians until repatriated via Vienna and Zurich in February 1916. Mr Parsons

Nursing in Serbia with Lady Paget in 1915

attended a meeting of the Serbian Relief Fund in London on 24th February 1916 and a final footnote to the adventure appeared in the minutes for 2nd February when Olive Hoare was thanked for rescuing the surgical instruments of the unit from the hands of the Austrian invaders.

Other Spheres of Activity : In addition to these above undertakings, the minutes of the executive committee of the SRF contain records of grants to various other projects in Serbia, including £1000 to the Berry Mission. Donations made by them in December 1914 included £1000 for blankets for the Serbian Red Cross and £1,500 for materials for the Serbian Red Cross in Nish. The following month there were donations of £2,519 to Madame Grujić and a grant of £2,600 to the Red Cross. There was also funding for overalls for Dr Bennett's Red Cross unit and a modest £250 towards the efforts of Miss Annie Christitch in Valievo. Miss Christitch, a distinguished Serbian feminist and journalist had given much help to the Scottish Women's Hospital unit in Kragujevatz.[299]

Not all such requests for money met with a favourable reception. In August 1915, when the wife of Admiral Troubridge asked for £1000 for the hospital in Belgrade which was run by her husband for the Naval Brigade and civilian population, she was told firmly that it was not in the committee's power to grant money to a Hospital run by the British Government. As late as October, a request from the Scottish Women's Hospital Committee for a grant towards a dispensary for women and children, was referred back to their own headquarters. The committee also refused to make a grant towards a hospital of four thousand beds, established in a former prison in Kragujevatz by Mrs Hankin Hardy, on the grounds that they were already supporting Mrs Stobart's unit there.

A newspaper article in the *Nottingham Express* issued on 14th April 1915 stated that the SRF had by this stage, expended some £20,000 on drugs, surgical accessories, blankets, clothing and disinfectants.[300] In addition, a depot at their premises in Cromwell Street had been lent to them as a store for receiving gifts in kind. Here they had received and packed for shipment to Serbia around 750 packages of hospital stores including no fewer than 100,000 garments. Although the Serbians were the great beneficiaries of this generosity, there were even those amongst the

Serbian Relief Fund

English staff who were grateful.... Ellen Chivers Davies when a prisoner in December 1915, confessed that most of her clothes had been obtained from the Red Cross stores in Nish or looted from luggage abandoned by the Stobart unit as well as *'Most of my underwear seems to have been sent out to the Serbian Relief Fund by a kind lady named Macgregor, and I bless her every day...'*[301]

By May 1915, total receipts by the SRF amounted to £85,965.6.5, of which £48,724.9.1 had so far been spent. The money had not only helped to equip and maintain the four Hospital units but also send out Dr Moon and a large number of fever nurses ; a sanitary engineer named Mr C J Jenkin and Dr Lefray, a consulting entomologist *'to deal with the fly question'*.

In June, the plans of Madame Pasitch, the wife of the Serbian Prime Minister for an English orphanage in Skoplje were approved. After a successful Flag Day in London, a grant of £1000 was offered for the establishment of the orphanage. Plans for the orphanage were not finalised before the outbreak of war brought a halt to all such endeavours.

Attention at this point, was turning towards civil relief work, particularly in the 'ravaged districts' North and West of Uzsitsi. On 30th June it was resolved : *'That this committee considers that, failing any present prospect of the resumption of the offensive by the Serbian army, the claims of civil relief should be considered prior to those of hospital extension.'* Accordingly in July, a grant of £500 was sent of Mr Greig for distribution in Monastir.

It was nonetheless agreed that Lady Paget should take out 4000 respirators for Serbian troops when she returned, although a decision by the War Office to send 150,000 such respirators rather overshadowed the effort.

In September, the committee received a cable from Sir Ralph Paget warning that it was inadvisable to send out fresh forces for relief owing to the *'political situation'*. The Committee became increasingly powerless as the situation developed, advising remaining units rather

Nursing in Serbia with Lady Paget in 1915

belatedly in January 1916 that they were *'free to return and cannot be helped financially towards the upkeep of their hospitals but that beyond this the decision rests with the Units corporately, though the Committee advises their return...'*

On 23 December 1915, the committee heard that Sir Ralph Paget and several members of the units had safely returned to England. Sir Ralph made his report on recent events in person on 30th December. Undeterred by the loss of the most of its hospital equipment in Skoplje and Belgrade, the committee now turned its attention to helping the Serbian refugees in Corsica, undertaking to maintain 2,300 refugees there for a period of three months. In January, the committee approved the appointment of Dr Lilias Hamilton of the Wounded Allies Relief Fund as a doctor to the refugee camps in Corsica. Their agreement in March to grant money to the Scottish Women's Hospital for work in Corsica heralded a period of close cooperation with that organisation in the refugee camps there.

From this date, the committee seems to have concentrated mostly upon the care of Serbian refugees and prisoners of war. A special committee of the Serbian Relief Fund, chaired by Mrs Carrington Wilde, oversaw the education of over three hundred Serbian refugee boys in England, establishing boys' hostels in Oxford, Cambridge, Aberdeen and elsewhere.[302] Extensive help was given in Corfu to the remnants of the army which had survived the disastrous retreat across the mountains. Important work was also carried out in Corsica amongst the thousands of Serbian women and children who had arrived there as refugees. Many had been placed in huge barracks with shelter and food but little else. Establishing its headquarters in Ajaccio, the SRF planted such refugees in family groups in the surrounding villages and opened schools, dispensaries, churches and workshops for them.

Francesca Wilson, an aid worker, was interviewed by Lady Grogan who selected staff for the SRF in April 1917 and sent out to Corsica where she worked in the mountain village of Bocagnano, hastily learning Serbian. With her brother Maurice, she later worked at the SRF camp in Bizerta in Tunisia, amongst thousands of disabled Serb soldiers. She wrote an account of her experiences in her autobiography *'In the Margins of*

Serbian Relief Fund

Chaos. Recollections of Relief Work in and between Three Wars' which was published in 1944.

As the Serbian army finally began to drive back the invaders there was activity once more in Serbia. In October 1918, when Dr Isobel Emslie and her staff of the America unit of the Scottish Women's Hospital were accompanying the victorious Serbian army as it advanced from Salonika back to Belgrade, they spent a night in Skoplje in the building that had been Lady Paget's Hospital. She found members of the Serbian Relief Fund clearing out the building in preparation for the reception of civilian patients.[303] The administrator of her unit, Mrs Mary Huges Green also recalled the visit:

'That night we got to Skoplje about dusk, and went to Lady Paget's old hospital where we found some of the Serbian Relief people busy getting the place into order. They were very kind and helped us to get hot water for tea, and we spent quite a comfortable night there... We were glad to find that the town had not been very much destroyed, but most of the railway bridges and telegraph and telephone systems were blown up, and there was useless and wanton waste everywhere...' [304]

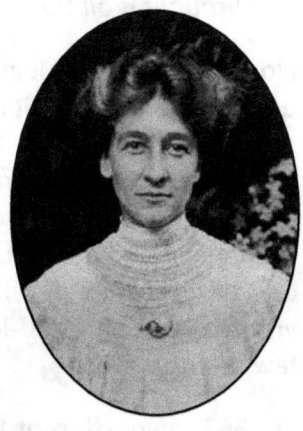

After the liberation of Serbia in 1918, the SRF played a prominent role in helping the civilian population. It was estimated that almost a quarter of the population had been lost during the war, leaving around 250,000 orphans. In the aftermath of this devastating conflict, staff of the Serbian Relief Fund worked with the new government of the Kingdom of Serbs, Croats and Slovenes to establish modern medical and social institutions for children, disabled war veterans and the sick. As part of this work, an English orphanage was opened in 1919 in a run down former poor house in Nish, under the charge of Florence Maw, a former Stobart orderly (above) and Jean Rankin, one of the fever nurses who had joined Flora at the typhus colony in April 1915. The pair had met whilst working amongst Serbian refugees in Corsica.

Nursing in Serbia with Lady Paget in 1915

The long business of winding up the Serbian Relief Fund was commenced in December 1920. All remaining assets were transferred to the Anglo-Serbian orphanage in Nish and helped to fund the erection of a purpose built modern orphanage in the grounds of St Pantaleon Church, not far from the town centre. The new building was opened on 7th November 1926 at a ceremony attended by Mrs Carrington-Wilde, as representative of the SRF.

Francesca Wilson visited the orphanage at Nish in 1929. She found it a *'fine building'* for fifty boys and girls between the age of five and twenty. She already knew Miss Maw : *'She was a slender woman with white hair, vivid smile, and a quaint, gay manner'*.[305] She was deeply impressed by the orphanage:

'The orphanage had a high reputation and was the only co-educational Home in Yugoslavia. Many of its boys and girls went on to university and technical schools, but they used to come back to it for their holidays, for they regarded it as their home. The English women who ran it had a great influence in the regions of Nish and were consulted by officials on all sorts of problems. Mrs Carrington Wilde visited it every second year and brought it all the support it needed from the English end....'[306]

Florence Maw and Jean Rankin continued to run the children's home until the building was taken over by the Gestapo in 1941 and ransacked. After the war, efforts to continue the work were hampered by the new Yugoslavian government which was suspicious of the emphasis placed upon the Orthodox Church. Maw and Rankin resigned and the orphanage was handed over to the city of Nish in 1946. The pair retired on a modest state pension to a little cottage in Dubrovnik.[307] After a final visit to Britain in 1951, Jean Rankin died in 1952, followed by Florence a few months later.

In 1953, ownership of the orphanage was transferred to the Yugoslav authorities on the condition that the building would serve its original purpose and set up a commemorative plaque on the wall of the Home. A marble plaque was, accordingly, placed on the building which read: *'To the glory of God and in memory of Florence Maw and Jean Rankin who*

Serbian Relief Fund

devoted their lives to the service of the children of Serbia, 1915-1947.'

The building remains today and since 1965 had been used as a hall of residence for high school students. A bust of Mrs Carrington-Wilde which was placed in front of the Home in 1938, was removed in 1948 but replaced in 2004. It bears the inscription in Serbian and English: '*A Friend of the Serbian People*'.[308]

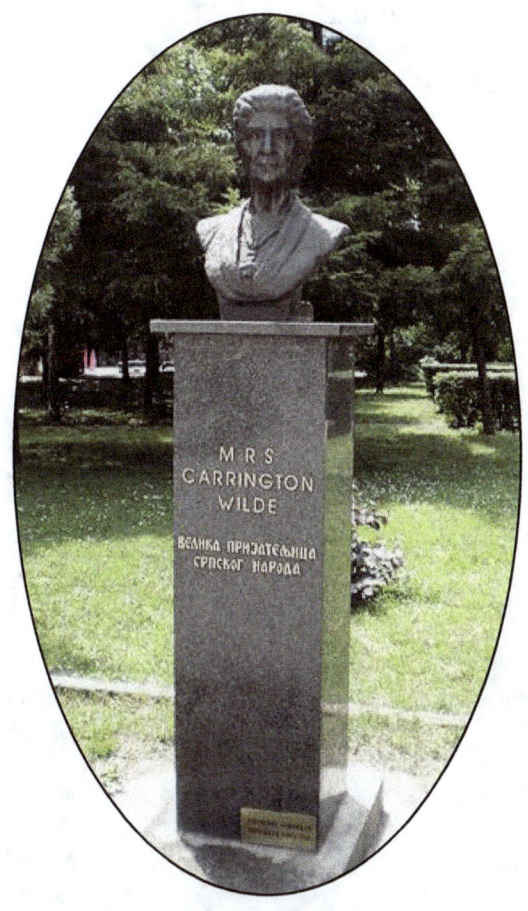

Image: courtesy of Intermedichbo, *2013.*

Nursing in Serbia with Lady Paget in 1915

Appendix 2

Staff of Lady Paget's Hospital

A List of Members of Serbian Relief Fund Unit 1

As contained in *With Our Serbian Allies* by Lady Paget, published by the Serbian Relief Fund, 28 July 1915

General Superintendent: Lady Paget

Surgical and Medical Staff: Professor Morrison F.R.C.S., surgeon in chief; Mr Walter Eaton M.B.; Mr W B Knobel M.D.; Mr T G Maitland M.D.

Secretary: Hon. R C F Chichester

Assistant Secretary: Mr J W Wiles

Matron: Miss F A Fry

Dispenser: Miss Skey

Nursing Sisters

Miss Dorothy Grierson	Miss Mary G C Heathcote
Miss Jennie Sibley	Miss Agnes M Macqueen
Miss Charlotte E Heinrich	Miss Alice Pell
Miss Edith J M Bowers	Miss Jean C G Donald
Miss Nellie Clark	Miss Marianne Eliz. Hall

Staff of Lady Paget's Hospital

Miss Elizabeth Mary Campbell

Miss Helen M Coleman

Miss Blanche Madden (additional)

Miss Gertrude Smith

Miss Florence E Burman

Madame Pavlovich

Ward Maids

Miss Eleanor Cave

Miss Dorothy K Benwell

Miss Olive Tremayne Miles

Miss K Isherwood

Miss Mabel Constance Pollard

Miss Presland

Dressers

Mr Frank Newey

Mr Edward B Alabaster

Mr Herbert W Hall

Mr Arthur Cloudesley Smith

Orderlies

Mr James Duncan Fry

Mr Ivan Stuart Campbell

Mr Edgar W Davies

Mr F H Markoe

Mr John Alexander Reekie

Mr Spearman C Swinburne

Mr Ian Maxwell Rattray

Mr Carlton Williams

Mr H Diprose

Mr T E Milligan Grundy

Mr H Fremlin Squire

Mr Rex William Jackson

Mr Richard Hunt

Mr Joseph Gasking

Assistant Baggage Master: Mr Robert Parr

Cook: Francesco D'Angelo

Nursing in Serbia with Lady Paget in 1915

Supplementary Members

Surgeon: Mr E F Eliot F.R.C.S.

Dispenser: Miss Lucy Grimes

Nursing Sisters

Miss Moore	Miss Jane E Peters
Miss L L Cluley	Miss Lilian Gerard
Miss F M Scott	Miss Ball
Miss D H Mackintosh	Miss Lüders
Miss Bonser	Miss Ridge
Miss Parsons	Miss Robinshaw
Miss Rankin	Miss Scammel
Miss Caldow	Miss Kelly
Miss Skertchley	Miss O'Neil
Miss Egerton	Miss Gowans
Miss Norman	Miss Sturt
Miss Bird	Miss Crombleholme
Miss Bullock	Miss Lyn Jones
Miss Mansell	Miss Round
Miss Hudson	Miss J C Pickering
Miss A Dorothea Beaton	

Staff of Lady Paget's Hospital

<u>Orderlies etc</u>

Mr Roland Bryce					Mr H Hardinge

Mr C Cooke-Taylor				Mr T J Grieve

Mr Collins						Mr Campbell

Additional information as reported in *The British Journal of Nursing*, 17th April 1915 [p313]:

'The following nurses left London on Sunday last for fever work in Serbia, under the Serbian Relief Fund.

Miss Louisa Ball, who in addition to holding the certificate of St Mary's, Paddington, had worked for seven years as a Queen's Nurse in Shoreditch; Miss Sara Bonser, trained at the Seamen's Hospital, Greenwich, who speaks French, German and Italian and has nursed in France, Germany and India; Miss Maud E Bullock, who trained at the Chesterfield Hospital, she has also had experience of fever nursing and nursed in Montenegro, and at Janina during the Balkan War; Miss Roberta Parsons, trained for three years at the Tabitha Hospital, Chicago, she has had much experience in nursing typhus and typhoid fevers; Miss E E Egerton, Miss Helen Smith, Miss Mary Michie Smith and Miss M E Skertchley all of whom have had both general and fever training; and Miss J S Rankin, trained at Stobhill Hospital, Glasgow, who has had five years' experience of private nursing. It will be realised that the nurses have been very carefully selected, and we wish them success in the onerous work before them.'

Nursing in Serbia with Lady Paget in 1915

Lady Paget's Unit in Serbia No II

As contained in *'With our Serbian Allies. Second Report'* by Lady Paget, printed for private circulation, 1916

Medical Staff

Medical Director: T Gwynne Maitland M A, B.Sc,M.D,C.M., D.Phil.

Surgeon in chief: Fergus Armstrong M.D., F.R.C.S.

Surgeon: Dr M Seedorff (Danish)

Assistant Surgeons: Dr Erik Himmelstrüp; Percy Wallice M.R.C.S., L.R.S.P.

Physicians: R M Morison M.B.; Dr A F Cornelius (American); Dr Erle D Forrest (American); Dr R V Brokaw (American)

Chancery Staff

Secretary: Mr Edgar Davies   Treasurer: Mr T E Milligan Grundy

Dispenser: Mr A Paterson   Radiographer: Mr J Lamb

Anaesthetists: Mr Ivan S Campbell; Mr E P Chapman

The following gentlemen were not official members of the Staff, but very kindly acted as voluntary workers:

Bacteriologists: Dr T H Plotz (American); Dr George Baehr (American)

Sanitary engineers: Dr Osborn; C E Fox (both American and members of the American Red Cross Sanitary Commission)

Nursing staff

Matron: Miss Louisa Ball

Housekeeper: Mrs Olive Jourdain

Staff of Lady Paget's Hospital

Masseuses: Miss G Polgreen; Mrs Ada Barlow

Sisters (British):

Miss Mabel Atkinson (NZ)	Miss M K Coleman
Miss Maud Bullock	Miss T Crombleholme
Miss Jean Caldow	Miss Eva E Egerton
Miss I Gray	Miss M T O'Neill
Miss I Hudson	Miss J S Rankin
Miss Dora Johnson	Miss Beatrice Robinshaw
Miss G Lynn Jones	Miss S A Round
Miss Alice Leveson	Miss Ethel Scammell
Miss Agnes Mann	Miss M M Sharpin
Miss Rosalie Mansell	Miss M E Skertchley
Miss C B Mellis	Mrs Percy Wallice

Sisters (Danish)

Miss Henny Gravesen	Miss Signe Möller
Miss Johnny Hendricksen	Miss Minna Wifstrand
Miss Thekla Madsen	

Nursing in Serbia with Lady Paget in 1915

Sisters (Dutch)

Miss Willy Forbes-Schmeltzer

Miss Van Der Vebn

Miss Marie Van Oyen

Sister (French)

Sisters (American)

Mlle. Villemon

Miss R Parson

Orderlies (British)

Storekeeper: Mr C R Cooke-Taylor

Chauffeur and carpenter: Mr J L Gasking

Mr H C M Hardinge

Orderlies (American)

Mr W W Eaton

Mr G B Logan

Mr F Klepal

Mr D Peters

Mr R Shellens

Mr M A Tancock

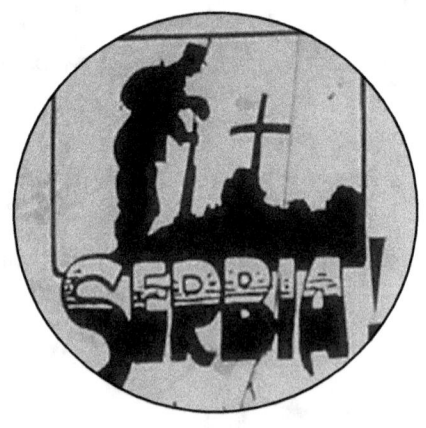

Staff of Lady Paget's Hospital

126 WITH OUR SERBIAN ALLIES

TABLE III.—LIST OF WORKERS AND PATIENTS AT LADY PAGET'S HOSPITAL ON NOVEMBER 6, 1915.

Workers.

   3 Serbian Interpreters.
   1 Austrian Engineer.
   1 Italian Mechanic.
   3 Serbian Nurses.
   3 Serbian Sewing-women.
 18 Serbian Washerwomen.
   1 Serbian Woman Cook.
311 Austrian Orderlies.
   5 Bulgarian Officers' Orderlies.
 23 Bulgarian Sentries.
   2 Bulgarian Intendants.
   1 Bulgarian Storekeeper.
   1 Serbian Barber.
   1 Serbian Groom.
  —
374

Patients.

354 Bulgarians.
 74 Austrians.
237 Serbians.
—
665

Total 1,039

A list of local staff and prisoners-of-war employed at the hospital (from Lady Paget's Second Report, 1916).

Nursing in Serbia with Lady Paget in 1915

THE SERBIAN RELIEF FUND
5 CROMWELL ROAD, S.W.

Patroness:
HER MAJESTY THE QUEEN.

President:
THE LORD BISHOP OF LONDON.

Vice-Presidents:

H.E. CARDINAL BOURNE.
THE EARL CURZON OF KEDLESTON.
THE LORD BISHOP OF OXFORD.
RT. HON. H. H. ASQUITH, M.P.
RT. HON. A. BONAR LAW, M.P.
RT. HON. AUSTEN CHAMBERLAIN, M.P. [M.P.
RT. HON. WINSTON CHURCHILL,

RT. HON. HERBERT SAMUEL, M.P.
RT. HON. D. LLOYD GEORGE, M.P.
MADAME GROUITCH.
REV. G. CAMPBELL-MORGAN, D.D.
REV. F. B. MEYER, D.D.
MR. NOEL BUXTON, M.P.

Chairman:
*THE LORD HENRY CAVENDISH BENTINCK, M.P.

Vice-Chairman:
*MR. GLYNNE WILLIAMS.

Committee:

*THE LORD CHARNWOOD.
THE LORD FITZMAURICE.
*THE LORD HAVERSHAM.
THE HON. BERNARD WISE.
*SIR EDWARD BOYLE, BART.
*SIR ARTHUR EVANS, LL.D., F.R.S.
*SIR VALENTINE CHIROL.
*HON. LADY WHITEHEAD.
*THE LADY RODNEY.
*LADY BOYLE.
*LADY GROGAN.
*LADY PAGET.

*MRS. NOEL BUXTON.
*MRS. BERTRAM CHRISTIAN.
MADAME CHRISTITCH.
*MRS. JAMES CURRIE.
*MISS AUBREY FLETCHER.
*MISS FRY.
MRS. H. R. GOTTO.
MRS. ARTHUR HARRISON.
MRS. GRICE HUTCHINSON.
DR. ELSIE INGLIS.
*MISS MACQUEEN.
*MRS. MASTERMAN.
MRS. SCARAMANGA RALLI.

(*Continued on page iii of Cover.*)

Above and right: Governing structure of the Serbian Relief Fund (from the cover of Lady Paget's Second Report, *1916)*

Staff of Lady Paget's Hospital

THE SERBIAN RELIEF FUND
5 CROMWELL ROAD, S.W.

(Continued from page ii of Cover.)

Committee *(continued)*:

*Mrs. SETON-WATSON.
*Mrs. CARRINGTON WILDE.
*Mr. W. A. ALBRIGHT.
*Mr. P. ALDEN, M.P.
Mr. JAS. BERRY, F.R.C.S.
*Mr. H. N. BRAILSFORD.
*Mr. R. M. BURROWS, D.Litt.
*Mr. BERTRAM CHRISTIAN.
Rev. PERCY DEARMER, D.D.
Mr. G. HANRAHAN.
Mr. C. L. GRAVES.

Mr. JOYNSON-HICKS, M.P.
Mr. JAMES F. HOPE, M.P.
Mr. HUGH LAW, M.P.
Mr. R. O. MOON, M.D., F.R.C.P.
*Mr. H. E. MORGAN.
Mr. T. P. O'CONNOR, M.P.
Mr. J. O'GRADY, M.P.
Mr. A. M. SCOTT, M.P.
Mr. J. ST. LOE STRACHEY.
*Mr. A. G. SYMONDS.
*Mr. G. M. TREVELYAN.

Hon. Treasurer:
*Rt. Hon. The EARL OF PLYMOUTH.

Hon. Secretary:
*Mr. R. W. SETON-WATSON, D.Litt.

Hon. Financial Secretary:
Mr. F. C. LINDO.

General Secretary:
Mr. F. M. SCOTT.

Bankers:
LONDON COUNTY & WESTMINSTER BANK, LTD.
St. James's Square, S.W.

Hon. Auditors:
Messrs. COLE, DICKIN & HILLS.

* Executive Committee.

Nursing in Serbia with Lady Paget in 1915

Sources

Most of the biographical information in this book has been taken from census returns, probate records and professional registers available on the family history websites Ancestry and Find My Past. Both sites are an invaluable tool for the biographer.

Primary Sources

British Library: Florence Maw. *The Chronicle of Her Lifework in Serbia* (1957) YA. 1995a. 26004

Imperial War Museum: Private papers of F M Scott. Document 77/15/1

Imperial War Museum: Private papers of Dr H F Squire. Document 3275

National Archives: Medal cards. WO372

Record Office for Leicestershire, Leicester & Rutland: Register of Nurses at North Evington Infirmary. DE3789/99

Record Office for Leicestershire, Leicester & Rutland: Leicester Building Plans, 1875. No. 10265

School of Slavonic & Eastern European Studies, University College, London. Papers of R W Seton-Watson. SEW7/7

Newspapers & Periodicals

British Journal of Nursing, 1914-1918

Illustrated Leicester Chronicle, 1914-1918

Illustrated War News, 1916

Kelly's Directory of Hampshire & the Isle of Wight, 1935

Leicester Chronicle & Leicestershire Mercury, 1914-1918

Leicester Daily Post, 1914-1918

Sources

Leicester Pioneer,1914-1918

London Gazette,1914-1918

Bibliography

Abraham, J Johnston, *My Balkan Log* (1922)

Armitage,FP, *Leicester 1914-1918 The Wartime Story of a Midland Town* (1933)

Askew, Alice & Claude, *The Strickenland. Serbia as We Saw it (1916)*

Berry, J, *The Story of a Red Cross unit in Serbia* (1916)

Burgess, Alan, *The Lovely Sergeant (1963)*

Corbett, Elsie, *Red Cross in Serbia* (1964)

Davies, Ellen Chivers, *A Farmer in Serbia* (1916)

Dearmer, Mabel, *Letters from a Field Hospital* (1915)

Gordon, Mr & Mrs Jan, *The Luck of Thirteen* (1916)

Hartnell-Beavis, J & Souttar, HS, *A Field Hospital in Belgium,* published in the British Medical Journal, 9 Jan 1916

Herbert, Lady Muriel, *Serbia & the Serbians* (1915)

Hutton, I Emslie, *With a Woman's Unit in Serbia, Salonika and Sebastopol* (1928)

Keegan, John, *The First World War* (1998)

Kerr, M H Munro, *Scottish Women's Hospital Work in Serbia,* reprinted from the Glasgow Medical Journal (1917)

King, Hazel, *One Woman at War. Letters of Olive King* (1986)

Kripner, Monica, *The Quality of Mercy. Women at War in Serbia* (1980)

Nursing in Serbia with Lady Paget in 1915

McLaren, Eva Shaw, *A History of the Scottish Women's Hospitals* (c1919)

Maglic, Konstantin, *The Dandy Hun* (1919)

Matthews, Caroline, *Experiences of a Woman Doctor in Serbia* (1917)

Mikić, Zelimar D, *Ever Yours Sincerely. The Life & Work of Dr Katherine MacPhail* (2007)

Miller, Louise, *A Fine Brother. The Life of Captain Flora Sandes* (2012)

Morrison, J T J, *Experiences in Serbia,* reprinted from The Lancet, 6 Nov 1915

Oxford Dictionary of National Biography (2004)

Paget, Lady, *With Our Serbian Allies. First Report (*July 1915)

Paget, Lady, *With Our Serbian Allies. Second Report (*May 1916)

Paget, Sir Ralph, *Report of the Retreat of Part of the British Hospitals from Serbia, Oct –Dec 1915* (1916)

Squire, Henry Fremlin, *Middle East Scrapbook*, 1997

Stanley, Monica M, *My Diary in Serbia April 1, 1915-November 1, 1915*, (1916)

Stobart, Mrs St Clair, *The Flaming Sword in Serbia and elsewhere, (1917)*

Wilson, Francesca M, *In the Margins of Chaos, (1944)*

Wilson, Francesca M, *Rebel Daughter of a Country House. The Life of Eglantyne Jebb* (1967)

Sources

RELIEF OF REFUGEES 127

TABLE IV.—REGULAR SUPPLIES NEEDED BY LADY PAGET'S HOSPITAL FOR THE MAINTENANCE OF 1,040 PERSONS, AND PROVISIONS GRANTED BY THE SERBIAN GOVERNMENT.

Daily—

Bread	1,000 loaves
Beef	150 kilos
Mutton	80 ,,
Chickens	20 ,,
Milk (to be delivered at 7 a.m.)	120 ,,
Sour Milk	120 ,,
Eggs	300 ,,

Weekly—

Sugar	400 kilos
Cognac	30 bottles
Kerosene	1,000 kilos
Soda	1 sack

The use of five pairs of oxen with carts daily, for bringing up food supplies.

Details of food supplied to refugees, 1915-1916 (from Lady Paget's Second Report, 1916*)*

Nursing with Lady Paget in Serbia in 1915

References

Introduction

1. *Illustrated Leicester Chronicle*, 18 Sep. 1915, p9

Chapter 1: Early years

2. *Leicester Daily Post*, 13 Jan.1915, p6

Chapter 2: The Serbian Relief Fund

3. Serbian newspaper quoted in *With our Serbian Allies First Report,* by Lady Paget (July 1915), p45

4. Francesca M Wilson, *Rebel Daughter of a Country House, The Life of Eglantyne Jebb* (1967)p129

5. Francesca M Wilson, ibid.p130

6. Francesca M Wilson, ibid.p130

7. Francesca M Wilson, ibid.p131

8. Jason Tomes, *Paget, Dame Leila Wemyss*, Oxford Dictionary of National Biography (2004)

9. Ibid.

10. SEW/7/7 Serbian Relief Fund executive committee minutes, 1914-1916 Papers of RW Seton-Watson, School of Slavonic and Eastern European Studies, University College, London

11. J Johnston Abraham, *My Balkan Log* (1922), p39

12. *Leicester Chronicle and Leicestershire Mercury,* 20 February 1915, p6

13. *Leicester Daily Post,* 18 June 1915, p1

14. *British Journal of Nursing,* 10 Apr. 1915, p293

15. Lady Paget, *With our Serbian Allies. First Report* (July 1915) p8

16. Henry Fremlin Squire, Middle East Scrapbook (1997),p165

17. bid. p159

18. J Johnston Abraham, *My Balkan Log (1922,) p59*

19. SEW/7/8 Serbian Relief Fund Press Cuttings Book, Apr 1915 Papers of RW Seton-Watson, School of Slavonic and Eastern European Studies, University College, London

20. J Johnston Abraham, *My Balkan Log (1922,) p61*

References

21. Ibid. p186

22. Ibid. p125

23. Ibid. p126

24. De Ruvigny's Roll of Honour 1914-19, vol 1, p82

Chapter 3: Journey to Serbia

25. Imperial War Museum, Private papers of Miss F Scott: 77/15/1

26. F May Dickinson Berry, *The Story of a Red Cross Unit in Serbia* (1916) p9

27. Royal College of Surgeons, Plarr's Lives of Fellows Online

28. *British Journal of Nursing*, 23 Jan. 1915, p69

29. J Johnston Abraham, *My Balkan Log* (1922,) p292

30. F May Dickinson Berry, *The Story of a Red Cross Unit in Serbia* (1916) p19

31. Mabel Dearmer, *Letters from a Field Hospital* (1915) p75

32. M H Munro Kerr, *Scottish Women's Hospital Work in Serbia*, reprinted from the Glasgow Medical Journal July-Aug 1917 (1917) p6

33. Dr Caroline Matthews, *Experiences of a Woman Doctor in Serbia* (1916) p7

34. F May Dickinson Berry, *The Story of a Red Cross Unit in Serbia* (1916) p19

35. Ibid. p20

36. Mabel Dearmer, *Letters from a Field Hospital* (1915) p95

37. F May Dickinson Berry, *The Story of a Red Cross Unit in Serbia* (1916) p21

38. J Johnston Abraham, *My Balkan Log* (1922,) p248

39. Miller, Louise, *A Fine Brother. The Life of Captain Flora Sandes* (2012) p58

Chapter 4: Lady Paget's Hospital

40. Alice & Claude Askew, *The Stricken Land. Serbia as we saw it* (1916) p56

41. J Johnston Abraham, *My Balkan Log* (1922) p146

42. Mr & Mrs Jan Gordon, *The Luck of Thirteen* (1916) p182

43. Monica M Stanley, *My Diary in Serbia April 1 1915 - Nov 1 1915* (1916) p88

44. Imperial War Museum, Papers of Dr H F Squire, diary entry Feb 1-7, Documents 3275

45. J Johnston Abraham, *My Balkan Log* (1922,) p185

46. J T J Morrison, *Experiences in Serbia*, reprinted from the *Lancet*, 6 Nov 1915 (1915) p4

47. J Johnston Abraham, *My Balkan Log* (1922,) p287

48. J T J Morrison, *Experiences in Serbia*, reprinted from the *Lancet*, 6 Nov 1915 (1915) p15

49. J Johnston Abraham, *My Balkan Log* (1922,) p75

50. J T J Morrison, *Experiences in Serbia*, reprinted from the *Lancet*, 6 Nov 1915 (1915) p10

51. Henry Fremlin Squire, Middle East Scrapbook (1997),p158

52. Henry Fremlin Squire, Middle East Scrapbook (1997),p172

53. Lady Paget, *With our Serbian Allies. First Report* (July 1915)

54. Mr & Mrs Jan Gordon, *The Luck of Thirteen* (1916) p25

55. Monica M Stanley, *My Diary in Serbia April 1 1915 - Nov 1 1915* (1916) p80

56. Alice & Claude Askew, *The Stricken Land. Serbia as we saw it* (1916) p23

57. Ibid. p27

58. *Leicester Daily Post,* 8 Apr 1915

Chapter 5: The Typhus Epidemic

59. Lady Paget, *With our Serbian Allies. First Report* (July 1915) p12

60. Želimir Dj Mikić, *Ever Yours Sincerely.The Life and Work of Dr Katherine MacPhail* (2007),p24

61. *Leicester Daily Post,* 8 Apr 1915

62. J Johnston Abraham, *My Balkan Log* (1922,) p194

63. Ibid. p225

64. Ibid. p75

65. Lady Paget, *With our Serbian Allies. First Report* (July 1915) p13

66. J Johnston Abraham, *My Balkan Log* (1922,) p264-265

67. Lady Paget, *With our Serbian Allies. First Report* (July 1915) p14

References

68. J Johnston Abraham, *My Balkan Log* (*1922,*) *p263*

69. Lady Paget, *With our Serbian Allies. First Report* (July 1915) p15

70. J Johnston Abraham, *My Balkan Log* (*1922,*) *p297*

71. Lady Paget, *With our Serbian Allies. First Report* (July 1915) p16

72. J Johnston Abraham, *My Balkan Log* (*1922,*) *p259*

73. Ibid. p225

74. *The British Journal of Nursing,* 22 May 1915, p439

75. J T J Morrison, *Experiences in Serbia,* reprinted from the *Lancet,* 6 Nov 1915 (1915) p17

76. Ibid.

77. J Johnston Abraham, *My Balkan Log* (*1922,*) *p66*

78. Ibid. p67

79. *The British Journal of Nursing,* 22 May 1915, p439

80. Ibid.

81. J Johnston Abraham, *My Balkan Log* (*1922,*) p297

82. Lady Paget, *With our Serbian Allies. First Report* (July 1915) p22

83. Ibid. p22

84. *The British Journal of Nursing,* 22 May 1915, p439

85. The *British Journal of Nursing ,*1 May 1915,p365

86. Lady Paget, *With our Serbian Allies. First Report* (July 1915), p18

87. *Leicester Daily Post,* 23 Apr 1915 , p8

88. Ibid.

89. *The British Journal of Nursing,* 17 Apr.1915,p324

90. Lady Paget, *With our Serbian Allies. First Report* (July 1915) p24

91. *The British Journal of Nursing,* 22 May 1915 , p439

92. Monica M Stanley, *My Diary in Serbia April 1 1915 - Nov 1 1915* (1916) p60

Nursing with Lady Paget in Serbia in 1915

93. SEW/7/7 Serbian Relief Fund executive committee minutes, 1914-1916 Papers of RW Seton-Watson, School of Slavonic and Eastern European Studies, University College, London

94. The British Journal of Nursing ,6 Feb 1915,p164

95. The British Journal of Nursing, 13 Feb. 1915, p128

96. Lady Muriel Herbert, Serbia and the Serbians (1915) p17

97. Ibid. p12

98. Ibid. p16

99. Ibid. p19

100. Internet source: WW1 Australian Women Doctors- Looking for evidence

101. SEW/7/7 Serbian Relief Fund executive committee minutes, 1914-1916 Papers of RW Seton-Watson, School of Slavonic and Eastern European Studies, University College, London

102. Lady Muriel Herbert, Serbia and the Serbians (1915) p21

103. J T J Morrison, Experiences in Serbia, reprinted from the Lancet, 6 Nov 1915 (1915) p25

104. SEW/7/7 Serbian Relief Fund executive committee minutes, 1914-1916 Papers of RW Seton-Watson, School of Slavonic and Eastern European Studies, University College, London, p22

105. The British Journal of Nursing, 10 Apr 1915, p292

106. The British Journal of Nursing, 17 Apr 1915, p313

107. Alice & Claude Askew, The Stricken Land. Serbia as we saw it (1916) p22

108. Lady Muriel Herbert, Serbia and the Serbians (1915) p26

109. Alice & Claude Askew, The Stricken Land. Serbia as we saw it (1916) p50

110. New York Times, 28 May 1915

111. Lady Paget, With our Serbian Allies. First Report (July 1915) p24

112. Mrs St Clair Stobart, The Flaming Sword in Serbia and Elsewhere (1917), p19

113. Monica M Stanley, My Diary in Serbia April 1 1915 - Nov 1 1915 (1916) p27

114. SEW/7/7 Serbian Relief Fund executive committee minutes, 1914-1916 Papers of RW Seton-Watson, School of Slavonic and Eastern European Studies, University College, London, p39

115. J Johnston Abraham, My Balkan Log (1922,) p145

116. Mr & Mrs Jan Gordon, The Luck of Thirteen (1916) p187

References

Chapter 6: Home to Leicester

117. Monica Krippner, *The Quality of Mercy* (1980), p39

118. Mabel Dearmer, *Letters from a Field Hospital* (1915) p64

119. Monica M Stanley, *My Diary in Serbia April 1 1915 - Nov 1 1915* (1916) p45

120. *Leicester Daily Post,* 8 June 1915 , p1

121. Imperial War Museum, Private papers of Miss F Scott: 77/15/1

122. *The Leicester Pioneer,* 8 Oct 1915, p3

123. J Johnston Abraham, *My Balkan Log (1922,) p291*

124. SEW/7/8 Serbian Relief Fund Press Cuttings Book, Apr 1915 Papers of RW Seton-Watson, School of Slavonic and Eastern European Studies, University College, London

125. Monica Krippner, *The Quality of Mercy* (1980), p75

Chapter 7: Lady Paget's Return

126. SEW/7/7 Serbian Relief Fund executive committee minutes, 1914-1916 Papers of RW Seton-Watson, School of Slavonic and Eastern European Studies, University College, London, p31

127. Ibid. p29

128. Ibid. p39

129. Ibid., p43

130. Lady Muriel Herbert, Serbia and the Serbians (1915) p32

131. Ibid.,p34

132. Ibid. p35

133. Ibid. p36

134. Ibid. P36

135. Ibid. p113

136. Lady Paget, *With our Serbian Allies. First Report* (July 1915) dedication

137. Lady Paget, *With our Serbian Allies,* Second Report (May 1916) p3

138. Monica M Stanley, *My Diary in Serbia April 1 1915 - Nov 1 1915* (1916) p75

139. Lady Paget, *With our Serbian Allies,* Second Report (May 1916) p4

Nursing with Lady Paget in Serbia in 1915

140. Ibid. p4

141. Ibid. p5

142. Letter of George B Logan, *Princeton Alumni Weekly*, vol 16 no 29,23 Feb 1916, p455

143. Lady Paget, *With our Serbian Allies,* Second Report (May 1916) p6

144. Ibid. p9

145. John Keegan, *The First World War* (1998) p269

146. Lady Paget, *With our Serbian Allies,* Second Report (May 1916) p12

147. Ibid. p13

148. Ibid. p14

149. Ibid. p15

150. Ibid. p16

151. Ibid. p17

152. Sir Ralph Paget, *Report on the Retreat of Part of the British Hospital Units from Serbia, Oct-Dec 1915*(1916), p6-7

153. *British Journal of Nursing,* 9 Jan. 1915, p30

154. J Johnston Abraham, *My Balkan Log* (*1922,) p240*

155. Sir Ralph Paget, *Report on the Retreat of Part of the British Hospital Units from Serbia, Oct-Dec 1915*(1916), p7

156. Lady Paget, *With our Serbian Allies,* Second Report (May 1916) p26

157. Ibid. p27

158. Letter of George B Logan, *Princeton Alumni Weekly*, vol 16 no 29,23 Feb 1916, p455

159. Lady Paget, *With our Serbian Allies,* Second Report (May 1916) p28

160. Ibid. p30-31

161. Ibid. p32

162. Ibid. p34

163. Letter of George B Logan, *Princeton Alumni Weekly*, vol 16 no 29,23 Feb 1916, p455

164. Lady Paget, *With our Serbian Allies,* Second Report (May 1916) p37

References

165. Ibid, p49

166. Ibid. p47

167. Ibid, p122

168. Ibid,p53

169. Ibid. p115

170. Ibid.p56

171. Letter of George B Logan, *Princeton Alumni Weekly*, vol 16 no 29,23 Feb 1916, p455

172. Lady Paget, *With our Serbian Allies,* Second Report (May 1916)   p51

173. Letter of George B Logan, *Princeton Alumni Weekly*, vol 16 no 29,23 Feb 1916, p455

174. Ibid.

175. Lady Paget, *With our Serbian Allies,* Second Report (May 1916) , p63

176. Ibid.p64

177. Letter of George B Logan, *Princeton Alumni Weekly*, vol 16 no 33,24 May 1916, p759

178. SEW/7/7 Serbian Relief Fund executive committee minutes, 1914-1916 Papers of RW Seton-Watson, School of Slavonic and Eastern European Studies, University College, London, p122

179. *Aberdeen Press & Journal,* 11 Mar 1916

Chapter 8: Nurse Scott after Serbia

180. Robin Jenkins, *The Base Hospital* (2022)

181. Constantin Maglic, *The Dandy Hun (1919),p187*

182. *The Leicester Pioneer,* 18 Mar. 1918, p8

183. F P Armitage, *Leicester 1914-1918 The War-time Story of a Midland Town* (1933), p287

184. *The Leicester Pioneer,* 5 Oct.1917

185. *The Leicester Pioneer,* 18 Mar.1918,p8

186. *The Illustrated Leicester Chronicle,*6 Apr. 1918

187. *The Illustrated Leicester Chronicle,*3 Aug. 1918

188. *Kelly's Directory of Hampshire and the Isle of Wight,* 1933

Nursing with Lady Paget in Serbia in 1915

189. F P Armitage, *Leicester 1914-1918 The War-time Story of a Midland Town* (1933), p286

190. Information supplied by Isle of Wight County Record Office

Chapter 9: The Cast of Characters

191. *Dictionary of Ulster Biography*

192. J Johnston Abraham, *My Balkan Log* (1922,) p301

193. Ibid. p310

194. Internet source: Plarr's Lives of the Fellows Online. Entry for Edward Alabaster

195. J T J Morrison, *Experiences in Serbia,* reprinted from the *Lancet,* 6 Nov 1915 (1915) p24

196. *British Journal of Ophthalmology*, Obituary, Oct 1971, p720

197. Alice & Claude Askew, *The Stricken Land. Serbia as we saw it* (1916) p22

198. Internet source: www.findagrave.com

199. Alan Burgess, *The Lovely Sergeant (1963),p19*

200. *British Journal of Nursing,* 9 Jan. 1915, p30

201. Mabel Dearmer, *Letters from a Field Hospital* (1915) p65

202. SEW/7/7 Serbian Relief Fund executive committee minutes, 1914-1916 Papers of RW Seton-Watson, School of Slavonic and Eastern European Studies, University College, London, 7th Jan 1915, p14

203. F May Dickinson Berry, *The Story of a Red Cross Unit in Serbia* (*1916*) p18

204. Elsie Corbett, *Red Cross Unit in Serbia 1915-1919* (1964) p18

205. Internet source: Plarr's Lives of the Fellows. Entry for James Berry

206. Lady Muriel Herbert, *Serbia and the Serbians* (1915) p53

207. Ibid. p101

208. Ibid. p113

209. Monica M Stanley, *My Diary in Serbia April 1 1915 - Nov 1 1915* (1916) p87

210. Internet source: http://www.HarrowSchool-WW1.org.uk

211. *The Leicester Chronicle and Leicestershire Mercury,* 20 Feb 1915, p6

212. *The Leicester Daily Post,* 18 June 1915, p1

References

213. National Archives: Medal card WO372/23/8211

214. Hazel King, *One Woman at War. Letters of Olive King (1986),p109*

215. Ibid. p133

216. Ibid. p148 and p174

217. Želimar Dj. Mikić, *Ever Yours Sincerely. The Life and Work of Dr Katherine S MacPhail (2007) p76*

218. Hazel King, *One Woman at War. Letters of Olive King (1986)*,p211

219. ROLLR DE3789/99: Register of Nurses at North Evington Infirmary, f50

220. Royal College of Nursing: Midwives Roll for 1920

221. *Leicester Daily Post*,4 Feb 1915,p6 and *Leicester Daily Post,* 8 Apr 1915

222. *Illustrated Leicester Chronicle,*12th June 1915, p7

223. National Archives: WO399/10455

224. St Clair Stobart, *The Flaming Sword in Serbia and Elsewhere (1917), p58*

225. Internet source: Plarr's Lives of the Fellows Online. Entry for James Berry

226. J T J Morrison, *Experiences in Serbia,* reprinted from the *Lancet,* 6 Nov 1915 (1915) p24

227. Imperial War Museum, Papers of Dr H F Squire, diary entry Feb 1-7, Documents 3275

228. J T J Morrison, *Experiences in Serbia,* reprinted from the *Lancet,* 6 Nov 1915 (1915) p24

229. J Johnston Abraham, *My Balkan Log (1922,) p93*

230. Ibid. p175

231. Ibid. p198

232. Ibid. p225

233. Ibid. p306

234. Dr J Hartnell Beavis and H S Souttar, '*A Field Hospital in Belgium*', published in *British Medical Journal*, 9 Jan 1915, p64

235. Alice & Claude Askew, *The Stricken Land. Serbia as we saw it* (1916) p22

236. Ibid. p125

237. Register of Civilian Deaths, 1939-1945

Nursing with Lady Paget in Serbia in 1915

238. I Emslie Hutton, *With a Woman's Unit in Serbia, Salonika and Sebastopol*'(1928) p37

239. Ibid.p39

240. Ibid. p49

241. Internet source: http://www.history.rcplondon.ac.uk/inspiring-physicians (Royal College of Physicians)

242. Internet source:http://www.plants.jstor.org (Natural History Museum)

243. Biographical information supplied by Nicholas Rogers, archivist of Sidney Sussex College, Cambridge

244. Internet source: letters transcribed in http;//www.livesofthefirstworldwar.iwm.org.uk

245. Imperial War Museum, Papers of Dr H F Squire, letter 15 Mar.1915, Document 3275

246. Internet source: www.facebook.com/groups/tracingthetribe [site for Jewish genealogy]

247. J T J Morrison, *Experiences in Serbia*, reprinted from the *Lancet*, 6 Nov 1915 (1915)p17

248. J Johnston Abraham, *My Balkan Log* (*1922*)p46

249. J T J Morrison, *Experiences in Serbia*, reprinted from the *Lancet*, 6 Nov 1915 (1915) p24

250. SEW/7/8 Serbian Relief Fund Press Cuttings Book, Apr 1915 Papers of RW Seton-Watson, School of Slavonic and Eastern European Studies, University College, London

251. Imperial War Museum, Papers of Dr H F Squire, letter 1 Mar.1915, Documents 3275

252. Elsie Corbett, *Red Cross in Serbia*, (1964) p1

253. Ibid. p3

254. Mrs St Clair Stobart, *The Flaming Sword in Serbia and Elsewhere (1917)*, p35

255. Zelimar Dj. Mikić, *Ever Yours Sincerely. The Life and Work of Dr Katherine S MacPhail (2007)*,p25

256. SEW/7/8 Serbian Relief Fund Press Cuttings Book. 23 Mar 1915. Papers of RW Seton-Watson, School of Slavonic and Eastern European Studies, University College, London

257. *Illustrated War News,* 10 May 1916, p6

258. *British Journal of Independent Medicine,* 1 Oct 1848

259. *London Gazette,*8 Sep 1916,p8811

260. Register of Merchant Seamen, 220346, Nov 1920

261. Dr Caroline Matthews, *Experiences of Woman Doctor in Serbia* (1916),p73

References

262. Ibid. p205

263. SEW/7/8 Serbian Relief Fund Press Cuttings Book, 4 Feb 1915 Papers of RW Seton-Watson, School of Slavonic and Eastern European Studies, University College, London

264. J T J Morrison, *Experiences in Serbia,* reprinted from the *Lancet,* 6 Nov 1915 (1915) p24

265. Internet source: Plarr's Lives of the Fellows. Entry for James T J Morrison

266. *London Gazette,* 29 Sep 1908, p7021

267. SEW/7/8 Serbian Relief Fund Press Cuttings Book, Apr 1915 Papers of RW Seton-Watson, School of Slavonic and Eastern European Studies, University College, London

268. J T J Morrison, *Experiences in Serbia,* reprinted from the *Lancet,* 6 Nov 1915 (1915) p24

269. *Oxford Dictionary of National Biography*: entry for Ralph Spencer Paget

270. Ibid.

271. Ibid.: entry for Dame Leila Wemyss Paget

272. National Archives Medal card: WO372/23/32985

273. Internet source: www.livesofthefirstworldwar.iwm.org.uk

274. Imperial War Museum, Papers of Dr H F Squire, diary and letters, Nov 1914-Feb 1915, Documents 3275

275. Internet source: www.211squadron.org/hf_Squire

276. Stanley, Monica, *My Diary in Serbia'* (1916), p20

277. Ibid. p51

278. Ibid. p63

279. Ibid. p91

280. Ibid. p110

281. Ibid. p120

282. Krippner, Monica, *The Quality of Mercy. Women at war Serbia 1914-1915* (1980), p20

283. Stobart, Mrs St Clair, *'The Flaming Sword in Serbia and Elsewhere'* (1917) p11

284. SEW/7/7 Serbian Relief Fund executive committee minutes, 1914-1916 Papers of RW Seton-Watson, School of Slavonic and Eastern European Studies, University College, London, p17

285. Krippner, Monica, *The Quality of Mercy. Women at war Serbia 1914-1915* (1980), p138

Nursing with Lady Paget in Serbia in 1915

286. J T J Morrison, *Experiences in Serbia*, reprinted from the *Lancet*, 6 Nov 1915 (1915) p3

287. *Leicester Daily Post*, 18 June 1915, p1

288. J Johnston Abraham, *My Balkan Log* (1922,) p285

289. Internet source: www.poolemuseumsociety.wordpress.com

Appendix 1

290. SEW/7/7 Serbian Relief Fund executive committee minutes, 1914-1916 Papers of RW Seton-Watson, School of Slavonic and Eastern European Studies, University College, London,

291. *British Journal of Nursing*, 13 Feb. 1915, p128

292. *British Journal of Nursing*, 10 Apr. 1915, p292

293. *British Journal of Nursing*, 3 Apr. 1915, p274

294. *Leicester Daily Post*, 3 Apr. 1915

295. *The Daily Chronicle*, 2 Apr. 1915

296. Monica M Stanley, *My Diary in Serbia April 1 1915 - Nov 1 1915* (1916) p73 and p78

297. Ellen Chivers Davies, *A Farmer in Serbia* (1916) p26

298. Monica M Stanley, *My Diary in Serbia April 1 1915 - Nov 1 1915* (1916) p112

299. *British Journal of Nursing*, 27 Feb. 1915, p168

300. SEW/7/8 Serbian Relief Fund Press Cuttings Book, Apr 1915 Papers of RW Seton-Watson, School of Slavonic and Eastern European Studies, University College, London

301. Ellen Chivers Davies, *A Farmer in Serbia* (1916) p176

302. Monica Krippner, *The Quality of Mercy. Women at War in Serbia* (1980), p177

303. Dr Isobel Emslie Hutton, *'With a Woman's Unit in Serbia, Salonika and Sebastopol* (1928), p153

304. Eva Shaw Mclaren, *A History of the Scottish Women's Hospitals*, reprinted in *Scottish Nurses in the First World War* (2013), p333

305. Francesca Wilson, *In the Margins of Chaos* (1944), p67

306. Ibid. p103

307. Monica Krippner, *The Quality of Mercy. Women at War in Serbia* (1980), p210

308. British Library, Florence Maw. The Chronicle of her Lifework in Serbia (1957) YA.1995a.26004

References

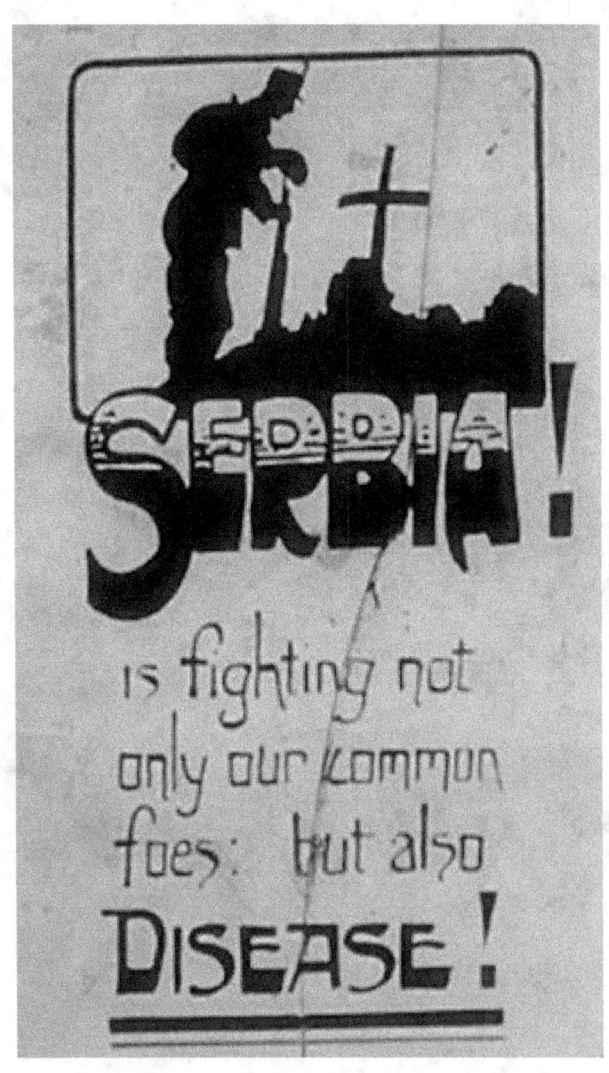

Nursing with Lady Paget in Serbia in 1915

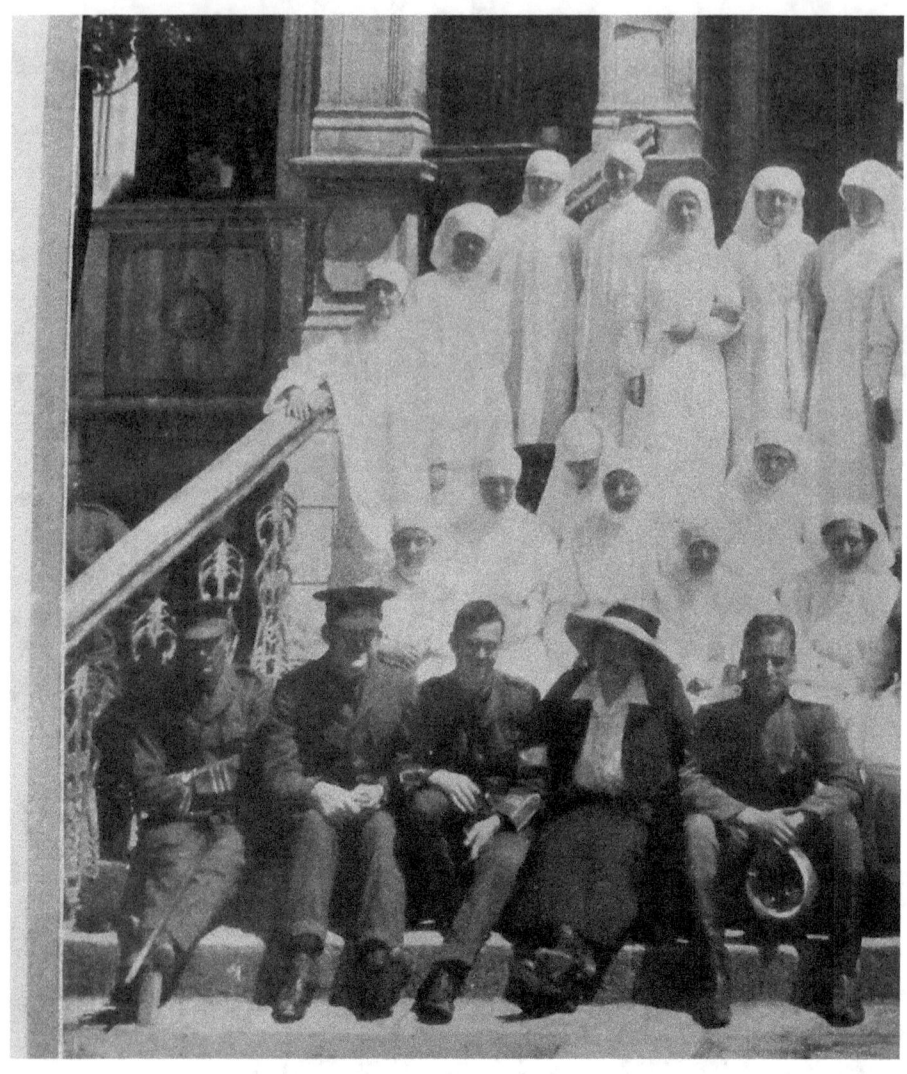

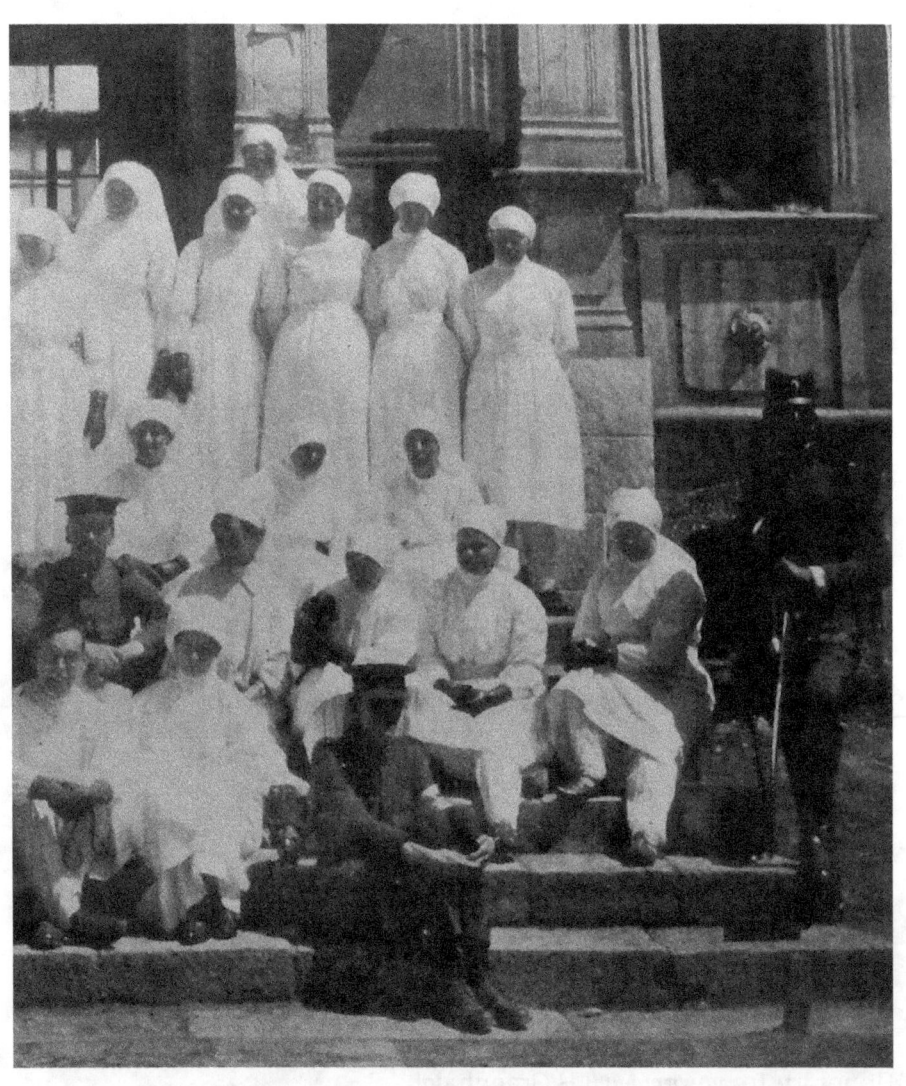

The staff of the typhus colony in May, 1915. Flora sits amidst the newly arrived fever nurses, third from the left in the second row from the front. (from Lady Paget's With our Serbian Allies First Report, *July 1915).*

Nursing in Serbia with Lady Paget in 1915

Serbian Relief Fund Unit 3

Stobart Hospital at Kragujevatz

List of Personnel

As contained in *The Flaming Sword in Serbia and Elsewhere* by Mrs St Clair Stobart, published 1917

Directress: Mrs St Clair Stobart

Surgical and Medical Staff: Mrs King-May Atkinson; Miss Beatrice Coxon; Miss Helen Hanson; Miss Mabel Eliza King-May; Miss Edith Maude Marsden; Miss Catherine Payne; Miss Isobel Tate

Nursing Sisters: Miss E V Bury; Miss Alice B Booth; Miss Alice Browne; Miss Ellen Collins; Miss F Clifton; Miss Isabelle Dickson; Miss Lorna Ferris; Miss Emily Hill; Miss Jessie Kennedy; Miss Alice Leveson; Miss Katherine Lawless; Miss Mary McGrow; Miss M MacLaverty; Miss Dorothy Newhall; Miss Ada Read; Miss Isabella Thompson; Miss Constance Willis; Miss Jessie de Wasgindt

Women Orderlies: Miss Anna J Beach; Miss Cissy Benjamin [head orderly];Miss Laura Bradshaw; Miss D E Brindley; [cook]; Miss A K Burton; Miss E M Cargin; Mrs Percy Dearmer [linen]; Miss Lorna A Johnson [laundry]; Miss Beatrice Kerr [sanitation]; Miss F B Maw; Miss Anne McGlade [secretary]; Miss D M Picton [cook]; Miss Monica Stanley [head cook]; Miss Phyllis Shakespeare [cook]; Miss Fairy Warren; Miss Minnie Wolsley [dispenser]

Honorary Treasurer: Mr J H Greenhalgh

Honorary Chaplain: Rev Dr P Dearmer

Men Orderlies: Mr Agar [Xray]; Mr Black [head chauffeur]; Mr Beck [refugee clothing]; Mr Colson [chauffeur]; Mr Korobenikoff [medical student] Mr Vooitch [interpreter]

Staff of Stobart's Unit

Dispensaries' staff

Surgical and Medical Staff: Miss H Cockburn; Miss H Hall; Miss A L Muncaster; Miss A J Macmillan; Miss G D Maclaren; Miss M Stewart; Miss Mary Iles

Dispenser: Mr E Stone

Nursing Sisters: Miss Bambridge; Miss Cockrill; Miss E Chapple; Miss Downes; Miss Gambier; Miss E B Giles; Miss Hall ; Miss Henley; Miss M Price; Miss Smith Lewis; Miss Stone; Miss M Stewart; Miss Wells; Miss Willis; Miss Wren

Women Orderlies [cooks]: Mrs Aldridge; Miss Barber; Miss Chesshire; Mrs Dawn; Miss Mansel-Jones; Miss Tatham; Miss Tubb

Man Orderly: Rev E S Rogers

Chauffeurs: Mr G D Boone; Miss E K Dickinson; Miss G Holland; Mr O Holmstrom; Mr Hulett; Mr Jordan; Rev J Little; Mr A Marshall; Miss Sharman

Nursing in Serbia with Lady Paget in 1915

Index

Illustrations are emboldened

Abbassieh, S S: 213

Aberdeen: 258

Abraham, Dr Johnston: 16,19,20,21,49,55,58,63,77-81,83,84,86-88,114,126,143,**178**,184,203,204,216,247,248

Accident: 32,33,43,104,111

Admiralty: 15,28

Adriatic: 122

Advice for sea voyages: 109

Aegean: 9,42

Aegusa: 222

Aeroplane: 135

Africa: 36

Agar, Mr: 292

Air raids: 135,209,240

Aitken, Mrs: 252

Ajaccio: 258

Alabaster, Edward B: 19,62,126,127,180,213,232,263

Albania: 110,131,140,158,162,182,183,234,245,253

Albanians: 10,55,145,146,192

Albright, W A: 271

Alden, P, MP: 271

Aldridge, Mrs: 293

Alexander, Ethel: 27

Alexandra Rose Day Ctte: 3

Allies: 136,137,138,141,162

Ambulances: 77,94,119,125,128,144,146,147,148, 152,156,**158**,159

America: 106,112,135,185,190,194,246,251,265

American Mission: 49

American Red Cross: 125,223

American Red Cross Sanitary Commission: 154,266

Americans: 49,77,83,119,125,126,146,151,154, 184,268

Anaesthetist: 28,100,200,252

Anglo-American unit: 142

Anglo-Serbian Children's Hospital, Belgrade: 194,224

Anglo-Serbian orphanage, Nish: 260

Animals: 26,48,50,70,108,113

Antwerp: 207,244,247,254

Arab: 48,54,114,212

Archduke Franz Ferdinand: 12

Aristocracy: 63,162

Armoury, Malta: 38

Armstrong, Fergus: 105,135,**181-182**,208,227,228,266

Army leave: 127

Army Service Corps: 138

Arran, Isle of: 8

Arrest: 123

Artillery: 147

Index

Asia Minor: 9,42,45

Askew, Alice & Claude: 70,105,181,182,**183**,184,208,240

Asquith, Herbert, MP: 14,250,270

Assassination: 12,235

Associated Press:106,157

Astley-Clark, Dr:170,**171**,172,173

Asylum, Mental, Leicester:1;7

Athens:40,41,42,100,213,220

Atkinson, Miss Mabel:252,267

Atkinson,Mrs King-May:253

Atrocities: 150,193

Australia: 102,196,197

Australian Serbian Canteens: 193

Austria-Hungary: 9,12,74,122,136

Austrians: 52,58,60,61,64,66,68,72,73,74,77, 81, 82,84, 92,97,98,99,100,106,110,111,112,117,119, 135,137,139,141,142,146,147,148,149,161, 162,179, 185,188,193,215,216,229,245,253

Austro-Hungarians: 135,161

Avonmouth: 28,31

Awards: 157,174,178,179,180,188,193,194,197, 208, 226,228,233,235,236

Bacon: 67,247

Bacteriologist: 100,196,252

Baehr, Dr George: 266

Bailey, Miss [later Mrs Elliott]: 122

Bailey, Mrs: 254

Balaclava helmets: 26,128

Balkan Committee: 10

Balkan States: 107

Balkan War, First: 10,13,58,77,151,228,244,247,265

Balkan War, Second: 12,136,228

Ball, Nurse Louisa: 104,264,265,266

Ballroom: 165,167

Bambridge, Nurse: 293

Band, military: 21,103,179,212

Bangkok: 13

Banjo: 30,33,41,188,205

Bank, National Bulgarian: 151

Bank, National Serbian: 138

Banks, Dr: 79,179,**215**,216

Banquet: 103,105

Barber, Miss 293

Barlow, Mrs Ada: 142,184-186,267

Barracks: 80,81,82,83,87,88,89,112,146,258

Barrie, Dr: 79,82,143

Barrington Ward, Mr: 100,101,131,252

Basements: 81,82,93,94

Bastia: 223

Bathroom: 152

Baths: 31,47,52,64,88,93

Battle: 145,147

Battlefield: 71,147

Bavaria: 13

295

Nursing in Serbia with Lady Paget in 1915

Bazaar: 45,54,**114**,237

Beach, Miss Anna J: 292

Beadle Mr A: 253

Beans, haricot: 68

Beaton, Nurse A Dorothea: 100,264

Beausite: 1,**2**,7

Beavis, Dr-see Hartnell-Beavis

Beck, Mr: 293

Bed sores: 65

Bedding: 16,25,26,37,57,61,65,96,162,169,256

Bedroom: 37,163

Beds: 46,52,59,60,64,96

Belarusians: 162

Belgium: 105,207,246,254

Belgrade: 10,11,12,13,21,62,101,108,122, 133, 137,188,194,215,223,224,229,241,246,248,254, 255,256,258

Bellingham Smith, Dr: 100,102,209,252

Bells: 37,38,51

Bengers Food, 26,64

Benjamin, Miss Cissy: 292

Bennett, Dr: 28,31,47,256

Bennett, Grace Emma: 8

Bentick, Lord Hen Cavendish: 270

Benwell, Miss Dorothy K: 263

Bergen: 156

Berlin: 106

Berry Unit: 31,47,55,187,188,200,205,206,237, 240,247, 255,256

Berry, Dr James: 28,29,30,31,32,33,43,49,175,186,**187**- 189,200,205,240,247,255,256,271

Berry, Mrs – see Dickinson, Dr F M

Berry, Nurse Vivyan: 241

Bicycles: 29,154,164

Biggs, Miss Marjory L: 174

Billesdon Convalescent Home: 25

Bird, Nurse Helena: 254,264

Birds: 25,48,70,88,118

Birmingham: 61, 85, 191, 193, 214, 232, 246

Birmingham Post: 19,126,217

Biscay, Bay of : 33,34,195

Biscuits: 26,41,68,95,110

Bishop, Miss: 252

Bizerta Tunisia: 258

Blaby: 195

Black, Mr: 292

Black, Mrs: 26

Bocagnano:258

Boer War: 230

Bolinchars, 147

Bombardment: 137, 224,241, 244, 255

Bombs: 135

Bonar-Law, Andrew MP: 14, 250, 270

Index

Bonser, Nurse Sara: 104, 264, 265

Book: 'Tragedy of Women of Serbia':154

Boone, G D: 293

Booth, Nurse Alice B: 292

Boots: 25,69,89,90,98,114,115

Bosnia Herzogovina: 9

Bottles, hot water: 26,43

Boulogne: 23,124,210,241,253

Bourne, Cardinal: 270

Bovril: 26,95

Bowers, Miss Edith J M: 262

Boyle, Sir Edward: 130,270

Boyle, Lady: 270

Bradshaw, Miss Laura: 292

Bran tub: 166

Brandy: 99

Brailsford, H N: 271

Brass: 114

Bray, Jean: 226

Bread: 41,42,45,50,67,68,95,110,111,169,193

Breakfast: 48,52,67,68,119,121,248

Bridges: 50,**119**,136,138,259

Brindisi: 100,122,184,231,246

Brindley, Miss D E: 292

British & Indian Steam Navigation Co. :31

British Farmer Red Cross Fund: 253

British Farmer's Unit: 253-256

British Farmer's Unit, 2nd: 255-256

British Journal of Nursing: 84,92,97,100,104,227,265

British Naval Mission, Belgrade: 137,138,256

British Red Cross: 15,16,19,20,31,49,77,78,79,81, 82,84,85,87,89,121,143,178,179,185,187,203, 212,215

Brockaw, Dr R V: 266

Browne, Nurse Alice: 292

Bryce, Roland: 265

Bucharest: 156,157,215

Budapest: 188,230

Buffalo: 111

Bugles: 112

Bulgaria: 10,12,50,136,152,165,241,244

Bulgarians: 55,137,140,141,145,146,147,148, 149,150, 151,153,154,155,157,162,186,208,252

Bullet holes: 147

Bullock, Nurse Maud E: 104, 264, 265, 267

Bullock's milk: 168

Bureaucracy: 80,120,123

Burgess, Miss E: 254

Burman, Miss Florence E: 263

Burnley: 186

Burrows, R M: 271

Burton, Miss A K: 292

Burton-on-Trent:5,125

Nursing in Serbia with Lady Paget in 1915

Bury, Nurse E V: 292

Butter: 68,110,111,169

Buxton, Charles: 9,10

Buxton, Mrs: 270

Buxton, Noel, MP: 9,14,270

Byzantine Empire: 54

Cadet School, Skoplje: 79,**80**.81,82,83,**88**

Cahan, Mr: 11

Cakes: 68,166,237

Calais: 208

Calcutta: 7

Caldow, Nurse: 264,270

Caledonien, SS: 39,40,41,**43**,44

Calendar: 59,107,111

Calendar, Gregorian: 59,107

Calendar, Julian:59,107

Calico suits: 237

Cambridge: 30,35,89,237,258

Cambridge Magazine:211-212,213,237

Campbell, Dr Adeline: 76,223

Campbell, Miss Elizabeth Mary:263

Campbell, Ivan Stuart: 263,266

Campbell, Mr:265

Campbell-Morgan, Rev G:270

Canada:8,98,109,175

Candles: 26,50,51,52.66.162

Canteens: 194

Cargin, Miss E M: 292

Carriage, horse:103,111,112,113,119

Carrington-Wilde, Mrs: 258,260,**261**,271

Cartridges:148

Cathedral:21

Cattle truck: 65,247

Cavan, Mr: 109,110

Cave, Miss Eleanor:263

Cemetery:71,77,150,193,212

Censorship: 59

Central Powers: 136

Ceramic, SS:228

Cess pits: 94

Ceylon: 120

Chalets: 123

Chalons-sur-Marno: 223

Chamberlain, Austen, MP: 14, 250, 270

Champagne:30,32,35,103

Chapel of Bones, Malta: 38,**39**

Chaplain: 99,134,198,240,253

Chaplin, Charlie: 169

Chapman, E P: 266

Chapple, Nurse E: 293

Charnwood, Lord: 270

Index

Chauffeurs: 105

Chef: 111

Cherbourg: 244,247

Cherry trees: 66

Chesshire, Miss: 293

Chichester, Hon Richard: 44,46,62,95,111.120,122, **129**,130,131,132, 134,189,**190**,191,209,213,262

Chickens: 56,57,67,69,110,168,169

Children: 138,145,148,154,223,225,258

Childs, Elmer Elsworth: 135

Chirol, Sir Ignatius Valentine: 14,270

Chocolate: 26,95,119

Cholera: 59,128,197

Christian faith: 108,109

Christian, Mrs: 270

Christian, Sir Bertram: 14,24,70,130,271

Christitch, Annie: 222,226,256,270

Christmas: 20,63,162-167,212,216,222

Church League for Women's Suffrage: 198

Church service: 19,53,198

Churchill, Winston: 14,248,250,270

Cigarette card: **158,159**

Cigarette case: 118,166

Cigarettes: 50,66,67,111,112,116

Cinema, Skoplje: 103,108,212

Cinema, Belgrade: 194

Cinema, Worksop: 165,167

Cinemas [picture houses]: 48,165,168,169

Citadel – see Grad Fortress

Civilians: 140,150,151,162,224,229,253,256,259

Clark, Nellie: 20,22,63,192,211,212,262

Clarke, Basil:122

Class distinction: 35

Classroom: 59

Cleaning: 16,17,61,82,259

Clements School for Girls: 1

Clemow, Dr:31,248

Clifton, Nurse F ['Ginger']:245,292

Closure of public places: 128

Clothing: 69,73,83,109,115,128,143,150,154, 156,158, 169,193,210,255,256,257

Cloudesley Smith, Arthur: 62,180,263

Cluley, Frances: 195

Cluley, Nurse Laetitia: 25,**27**,33,72,77,115,124,195, 196,264

Coaling, Miss K M: 254

Cocoa: 26,64,95

Cockburn, Dr H: 293

Cockrill, Nurse: 293

Coffee: 41,67,68,190

Coffins: 76,77,99,193

Cold conditions: 52,57,61,96

Nursing in Serbia with Lady Paget in 1915

Coleman, Alderman G T: 17,191

Coleman, Helen M: 17,191,**192**-195,247,263

Coleman, M K: 104,267

Collins, Mr: 265

Collins, Nurse E: 292

Colson, Mr: 292

Columbia University: 135

Columna Restaurant, Nish: 126,247

Comitadji:141,145

Commandant, Bulgarian: 147,148

Committee of Mercy of New York, 134

Committees to alleviate local distress: 129,131

Condensed milk: 111

Confusion of dates: 59,104,106,107

Constantinople: 9,32,40,42,54,197

Consul, British: 11,21,37,120,124,212,237

Consul, French: 120

Consul, Italian: 62,120,247

Consul, Russian: 37

Consul, Serbian: 237

Convicts, 36

Cook, Thomas, Tour Operators: 41

Cooke-Taylor, C R: 265,268

Cook: 95,105,111,118,213,238-242

Corah, Mrs: 26,108

Corbet, Miss Elsie: 188,220

Corfu: 155,156,183,258

Cornelius, Dr A F: 266

Corsica: 162,186,223,234,243,258,259

Costumes: 17,45,50,56,116,192,193

Cotton, Eliz: 5

Cotton, Miss: 125

Courtney, Kathleen: 223

Cowdray, Lady: 121

Coxon, Dr Beatrice: 253,292

Crackers: 166

Cripples, Guild of: 3

Croatians: 149,151

Cromblehome, Nurse T: 104,264,267

Crops: 193

Crosley, Mrs: 26

Cross of St Sava: 174,175

Crown Prince of Serbia: 20,134,224

Cunliffe Owen, Colonel: 36

Currie, Mrs James: 270

Curzon, Earl of: 270

Czar Ferdinand: 153

Czechoslovakia: 14,213

Czechs: 149

Daily Chronicle: 184, 254

Daily Express: 70,105.183

Index

Daily Mirror: 110

Dalyell, Dr Elsie Jean: 100,102,196-**197**,209,252

Dancing:103,114,174

Dandy Hun, The: 161

D'Angelo, Francesco: 263

Danish: 104,146,267

Dardanelles: 39

Davidson, Miss: 252

Davies, Edgar W: 263,266

Davies, Ellen Chivers: **255**,257

Davies, Miss Eleanor: 252

Davies, Miss M G: 252

Davies, Mr: 139

Dawn, Mrs: 293

De Montfort Hall, Leicester: 109

Dearmer, Mabel: 35,45,121,134,185,197-**198**,199,240,241,253,292

Dearmer, Percy: 99,134,198,240,253,292

Deaths: 20,76,78,85,88,97,106,132,134,185,240

Declaration of war: 122,124

Delirium: 90,91,92,93

Denmark: 251

Derby: 168

Derbyshire Advertiser: 110

Dervishes: 114

Des Gras, Sir Charles: 248

Dickinson, Annie: 200

Dickinson, Miss E K: 293

Dickinson, Dr Frances May [Mrs Berry]: 29,30,41,44,49,187,188,199-**200,** 205

Dickson, Nurse Isabelle: 292

Diet: 68

Dilwara, SS: 28,**31**,33,41,188

Dinars:115,151

Dining room: 58

Diptheria: 78,85,97,204

Diprose, H: 263

Disabled: 170,176,258,259

Discharge from hospital: 73

Discipline, harsh: 149

Disinfectant: 93, 256

Disinfection: 60,79,82,83,93,125,127,128

Dispensary: 151,253,256,258

Distress of local population: 129,190,209,257

Distribution, Centre for: 150,151

Dr Munro's Ambulance Corps: 208

Dogs: 26,71,113,125,141,144,163,165

Donald, Miss Jean C G: 262

Dongola, SS: 15,**251**

Donington Hall: 161

Donkeys: 48,52,54,66,70,164

Donnolly, Dr James: 49

301

Nursing in Serbia with Lady Paget in 1915

Downes, Nurse: 293

Drainage: 18,58

Dressers: 62,126,180,188,213,232,237,247

Dressings: 60,64,152

Drinks: 90-94,97,98,99

Drying room: 58

Dunkirk: 208

Dunraven Nursing Home, Ryde: 175

Durazzo: 182

Dutch: 251,268

Dysentery: 97

Eagle: 59.70

Earthquake: 54,123,228

Easter: 111,161

Eastridge Court, Ryde: 175,176

Eastwood: 168

Eaton, Dr W M: 200-201,262

Eaton, W W: 268

Education of Serbian boys: 258

Egerton, Nurse Eva E: 104,264,265,267

Eggs: 50,68,111,168

Egypt: 36,100,179,193,238

Electrical treatment: 171

Electricity: 58

Eliot, Dr E F: 30.57,201-202,213,232,264

Elliot, Mrs [formerly Miss Bailey]: 122

Embroidery: 164

Emslie Hutton, Dr Isobel:209,259

Enemies: 152,153

Engineer, sanitary: 94,257

Enteric fever -see typhoid

Entertainments: 164, 167,168,169,174,188,194, 212,221,240

Entomologist: 257

Epidemic: 76-78,85,221

Erin, steam yacht: **120**,121,213,219,222,237

Evacuation: 138,139,141,207,210,229,241,255

Evans, Sir Arthur: 14,270

Exhibition: 17,193

Exhumation: 150

Factory: 84,85

Famine: 150,155,162

Farewell party: 118

Fatalities: 83,85,97,106

Ferdinand, Czar: 153

Ferris, Nurse Lorna: 134,199,240

Fever: 58,63,74,83,85,97,192,212,241,254,265

Fever Hospital, Belgrade -see Hospital, British Fever

Fever Hospital, Skoplje- see Isolation Hospital

Fever, scarlet: 63,85,97,192,212

Index

Findlay, Lady Sybil Landsborough: 105,208

Findlay, Dr G Landsborough: 105,208

Fire of Salonika: 46,194

First, Dr Fabian: 253

Fish: 111,209

Fitch, Nurse K N: 104

Fitzmaurice, Lord Gerald: 14,270

Flag days: 1,124,**250**,257

Flags: 28,124,136,154,164,193

Fletcher, Mrs Aubrey: 270

Flies: 240,257

Floods: 59

Flour: 150,151,154

Flowers: 28,33,37,66,119,147,156,161,164,241

Flying Field Hospital: 245

Folkstone:124,253

Food: 14,26,41,58,67,68,95,110,117,122,145,158, 164,169,209,240

Food shortage: 61,74,93,95,96,142,150,151,152, 154,155,169, 193

Footwear: 27,69,73,115

Forbes-Schmeltzer, Nurse Willy: 268

Ford car: 182

Formalin: 49

Forrest, Dr Erle D: 266

Fortress -see Grad Fortress

Fox, Charles E: 154,266

France: 24,25,30,36,68,81,163,184,223,237,265

Franco-Prussian War: 162

Francs: 151

Frantz, Angus M: 135

Freeman, Rev J D:4

French: 41,43,44,103,122,123,136,137,138, 154, 210, 241,251,268

Friends, Society of: 223

Friends' War Victims Relief Committee: 162

Frontier: 48,255

Frost, Nurse: 252

Fruit: 26,35,37,38,41.166

Fry, Sister F A: 84,87,89,92,179,202-204,262, 270

Fry, James Duncan: 84,179,203,204,263

Fuel: 150,152

Fund raising: 184,185,193,194,223,225,250

Funerals: 20,134,193,211,234,241

Furnes: 207

Furnishings: 163,164

Furniture: 52,64,164

Gales: 32,33,34,42,**43**,44

Gallipoli: 136,199

Gambier, Nurse: 293

Gangrene: 16-18,60,65,69,79,85

Garrould's Nurses Department: 25

Nursing in Serbia with Lady Paget in 1915

Gasking, Joseph L: 263,268

Gendarmes: 145

Generals: 103,141,138,241

Gerard, Nurse Lilian: 100,264

Germans:100,111,135,136,137,**153**,154,156, 157,162,244

German language:111,216

Germany: 9,214,265

Germijan: 224

Gestapo,260

Ghevgeli: 48,49,138,210

Gibraltar: 31,35,36

Gifts:26,118,166,256

Giles, Nurse E B: 293

Glasgow: 120,221,223,265

Glass eye: 73

Glenfield: 172

Gloves, rubber: 89,90

Goats: 38,48,110,111

Goddard, Joseph: 1

Goddard, Major: 28

Gold: 31

Golders Green: 170,171

Gordon, Cora: 30,55,115,205-**206**

Gordon, Jan: 30,33,41,55,115,188,205-**206**

Gotto, Mrs H R: 270

Government, Serbian: 14,79,127,145,193,232,251

Governor, Bulgarian:150.151

Governor, Turkish: 80

Governor of Malta: 39

Governor of Skoplje: 135,138,212

Gowans, Nurse C: 104,264

Grad Fortress: 55,56,80,**101**,142,**144**,145,213,252

Graham, W P G:100,101,102,129,130,252

Granary: 58

Gratitude of patients: 73,92,95,96,98,99,128,157, 195,216

Graves: 21,50,51,71,77

Graves, C L :271

Grave's Disease: 20,63

Gravesen, Nurse Henny: 267

Gray, Nurse I :267

Greece: 9,10,36,42,107,136,137,162,220,238

Greeks: 21,77,78,100,106,143,146,148,212

Green, Mrs Mary Hughes: 259

Greenhalgh, J H :240,243,253

Greeve – see Grieve

Gregory, Pope (XII): 107

Greig, Mr: 257

Grierson, Nurse Dorothy: 262

Grieve, Mr T J:213,265

Grimes, Miss Lucy: 264

Index

Grogan, Lady: 15,28,223,258,270

Grujic, Mabel: 12,13,29,142,184,187,256,270

Grundy, T E Milligan: 263,266

Guentchitch, Colonel: 221

Gun boat: 44

Gunfire: 111,123,138,245

Guslar: 66,188

Gwynn, Stephen: 253

Hagerauch: 156

Haig, Dr V A: 223

Hair: 117

Halifax Royal Infirmary: 6

Hall, Dr H: 293

Hall, Herbert W 62,180,263

Hall, Sister Marianne Elizabeth: 212,262

Hall, Nurse: 293

Hamilton, Dr Lilias: 258

Hanrahan, G: 271

Hanson, Dr Helen: 253

Harbour: 37,**40**,42,45

Hardinge, H C M: 265,268

Hardy, Mrs Hankin: 104,256

Harrison, Mrs Arthur: 270

Harrison, Colonel:248

Hartnell-Beavis, Dr J: 70,105,108,113,181,183,**207-**
209,213,227,253

Hartney, Mrs: 184

Haversham, Lord: 270

Hazlerigg, Sir Arthur: 176

Headaches:33,34

Heathcote, Nurse Mary G C: 262

Heinrich, Nurse Charlotte E: 262

Henderson, John: 5

Hendricksen, Nurse Johnny: 267

Henley, Nurse: 293

Henry, Nurse: 82,90

Herbert, Lady Muriel:
101,102,105,130,131,132,189,190,209-211,252

Herbert, Samuel: 250

Hermann, Lipel: 92

Hewitt, Mr, newspaper proprietor:26

Hewitt, Mrs: 26

Hill, Nurse Emily: 292

Himmelstrüp, Dr Erik: 266

Hinckley:8

Hoare, Olive: 256

Hodge, John MP: 173

Hodges, Miss:10

Holland, Miss G: 293

Holmes, Dr: 179,204

Holmstrom, Mr O: 293

Nursing in Serbia with Lady Paget in 1915

Home Hospital, Leicester: 7

Home Hospital, Ryde: 175

Home of Recovery see Leicester Frith

Home of Recovery, Golders Green: 170,171

Homeless: 46

Honey: 67

Hope, James F, MP: 271

Horses: 48,104,112,246

Hospital, 5th Northern General, Leicester: 161,168,196

Hospital, British Fever, Belgrade: 133,241,254

Hospital, Crown Prince Alexander's, Salonika: 224

Hospital, Disabled Soldiers & Sailors, Nottingham: 162

Hospital, Eastwood VAD: 168

Hospital, First British Field, Serbia: 105,135,181,182,183,207,208

Hospital, First British Field, Belgium: 207

Hospital, First Reserve, Kragujevatz: 143

Hospital for Neurasthenics, Leicester: 170-174

Hospital, Isolation, Skoplje [Polymesis]: 77,78,87, 100,102,104,131,133,145,147,179

Hospital, Lady Paget's: passim, 15,20,**53**,57,58,102, 131,185,215,241,259

Hospital, North Evington Poor Law Infirmary, Leicester: 25,195,196

Hospital, St George's: 60

Hospital, Typhus, Skoplje see Typhus Colony

Hospital, Welbeck Auxiliary, Worksop: 162-167

Hospitals: 19,39,76,77,82,56,121,133,224,245

Hotel Liberty, Skoplje: 102

Hotel, Olympus Palace, Salonika: 44

Hotels: 37.41,44,128,175

Howe, T G: 254

Hudson, Nurse I R: 254,264,267

Hulett, Mr: 293

Humour: 66,69,89,110,168,169,189,199,220,221

Hungarian: 148,149,155,157

Hungary: 229

Hunt, Richard: 263

Hunter, Colonel William: 126,**127**,248

Hurricane: 240

Hutchinson, Dr Alice: 228-229

Hutchinson, Mrs Grice: 270

Hydrogen peroxide: 60,61,93

Hygiene: 60

Ice: 82,91,92

Iles, Dr Mary G: 293

Ill health: 18,22,31,45,59,61,62,74,103,116, 175,192, 193,194,219,229,237,241,245,247,255

Illustrated Leicester Chronicle: 160,172

Imperial War Museum: 26,57,92,109,124,176, 206,211,237

India: 28,31,37,230,265

Inglis, Dr Elsie: 175, 223,270

306

Index

Ingram, Dr Mabel Marian: 188

Instruments, medical: 64,256

Interpreter: 62,67,105,193,215,222,246,292

Interview: 24

Invasion: 136,137,162,208

Iodoform: 65

Ireland: 78,120,128,178

Irma, SS: 156

Isherwood, Nurse K: 82,90,91,97,263

Isle of Wight: 175,176

Isolation: 78

Italians: 36,100,122,124,224

Italy: 120,122,136,184,220,225,231,234

Jackson, Miss H M: 254

Jackson, Rex William: 211-214,220,263

Jagodina: 255

Jealousy: 117,150

Jebb, Eglantyne: 10,11,14

Jenkin, C J: 257

Jex-Blake, Dr A J: 210

John: 112

Johnson, Agnes Fielding: 27

Johnson, Nurse Dora: 267

Johnson, Miss Lorna A: 292

Jones, Edmund B: 100,252

Jones, Nurse G Lynn: 104,264,267

Jourdain, Mrs Olive: 266

Jordan, Mr: 293

Jordan, Sister Louisa: 76,223

Joynson-Hicks, MP: 271

Julian Calendar: 107

Justinian, Emperor: 54

Kadisch, Esther: 20,84,85,86,179,185,214,**215**,216

Kaimak [cream cheese]: 68

Kelley, Nurse L: 104,264

Kennedy, Nurse Jessie: 292

Kerr, Beatrice: 292

Kerr, Margaret Munro: 37

Kettles: 51

Khaki: 50,124,220

King of Greece: 137

King Peter of Serbia: 174

King, Olive: 194

King-May- see also Atkinson

King-May, Dr Mabel Eliza: 253,292

Kingdom of Serbs, Croats and Slovenes:259

Kitchen:82

Klepal, F:268

Knobel, Dr W B: 79,82,91,95,217-218,227,231,262

Korobenikoff, Mr: 292

Kossovo, Battle of: 12

Nursing in Serbia with Lady Paget in 1915

Kragujevatz: 15,46,76,107,143,184,194,199,220, 221,222,223,240,241,245,253,256

Kremlin: 156

Krivolak, Battle of :154

Kumanovo: 79

Kumanovo, Battle of :10

Lamb, J: 266

Lamp posts: 136

Lamps: 58

Lancet, The: 61,233

Landsborough - see Findlay

Language: 67,72,86,87,98,112,113

Lanterns: 136

Lapovo: 255

Laundry: 69,82,98

Lauvenuvitch, General: 122

Law, Hugh, MP: 271

Lawless, Nurse Katherine: 292

Lead Kindly Light: 21

Lefray, Dr: 257

Leicester: 1,**4**,7,17,23,30.109,124,128,170,171 191,193,195

Leicester Borough Council: 174

Leicester Chronicle & Leicestershire Mercury: 191

Leicester Daily Post: 7,17,26,77,94,95,96,110,122, 124,191,193,195

Leicester Frith Home of Recovery: 170-174

Leicester Frith House: 172

Leicester Mercury: 26

Leicester Pioneer: 125,170,172

Leicester Pioneers: **160**

Lemon: 37,66,71,94

Lemonade: 50,110

Letters: 29,98,109,110,153,191,209,211,213,220, 236,238

Letters of thanks: 124,125,128,157

Levas:151,152

Leveson, Nurse Alice: 267,292

Lice: 74,75,78,79,89,93,128

Lichfield, Lord & Lady:166

Lighting: 58

Lindo, F C: 271

Lindon, Elia: 131,189,209,210

Linen:103,104,292

Lipton, Sir Thomas: 47,120,**121**,185,218,**219**-222,237

Little, Rev J: 293

Little Dalby Hall: 27

Liverpool: 105,252

Lloyd George, David MP:270

Loan: 151,156

Logan, George B: 135,145,146,147,152,153,154,1 56,268

London: 234,246,253,255,257

London, Bishop of: 270

308

Index

Long, Miss Ethel Mary: 208

Lorries: 138

Lüders, Nurse V: 104,264

Luggage: 48,49,53,68,119,240,257

Macaroni: 68

Macedonia: 9,10,12,54,63,133,136,137,152,190

Macedonian Relief Fund: 10,11,14

Macedonians:10,54,150,151,192

Mackintosh, Nurse D H: 30,264

Macgregor, Ms: 257

MacLaren, Dr G D: 179,293

MacLaverty, Nurse M:292

Macmillan, Dr A J:293

MacPhail, Isobel: 224

MacPhail, Katherine: 76,194,221,**222**,223-226

MacQueen, Nurse: 262

Madden, Nurse Blanche: 263

Madsen, Nurse Theckla: 267

Magazines,145,148

Maglic, Konstantin: 161,162

Mail: 122,153

Maitland, Dr T G: 79,81,82,94,95,98,100,102,106, 139,142,146, 150,182,196,209,213,217,266

Maize: 209

Malta: 15,28,31,33,36-40,100,195,197,202,222

Manchester: 186

Mann, Nurse Agnes: 184,267

Mansel, Nurse Rosalie: 104,264,267

Mansel-Jones, Miss:293

Map: 52

March:141,143

Marco: 138

Marines: 138

Market: **54**,115,191

Markoe, F H: 263

Marsden, Dr Edith Maude: 253,292

Marseilles: 39,121,210,219,220,241,253

Mascot: **160**

Massage:171

Masseuses: 143

Masterman, Mrs: 270

Matches: 26

Matron: 162,167,168,170,172,**173**,174,203

Matthews, Dr Caroline: 228-**229**,230

Mattress: 57,65

Maw, Florence:259,260,292

Mayor of Leicester: 2-4,170-**171**,176

Mayor's Fund for Serbia:186

McEwan, Miss: 184

McGlade, Miss Anne: 292

McGrow, Nurse Mary: 292

McLaren, Barbara: 157,158

Nursing in Serbia with Lady Paget in 1915

McMillan, Dr: 173

McQueen, Miss: 10,11,14,15,24,270

Meals: 36,37,38,41,45,48,50,67,68,95,103,111,118, 164,166,208,213,216,221,216,221,235,236,247

Medals- see Awards

Medical Officer of Health, Skoplje: 62,79,141

Medical Officer, Bulgarian:154

Medical students: 30,62,233,237,254

Medication: 97,99

Mediterranean: 35,47,220

Mellis, Nurse C B: 254,267

Menu card: 103

Messagerie Line: 39

Messenger: 67

Messina: 122-**123**,228

Meyer, Rev F B: 270

Mice: 52,53

Mick: 98

Milan: 122

Miles, Dolly: 210

Miles, Miss Olive Tremayne: 263

Milk: 38,68,95,110,111,169

Mines: 122

Ministry of Pensions: 171,173

Mirror: 53,71

Misogyny: 63

Mistakes: 62,99,110

Mittins: 26

Mitrovitza: 139

Mladenovatz: 139,208,213,255

Möller, Nurse Signe: 267

Monastir: 11,14,139,210,224,257

Money: 74,115,116,151,154,224

Monkey :160

Montenegro: 10,31,116,131,205,206,228,245, 253,265

Montreal: 98,175

Moon: 40,100,103

Moon, Dr R O: 91,230-231,257,271

Moore, Nurse: 30,264

Moore, Mrs Arthur: 253,254

Moravians: 149

Morgan, H E: 271

Morison, Dr R M: 253,266

Morrison, Professor J T J: 15,17,59,61,62,63, 85,86,103,180,191,201, 202,212,214,217,231-233,237,246,247,262

Mortuary: 99

Moscow: 156,216

Moslem: 11

Mosques: 56,71,79

Mosquito net: 37

Mossoul, SS: 210

Motor vehicles: 119,125,128,138,142,144,145,

Index

147,153,155,156,**158**,159,163,164,167,207,223

Mountains: 45,48,50,53,71,88,103,143,162,224, 245

Mozley, Nurse: 254

Mud: 71,73,81,82,88,89,139,140,154,179,255

Mud houses: 50

Muncaster, Dr A L: 293

Munro, Dr Hector: 182,208

Music: 32,66,166,167,188,190,205,216,221

Music room: 32

Naples: 123,220

Nassau Literary Magazine: 135

Naylor, Stanley: 221

Naval Brigade – see British Naval Mission

Neill-Fraser, Margaret 'Madge': 76,223

Neurasthenics: 170

New Serbia, 15,55

New York Times: 106

Newcastle: 156

Newey, Frank: 62,180,213,263

Newhall, Nurse Dorothy: 292

Newnham & Girton Unit: 209

Newspapers: 26,29,72,99,109,157,173,186,221,228

Nish:15,47,79,81,100,101,102,104,126,132, 138,142,143,184,185,193,213,220,221,228, 241,247,252,256,257,259,260

Norman, Nurse C L: 104,264

North, Jonathan: 170,**171**

Norway: 156

Norwegian: 104

Nottingham: 8,163,165,167,168

Nottingham Express: 256

Novi Bazar: 131,189,190,191

Novi Sad: 224

Nursing Conditions: 12,19,25,59,185,203,210

Nursing Home: 1,23,25,124,160,162,167,175, 176,195

Nursing Kit:24,25

Nursing Sisters: passim, 116,117,128,140,157,158

O'Brien, Miss: 184

O'Connor, T P, MP: 271

O'Grady, J, MP: 271

Omelette: 67,68,107

O'Neil, Nurse M T:104,264,267

Onions: 154

Oranges: 37,66,71,94

Order of St Johns: 15,23,61,237

Order of St Sava: 174-175,179,188

Orderlies: 18,19,35,52,57,60,68,72,84,85,87,94, 98,101, 105,119,135,142,146,147,148,149,162,198, 199,203,209,219,232,236,241,255,259

Orphanages: 154,254,257,259,260

Osborn, Dr Stanley H: 147,154,266

Ottoman Empire: 55,63

311

Nursing in Serbia with Lady Paget in 1915

Overcrowding: 78,85

Oxen: 48,76,86,96,110

Oxford: 220,258

Oxford, Bishop of: 270

Packing cases: 26,47,52,64,112

Pacifism: 199

Paddington Station: 28

Paget, Lady Leila: passim: 12,**13**,14 15,18,24,34,44,52,57,62,63,81 82, 102,130,134,**140**,157.175,223,233-235,241,257,262,270; appointment as superintendent:15,62; argument at Isolation Hospital:148;authority over passengers: 139;captured by Bulgarians: 149,210; convalescence: 106,107,132,134;critiscism: 152,153,154,157; death reported: 106,235;dispute with medical staff: 63,135,232; falls ill with typhus: 90,91,213; instructed to return: 102;returns to England: 106,107,156; returns to Skoplje: 129-159; tours hospitals: 133,135;visit to Salonika: 138,241

Paget, Lady Mary [mother]: 106,110,233

Paget, Sir Ralph Spencer: 11,13,15,**16**,58,59,68,81,1 07,120,122,126, 130,133,134,142,144,206,220,233-235, 241,246,257,258; appointed British Commissioner: 15,234; death: 235

Paget, Sir Arthur Fitzroy: 13,233

Palace: 156

Palanka: 223

Pancakes: 118

Panic: 138

Pantelleria, Isle of: 36

Para: 74,116

Paris: 124,197,234

Parr, Robert: 263

Parrafin: 49,89

Parrafin tins: 60,64

Parrots: 26

Parsons, Mr: 255

Parsons, Nurse Roberta: 104,264,268

Pasitch, Mr [Serbian Prime Minister]: 81,190,215,247

Pasitch, Mrs: 254,257

Pass: 168,169

Passports: 48,120,122,123,167

Paterson, Mr A: 266

Patients: 59,66,73,90,269

Patrons: 250

Pavlovich,Madame:263

Pay:116,131

Payne, Dr Catherine:253,292

Peckham,Mr [British Consul, Skoplje]: 11

Pell Smith, Elinor: 7,27,176

Pell, Miss Alice: 17,262

Peters, Mr D: 268

Peters, Nurse Jane E: 100,264

Petrograd: 156,157,215,216

Petroleum:89

Pets: 26,34,70,108

Photographs: 29,69,123,150,156,173,193,220

312

Index

Pickering, Frances: 28,236

Pickering, Nurse Ivy: 25,**27**,33,43,108,115,116, 124,236,264

Picture Houses – see cinemas

Pigs: 110

Piraeus: 41,122,210

Pirot: 208,245

Plotz, Dr T H: 266

Plymouth, Earl of : 271

Pneumonia:79

Polgreen, Miss G: 267

Police: 124

Pollard, Miss Mabel Constance: 263

Polymesis -see Hospital, Isolation, Skoplje

Ponies: 112

Popovitch, General: 133,221

Poppies: 119

Pork: 67

Porridge: 67,220

Portland, Duchess of: 162,164,165,166,167

Portland, Duke of: 165,166

Portugal: 39,179,209

Posharevatz: 255

Postal Service: 34,49,70,108

Postcards :96,108,225

Pot holes: 48,69

Potassium permanganate: 38

Potato famine: 120,218

Potatoes: 154,169

Prague: 216

Prejudice: 63,143

Presbyterian Church: 26,109

Presland, Miss: 263

Press Association: 106,157

Price, Nurse M: 293

Prices: 115

Prickett, William: 135

Prime Minister, Greek: 136,137

Prime Minister, Serbian: 81,190,215,247

Prince, Serbian: 220,221

Princetown University: 135

Princip, Gavrilo: 12

Prishtina: 139,140,141,145

Prison: 256

Prisoners of war: 52,60,61,64,72,73,**74**,77,78,81, 82,84.87, 88,97,98,99,110,111,112,135,139,147, 149, 153,155,157,158,161,186,188,216,229,245, 255,257,258,269

Propaganda: 150

Protective clothing: 89,**90**

Protestant: 107

Public places, closure of: 79,128

Puddings: 68,111,118,166,168,212

Pump: 94

Nursing in Serbia with Lady Paget in 1915

Pupin, Professor: 135

Pybus, Miss E L: 254

Pyjamas: 20,65,**90**,104,115,122

Quaker: 162,223

Quarantine: 127

Queen Elionora of Bulgaria: 151,152,155

Queen Marie of Romania: 156,182

Queen Mary: 14,250,270

Queen of Norway: 156

Race course: 240,245,253

Raids: 50

Railway carriages: 48,49,127,128,139

Railway communications: 127,128,138,148,150,156,259

Rain: 36,71,84,115,139,240

Ralli, Mrs Scaramanga: 270

Rankin, Jean S: 259,260,264,265,267

Rationing of food: 151,164,169,193

Rats: 88

Rattray, Ian Maxwell: 263

Read, Nurse Ada: 292

Receiver: 60,64,183,236,256,257

Recreation room: 58

Red Cross: 183,236,256,257

Red Cross, Belgian: 244

Red Cross, Bulgarian: 151,156

Red Cross, French: 23,244,247

Red Cross, Italian: 124,128

Red Cross, Serbian: 47,62,78,82,183,184,256

Red Cross, uniform: 38,46,124

Reekie, John Alexander: 263

Refrigerator carts: 125

Refugees: 10,11,42,45,138,143,150,151,154, 155,156,162,186,209,215,223,234,235,238,240,241,245, 254,255,258,259

Register, national emergency: 176

Reggio Calabria:123

Reinforcements: 138

Relapsing fever: 58,63,78,86,203

Relief of destitute: 131,151,189,209,257

Rent: 154

Repatriation: 148,156,186,188,225,230,245,252, 255

Reporters: 121,220,228,245

Respirators: 257

Rest station, Nish: 241

Restaurants: 126,128,248

Retreat: 140,141,144,162,183,208,234,245, 246, 253,258

Revolution, Russian: 162

Rice: 26,58,68,110,150,154,209

Ridge, Nurse R M: 104,264

Index

Riding: 112,213

Rifles: 146

Riga: 214,215,216

Roads: 69,103,115

Roberts, Miss Eveline: 252

Robinshaw, Nurse Beatrice L: 104,264,267

Robinson, Times correspondent: 220,221

Rochester, St Bartholomew Hospital: 7

Rodney, Lady: 270

Rogers, Rev E S: 293

Rolling stock: 139

Roman Catholics: 151

Rome: 234,246

Roodhouse, Miss: 254

Roof: 88

Ross, Dr Elizabeth: 76,199

Round, Nurse S A: 90,91,264,267

Routine: 67

Rowntree, Sister – see Fry, Sister F A

Roy family: Keith Cotton: 7; Philip Scott: 7

Sannyasi Charan: 7; Theodore Cotton: 7

Royal Army Medical Corps: 126,197,202,211, 218,227

Royal College of Nursing: 6,167

Royal Free Hospital, London: 29

Royal Hotel, Malta: 37

Royal visit: 20

Royaumont Abbey, France: 197

Rumania: 162,167,188,189

Ruski Tzar, Nish: 248

Russia: 107,162,167,188,189,214,215

Russians: 20,44,68,77,84-86,162,185,214-216,253

Ryan, Dr James: 223

Ryde, Isle of Wight: 175,**176,177**

Saideh, SS: 105,240,252

Salford: 186

Salonika: 15,36,44,44,45,**46-47**,50.95,100, 101,103,105,107,118,120,121,122,133,136,**13 7**138,139,140,141,154,156,184,194,197,208, 210,219,222,224,241,245,253

Salonika, fire of: 46,194

Samuel, Herbert MP: 270

San Giovanni di Madeua: 246

Sandes, Flora: 142,184,185

Sanitary Mission: 81

Sanitation: 94,95,100,133,252

Sarajevo: 12

Scammel, Miss Ethel: 254,264,267

Scarlet fever: 97,212

Scenery: 71,89,108,213

Schellens, Richard: 154,268

Schools: 15,16,17,52,57,58,59,62

Scotland: 223,224

Nursing in Serbia with Lady Paget in 1915

Scott, A M, MP: 271

Scott family: Agnes Morwood: 6,112,167,176;Contstance Annie: 6,176; Elizabeth: 5; Gertrude Mary: 6,7,175,176;Jessie Sophie: 6,7; Sydney: 5,6,8,24,175; William: 5,6

Scott, Flora: **vi,27,160**,264;accident on ship:32,43; alone in charge: 91,97; appointment to Leicester Frith: 170,**173**; arrival in Skoplje: 51; birth: 5; death: 177; leaves Serbia: 118; resignation: 174; returns to England: 118; volunteers for typhus work: 87,90

Scott, F M: 271

Scott, Miss Monsie: 101,252

Scott, Robert Falcon: 101,252

Scottish Women's Hospitals: 37,39,76,175,194,197,209,221,222-223,228-230,241,255,256,258,259

Seal: 120

Searchlights: 40

Searle, Miss P: 254

Seasickness: 30-32,34,43,156

Seedorff, Dr M: 266

Sentries: 50,58,72,247

Septic wounds: 16-18,85,215

Serbia: 9,10,12,13,15,23,136

Serbia, strategic position: 9

Serbian army: 135,137,142,162,182,183,189,194, 208,222, 224,227,228,245,253,259

Serbian army, second: 105,213,214

Serbian Fever Hospital, Kragujevatz: 76

Serbian Flag Day: 2,**3**,124,**250**

Serbian Funeral March: 21,179

Serbian girls, scholarships for: 200

Serbian ladies: 84

Serbian language: 19,30,63,66,67,72,103,113,195, 237,240,241, 247,258

Serbian Medical Corps: 223

Serbian minister in London: 24

Serbian National Anthem: 2,3,241

Serbian Relief Fund: 14,61,94,107,129,132,134,15 1,175,197,213, 217,223,224,232,234,245,249,250-261,270-271; expenditure: 129,256,257; receipts: 129,257; resignation of chairman: 130; subscriptions to: 14,129,250; winding up: 260

Serbian Relief Fund Committee: 24,100,102,104,107,225,246,257,270-271

Serbian Relief Fund Unit, 1st [Lady Paget's]: 15,251,252,262-265,266-269

Serbian Relief Fund Unit, 2nd [Lady Wimborne's]: 100,101,102,108,129,130,142,179,187,189,196, 209,249,252

Serbian Relief Fund Unit, 3rd [Stobart]: 102,105,107,121,134,198,230,240,242-246,249,252-253,256,257,259,292-293

Serbian Relief Fund Unit, 4th [British Farmers']: 241,252,253-256

Serbian Relief Fund Unit, 4th [2nd British Farmers']: 241,255-256

Serbians: 66,**75**,77,85,100,106,112,128,135,144, 146, 155,188,192,245

Seton-Watson, Robert William: 14,15,271

Seton-Watson, Mrs: 271

Sewing: 11,26

Index

Shakespeare, Miss Phyllis: 292

Sharman, Miss: 293

Sharpin, Nurse MM: 267

Shaving: 61,79,93

Sheep: 61,79,93

Shellens, R: 268

Shell shock: 170,173

Shells: 146

Shepherds: 48,50

Ship cabins: 109

Shoes: 73,115

Shopping: 71,72,114,115,192

Shoring, Miss F M: 254

Shrapnel: 16,65,147,148,152

Sibley, Miss Jennie: 262

Sicily: 122

Sightseeing: 113

Silver ware: 114,115

Sim, Gerald: 105,208

Simmonds, Miss Emily: 184,185

Sinclair, Dr GH: 100,209,252

Sinclair, Miss: 252

Skertchley, Nurse ME: 105,264,265,267

Sketchley, Miss: 252

Skey, Miss: 262

Skoplje: 10,11,15,19,51,**54**,55,56,100,**101**,105,110, **114**,115,**119**,137,144,228,252,259

Sleeping bags: 51

Sleigh ride: 156

Slippers: 65,104

Slovenes: 149

Smallpox: 45,85,97

Smells: 56,57

Smith, Miss Gertrude: 96,263

Smith, Miss Mary Michie: 265

Smith, Nurse Helen: 104,265

Smith Lewis, Nurse: 293

Smoking: 35

Snipers: 146

Snow: 53,61,82,96,97,103

Soap: 26,65,108

Socks: 26,28,104

Sofia: 152,156,157

Soldiers: 50,58,59,66,73,75,128,143,168,169,194,245

Soltau, Dr Eleanor: 76,222,223

Sorović: 224

Soubotitch, Colonel: 83

Soup: 45,95,107

South Africa: 201,243

Southampton: 15,177

Spain:35

Nursing in Serbia with Lady Paget in 1915

Spirit lamps: 51

Spying: 149,229

Squire, Henry Fremlin: 18,19,57,63,202,211,212,213,219,236-238,263

Sremska Kamenica: 224

St John Ambulance Association: 232,237,244,247,251

St John of Jerusalem: 39

St Pantaleon Church: 260

Stables: 81,82,146

Staff room: 82

Stallash: 247

Stammers, Major: 126

Stanley, Monica: 56,69,99,107,133,238,**239**-242,253254,255,292

Station, railway: 119,136,138,139,142,145,165,215,223

Sterilization: 60,64,127

Stevens, Mary Paran: 13

Stewart family: Alban, 8: Ellen,8; Neil Cook, 8

Stewart, Dr M: 293

Stewart, Nurse M: 293

Stobart Unit- see Serbian Relief Fund, 3rd unit

Stobart, Mabel St Clair: 35,56,102,107,198,220,230,240,242,**243**-246,252,254,256

Stockings: 65,73,166

Stone, Nurse: 293

Storeman: 64

Stores: 47,140,141,144,145,151,152,156,157,208, 209,251,253,254,256,257

Storks: 118

Storm: 33,43

Stoves: 51,52,64,95,96

Strachey, Mr J St Lee: 271

Stretchers: 152

Stretton, Dr: 58

Sturt, Nurse L: 104,264

Submarines: 109

Suffrage, Church League for: 198

Suffrage, women's: 198,199,244

Suffragettes: 121,185

Sugar: 26,68,145,169

Sunrise: 48

Sunset: 40

Supplies: 26,47,104,121,133,141,150,152,237, 240,256

Suskalovitch, Major: 62,78,79,86

Sweden: 156

Sweden, Crown Princess of: 156

Sweets: 26,160

Swim: 122,237

Swinburne, Spearman C:263

Swiss: 146

Switzerland: 23,124,188

Index

Sydney, Australia: 102,194,196,197

Sydney, SS:241

Symonds, AG:271

Tables: 58

Tableware: 58,108

Tancock, Montague A: 135,147,268

Tate, Dr Isabel: 253,292

Tatham, Miss: 293

Taylor, Hugh Watts: 254

Tea: 26,41,42,45,51,67,68,110,120,145,166,167, 169,259

Teeth: 26,66

Tekkah [saint's tomb]: 80

Telegrams – see Cables

Telegraph and telephone lines: 138,142,259

Templemore, Lord and Lady: 46,132,190

Tents: 78

Terry, Nurse M: 254

Theatre, operating: 97,135,137

Theresa, Mother: 56

Thompson, Nurse: 252

Thompson, Nurse Ethel: 252

Thompson, Nurse Isabella: 292

Thompson, Nellie: 27

Timsons Removal Co: 26

Tins: 52,60,64,68,88

Tiny, Irish Wolfhound: 26,98,108,163,164,165

Toasts: 98,212,216

Tobacco warehouses: 15,20,84

Tonsilitis: 63

Torcello, SS: 253

Trains: 17,28,30,41,48,49,50,51,79,119,122,124, 127,128,136,137,138,142,145,156

Train, ambulance: 128

Transfer of staff: 134

Transfer of territory: 136

Transport: 15,28,121,139

Treaties: 136

Trekking: 131,**132**,189,190,209

Trendell, Miss L: 254

Trevelyan, GM: 271

Tricks: **168**,169,220

Triumphal procession: 147,156

Troubridge, Admiral: 224,241,253,256

Trousers: **69**,115,117

Tubb, Miss: 293

Tunisia: 258

Tunnels: 39,165

Turkey: 40,42,54

Turkey [poultry]: 67,166,212

Turks: 9,10,54,55,56,71,100,114,145,147,192

Nursing in Serbia with Lady Paget in 1915

Turtle, Nurse: 25

Typhoid: 78,132,134,154,190,199,240,241,254

Typhus: 46,49,75,76,78,79,81,85,87,91,92,101,157, 204,213,215,218,220,221,223,227,244,246, 247

Typhus Colony, Skoplje: 79,80,87,89,97, 102,116, 196,213,218,251,**290-1**

Typhus Commission: 86,247

Typhus epidemic:

76-117,126,193,195,221,223,230;

Typhus symptoms: 90,91,92

Ulster :120,218

Understaffing: 19,237

Uniforms: 25,38,50,73,81,82,85,118,124,126, 151,193,210

University, Belgrade: 62,194,246,247,254

Urinals: 60

Uscub- see Skoplje

Uscubitis: 63,86,101

Uzsitsi: 229,257

Valetta, Malta: 37,38,**40**

Valjevo: 135,223,229,241,256

Van Der Vebn, Nurse: 268

Van Oyen, Nurse: 268

Vanity, pet dog: 108,113

Vardar river: 50,80,136,**119**

Vegetables: 38,68,110

Veles: 138

Venezelos, Eleutherios: 136,137

Ventilation: 60

Victoria Rd, Leicester[Flora's home]: 1,7,**8**,23,25,53, 108,124,160,161,167

Vienna:10,255,188,197,230

Viles, Mrs: 108

Villa Velika, Skoplje: 189

Villemon, Nurse: 268

Vooitch, Mr: 293

Volcano: 135

Volga region: 162

Voluntary Aid Detachment [VAD]: 164,167,184

Vranja: 138

Vrintski: 179

Vrnjatchka Banja: 29,31,188,206,247,255

Vulture: 70

Wallice, Mrs Percy: 267

Wallice, Percy: 266

War crime: 150

War Office: 23,39,257

Wards: 59,60,**65**

Warren, Miss Fairy: 292

Warship: 36,122-123

Index

Wasgindt, Nurse Jessie de: 292

Washing: 25

Water: 94,98,110

Water spouts: 36

Water supply: 18,58,64,93,94

Welbeck Abbey: 162,**164,165**

Wells, Nurse: 293

Wheelchairs: 164,173

Whitehead, Lady: 270

Whitwick: 5

Wifstrand, Nurse Minna: 267

Wigston Magna: 8

Wiles, JW: 62,246-248,262

Wilkinson, Lady Beatrix: 209,252

Williams, Carlton :263

Williams, Glynne: 270

Williamson, William: 109

Willis, Nurse Constance: 292

Willis, Nurse: 293

Wilman, Dr J: 253

Wilman, Nurse :254

Wilson, Francesca: 226,258,260

Wilson, Maurice: 258

Wimborne Unit – see Serbian Relief Fund, 2nd

Wimborne, Lady Cornelia: 100.130,248-**249**

Windows: 60,85,168

Wine: 50,103,110,144,247

Winter: 152-154

Wise, Bernard: 270

Wolseley, Miss Minnie: 292

Wolves: 103,113

Women: 114,124,155,186,258

Women's Imperial Service League: 244,247,252

Women's Sick and Wounded Convoy Corps: 244

Women's World: 174

Wood: 96

Workshops: 258

Worksop: 162

Wounded: 16,17,59,60,65,66,85,137,138,140, 142,143,146,148, 152,185,195,244

Wounded Allies Relief Fund: 253,255,258

Wren, Nurse: 293

Wycliffe Society for helping the Blind: **124**

Wynch, Mr LM: 253,255

X-Ray equipment: 218,252

Yacht, Steam: **120**,121,213,219,220,222

Yovannovitch, Captain: 221

Yugoslavia: 225,226,234,235,238,248,260

Zurich: 230,255

Nursing in Serbia with Lady Paget in 1915

Zurinsky's restaurant, Skoplje: 190,209

www.ingramcontent.com/pod-product-compliance
Lightning Source LLC
Chambersburg PA
CBHW072045110526
44590CB00018B/3044